BASIC AND CLINICAL SCIENCE COURSE

Lens and Cataract

Section 11

2009–2010

(Last major revision 2008–2009)

AMERICAN ACADEMY OF OPHTHALMOLOGY
The Eye M.D. Association

LEO
LIFELONG EDUCATION FOR THE OPHTHALMOLOGIST®

LEO

The Basic and Clinical Science Course is one component of the Lifelong Education for the Ophthalmologist (LEO) framework, which assists members in planning their continuing medical education. LEO includes an array of clinical education products that members may select to form individualized, self-directed learning plans for updating their clinical knowledge. Active members or fellows who use LEO components may accumulate sufficient CME credits to earn the LEO Award. Contact the Academy's Clinical Education Division for further information on LEO.

The American Academy of Ophthalmology is accredited by the Accreditation Council for Continuing Medical Education to provide continuing medical education for physicians.

The American Academy of Ophthalmology designates this educational activity for a maximum of 30 *AMA PRA Category 1 Credits*™. Physicians should only claim credit commensurate with the extent of their participation in the activity.

Printed in Singapore

Basic and Clinical Science Course

Gregory L. Skuta, MD, Oklahoma City, Oklahoma, *Senior Secretary for Clinical Education*
Louis B. Cantor, MD, Indianapolis, Indiana, *Secretary for Ophthalmic Knowledge*
Jayne S. Weiss, MD, Detroit, Michigan, *BCSC Course Chair*

Section 11

Faculty Responsible for This Edition

James C. Bobrow, MD, *Chair,* Clayton, Missouri
Mark H. Blecher, MD, Philadelphia, Pennsylvania
David B. Glasser, MD, Columbia, Maryland
Kenneth B. Mitchell, MD, Columbia, South Carolina
Lisa F. Rosenberg, MD, Chicago, Illinois
Edward K. Isbey III, MD, Asheville, North Carolina
Practicing Ophthalmologists Advisory Committee for Education
Joseph Reich, MD, *Consultant,* Toorak, Australia

The authors state the following financial relationships:

Dr Blecher: Advanced Medical Optics, grant recipient

The other authors state that they have no significant financial interest or other relationship with the manufacturer of any commercial product discussed in the chapters that they contributed to this course or with the manufacturer of any competing commercial product.

Recent Past Faculty

Cynthia A. Bradford, MD
Steven I. Rosenfeld, MD

In addition, the Academy gratefully acknowledges the contributions of numerous past faculty and advisory committee members who have played an important role in the development of previous editions of the Basic and Clinical Science Course.

American Academy of Ophthalmology Staff

Richard A. Zorab, *Vice President, Ophthalmic Knowledge*
Hal Straus, *Director, Publications Department*
Carol L. Dondrea, *Publications Manager*
Christine Arturo, *Acquisitions Manager*
D. Jean Ray, *Production Manager*
Stephanie Tanaka, *Medical Editor*
Steven Huebner, *Administrative Coordinator*

AMERICAN ACADEMY OF OPHTHALMOLOGY
The Eye M.D. Association

655 Beach Street
Box 7424
San Francisco, CA 94120-7424

Contents

General Introduction xiii

Objectives **1**
Introduction **3**

1 Anatomy **5**
Normal Crystalline Lens 5
Capsule 7
Zonular Fibers 8
Lens Epithelium. 8
Nucleus and Cortex 9

2 Biochemistry **11**
Molecular Biology 11
Crystallin Proteins 11
Membrane Structural Proteins and Cytoskeletal Proteins 12
Increase of Water-Insoluble Proteins With Age 13
Carbohydrate Metabolism 13
Oxidative Damage and Protective Mechanisms 16

3 Physiology **19**
Maintenance of Lens Water and Cation Balance. 19
Lens Epithelium: Site of Active Transport. 19
Pump-Leak Theory 20
Accommodation 22
Presbyopia. 23

4 Embryology **25**
Normal Development 25
Lens Placode 25
Lens Pit 25
Lens Vesicle 25
Primary Lens Fibers and the Embryonic Nucleus 25
Secondary Lens Fibers 27
Lens Sutures and the Fetal Nucleus 28
Tunica Vasculosa Lentis 29
Zonules of Zinn. 29
Congenital Anomalies and Abnormalities 30
Congenital Aphakia 30
Lenticonus and Lentiglobus. 30
Lens Coloboma 31
Mittendorf Dot 31

Epicapsular Star 31
Peters Anomaly 32
Microspherophakia 32
Aniridia 33
Congenital and Infantile Cataract 34
Developmental Defects 39
Ectopia Lentis 39
Marfan Syndrome 40
Homocystinuria 41
Hyperlysinemia 41
Sulfite Oxidase Deficiency 41
Ectopia Lentis et Pupillae. 42
Persistent Fetal Vasculature 42

5 Pathology. 43
Aging Changes 43
Nuclear Cataracts 43
Cortical Cataracts 45
Posterior Subcapsular Cataracts 46
Genetic Contributions to Age-Related Cataracts. 50
Drug-Induced Lens Changes 52
Corticosteroids 52
Phenothiazines 52
Miotics 53
Amiodarone 53
Statins 53
Trauma 53
Contusion 53
Perforating and Penetrating Injury. 55
Radiation 55
Chemical Injuries 57
Intralenticular Foreign Bodies 57
Metallosis 57
Electrical Injury. 58
Metabolic Cataract 59
Diabetes Mellitus 59
Galactosemia 60
Hypocalcemia 61
Wilson Disease 61
Myotonic Dystrophy. 61
Effects of Nutrition and Smoking 62
Cataract Associated With Uveitis 63
Cataracts Associated With Ocular Therapies 64
Pseudoexfoliation Syndrome 65
Cataract and Skin Diseases. 66
Atopic Dermatitis 66
Phacoantigenic Uveitis 66

Lens-Induced Glaucoma 67
Phacolytic Glaucoma 67
Lens Particle Glaucoma 67
Phacomorphic Glaucoma 67
Glaukomflecken 68
Ischemia. 68
Cataracts Associated With Degenerative Ocular Disorders 68

6 Epidemiology of Cataracts 71

7 Evaluation and Management of Cataracts in Adults . . . 75
Clinical History: Signs and Symptoms 75
Decreased Visual Acuity 75
Glare 76
Altered Contrast Sensitivity. 76
Myopic Shift 77
Monocular Diplopia or Polyopia 77
Medical Management 77
Low Vision Aids for Cataract 78
Indications for Surgery 78
Preoperative Evaluation 79
General Health of the Patient 79
Pertinent Ocular History 80
Social History 81
Measurements of Visual Function 81
Visual Acuity Testing 81
Refraction 81
Brightness Acuity 81
Contrast Sensitivity 82
Visual Field Testing 82
External Examination 82
Motility 82
Pupils 82
Slit-Lamp Examination 83
Conjunctiva 83
Cornea 83
Anterior Chamber. 84
Iris 84
Crystalline Lens. 84
Limitations of Slit-Lamp Examination 85
Fundus Evaluation 85
Ophthalmoscopy 85
Optic Nerve 85
Fundus Evaluation With Opaque Media 86
Special Tests 86
Potential Acuity Estimation. 86
Tests of Macular Function 87

Preoperative Measurements 88
Biometry. 88
Corneal Topography. 88
Corneal Pachymetry. 88
Specular Microscopy 88
Patient Preparation and Informed Consent. 88

8 Surgery for Cataract 91
The Remote Past 91
Ancient and Medieval Techniques 91
Early Extracapsular Cataract Extraction 92
Early Intracapsular Cataract Extraction 94
The Recent Past 94
Modern Advances in Intracapsular Surgery 94
The Renaissance of Extracapsular Extraction 96
The Modern ECCE Procedure 97
Ophthalmic Viscosurgical Devices 98
Physical Properties 99
Characteristics of OVDs 99
Anesthesia for Cataract Surgery. 100
Phacoemulsification. 104
Ultrasonics Terminology 104
Vacuum Terminology 106
Phaco Instrumentation. 106
Phaco Power Delivery 108
Irrigation 110
Aspiration 110
Making the Transition 111
A Basic Phaco Procedure Outline 113
Exposure of the Globe 113
Paracentesis 113
Scleral Tunnel Incisions 113
Clear Corneal Incision 116
Continuous Curvilinear Capsulorrhexis 119
Hydrodissection 120
Hydrodelineation 121
Nuclear Rotation 121
Instrument Settings for Phacoemulsification 121
Strategies for Irrigation and Aspiration. 122
Location of Emulsification 123
One-Handed Technique of Nucleus Disassembly 125
Two-Handed Techniques of Nucleus Disassembly 126
Advances in Energy Delivery 130
Alcon Infiniti. 130
AMO Sovereign With WhiteStar 130
Bausch & Lomb Millennium 131
STAAR Surgical Sonic WAVE. 131

Alternate Technologies for Nucleus Removal . . . 131
  Sutureless Nonphaco Cataract Surgery . . . 131
  Laser Photolysis. . . . 132
  Water Jet Phacolysis . . . 132
Antimicrobial Prophylaxis . . . 132
  Before Surgery . . . 132
  In Surgery . . . 133
  After Surgery . . . 134
Modification of Preexisting Astigmatism. . . . 134
  Incision Size and Location . . . 135
  Astigmatic Keratotomy. . . . 135
  Limbal Relaxing Incisions . . . 135
  Toric IOLs . . . 136
Special Circumstances. . . . 136
  Cataract Surgery in the Patient Taking Anticoagulants . . . 136
  Cataract Surgery in the Patient Taking Tamsulosin. . . . 137
  Use of Capsule Staining . . . 137
  Use of Pupillary Expansion . . . 137
  Capsulorrhexis Issues . . . 138
  Loose Zonules . . . 138
  Mature Cataracts . . . 139
  Posterior Capsule Rupture . . . 140
Pars Plana Lensectomy . . . 142
  Indications . . . 142
  Contraindications . . . 142
Intraocular Lens Implantation . . . 142
  Historical Perspectives . . . 142
  Posterior Chamber IOLs . . . 144
  Multifocal Lenses . . . 146
  Other Designs . . . 148
  IOL Power Determination . . . 149
  Phakic IOLs . . . 153
  Techniques of Lens Implantation . . . 154
  Procedure . . . 154
  Secondary IOL Implantation . . . 155
  Relative Contraindications to Lens Implantation. . . . 156
Outcomes of Cataract Surgery . . . 156
Appendix . . . 157
  The Modern Intracapsular Cataract Surgical Procedure. . . . 157
  The Modern Extracapsular Cataract Surgical Procedure . . . 160

9 Complications of Cataract Surgery . . . 163

Corneal Edema. . . . 163
  Brown-McLean Syndrome . . . 165
  Vitreocorneal Adherence and Persistent Corneal Edema . . . 165
Corneal Complications of Ultrasound . . . 166
Detachment of Descemet's Membrane . . . 166

Induced Astigmatism . . . 167
Corneal Melting . . . 167
Incision Leak or Inadvertent Filtering Bleb . . . 168
Epithelial Downgrowth . . . 168
Toxic Solutions . . . 169
Conjunctival Ballooning . . . 170
Shallow or Flat Anterior Chamber . . . 170
  Intraoperative . . . 170
  Postoperative . . . 171
Elevated Intraocular Pressure . . . 172
Intraoperative Floppy Iris Syndrome . . . 173
Iridodialysis . . . 174
Cyclodialysis . . . 174
Ciliary Block Glaucoma . . . 174
Chronic Uveitis . . . 175
Retained Lens Material . . . 175
Capsular Rupture . . . 176
Vitreous Prolapse . . . 178
Complications of IOL Implantation . . . 178
  Decentration and Dislocation . . . 178
  Pupillary Capture . . . 180
  Capsular Block Syndrome . . . 180
  Uveitis-Glaucoma-Hyphema Syndrome . . . 181
  Pseudophakic Bullous Keratopathy . . . 181
  Incorrect IOL Power . . . 181
  IOL Design, Glare, and Opacification . . . 182
Capsular Opacification and Contraction . . . 182
  Posterior Capsule Opacification . . . 182
  Anterior Capsule Fibrosis and Phimosis . . . 184
Nd:YAG Capsulotomy . . . 184
  Indications . . . 184
  Contraindications . . . 184
  Procedure . . . 185
  Complications . . . 187
Hemorrhage . . . 187
  Retrobulbar Hemorrhage . . . 188
  Suprachoroidal Effusion or Hemorrhage . . . 188
  Expulsive Suprachoroidal Hemorrhage . . . 189
  Delayed Suprachoroidal Hemorrhage . . . 190
  Hyphema . . . 190
Endophthalmitis . . . 190
  Diagnosis . . . 191
  Treatment . . . 191
Cystoid Macular Edema . . . 193
Retinal Light Toxicity . . . 195
Macular Infarction . . . 195
Retinal Detachment . . . 196

10 Cataract Surgery in Special Situations 199

Cataract in Children . . . 199
 Surgical Planning . . . 199
 Surgical Technique . . . 200
 Postoperative Care . . . 202
 Complications . . . 202
 Prognosis . . . 202
 Correction of Aphakia . . . 203
Psychosocial Considerations . . . 204
 Claustrophobia . . . 204
 Dementia or Other Mental Disabilities . . . 205
 Inability to Communicate With the Patient . . . 205
Systemic Conditions . . . 205
 Anticoagulation Therapy or Bleeding Disorders . . . 205
 Arthritis . . . 206
 Chronic Obstructive Pulmonary Disease . . . 207
 Diabetes Mellitus . . . 208
 Obesity . . . 209
Ocular Conditions . . . 210
 External Eye Disease . . . 210
 Corneal Conditions . . . 211
 Mature Cataract/Poor Red Reflex . . . 214
 Cataract Following Refractive Surgery . . . 215
 Developmental Abnormalities . . . 216
 Increased Risk of Expulsive Hemorrhage . . . 219
 Glaucoma . . . 221
 High Refractive Error . . . 224
 Hypotony . . . 226
 Uveitis . . . 226
 Retinal Disease . . . 227
Trauma . . . 228
 Visualization . . . 228
 Inflammation . . . 228
 Retained Foreign Matter . . . 229
 Damage to Other Ocular Tissues . . . 229
 Zonular Dehiscence With Lens Subluxation or Dislocation . . . 230
 Lens Implantation . . . 231

Basic Texts . . . 233
Related Academy Materials . . . 234
Credit Reporting Form . . . 237
Study Questions . . . 241
Answers . . . 249
Index . . . 255

General Introduction

The Basic and Clinical Science Course (BCSC) is designed to meet the needs of residents and practitioners for a comprehensive yet concise curriculum of the field of ophthalmology. The BCSC has developed from its original brief outline format, which relied heavily on outside readings, to a more convenient and educationally useful self-contained text. The Academy updates and revises the course annually, with the goals of integrating the basic science and clinical practice of ophthalmology and of keeping ophthalmologists current with new developments in the various subspecialties.

The BCSC incorporates the effort and expertise of more than 80 ophthalmologists, organized into 13 Section faculties, working with Academy editorial staff. In addition, the course continues to benefit from many lasting contributions made by the faculties of previous editions. Members of the Academy's Practicing Ophthalmologists Advisory Committee for Education serve on each faculty and, as a group, review every volume before and after major revisions.

Organization of the Course

The Basic and Clinical Science Course comprises 13 volumes, incorporating fundamental ophthalmic knowledge, subspecialty areas, and special topics:

1 Update on General Medicine
2 Fundamentals and Principles of Ophthalmology
3 Clinical Optics
4 Ophthalmic Pathology and Intraocular Tumors
5 Neuro-Ophthalmology
6 Pediatric Ophthalmology and Strabismus
7 Orbit, Eyelids, and Lacrimal System
8 External Disease and Cornea
9 Intraocular Inflammation and Uveitis
10 Glaucoma
11 Lens and Cataract
12 Retina and Vitreous
13 Refractive Surgery

In addition, a comprehensive Master Index allows the reader to easily locate subjects throughout the entire series.

References

Readers who wish to explore specific topics in greater detail may consult the references cited within each chapter and listed in the Basic Texts section at the back of the book. These references are intended to be selective rather than exhaustive, chosen by the BCSC faculty as being important, current, and readily available to residents and practitioners.

Related Academy educational materials are also listed in the appropriate sections. They include books, online and audiovisual materials, self-assessment programs, clinical modules, and interactive programs.

Study Questions and CME Credit

Each volume of the BCSC is designed as an independent study activity for ophthalmology residents and practitioners. The learning objectives for this volume are given on page 1. The text, illustrations, and references provide the information necessary to achieve the objectives; the study questions allow readers to test their understanding of the material and their mastery of the objectives. Physicians who wish to claim CME credit for this educational activity may do so by mail, by fax, or online. The necessary forms and instructions are given at the end of the book.

Conclusion

The Basic and Clinical Science Course has expanded greatly over the years, with the addition of much new text and numerous illustrations. Recent editions have sought to place a greater emphasis on clinical applicability while maintaining a solid foundation in basic science. As with any educational program, it reflects the experience of its authors. As its faculties change and as medicine progresses, new viewpoints are always emerging on controversial subjects and techniques. Not all alternate approaches can be included in this series; as with any educational endeavor, the learner should seek additional sources, including such carefully balanced opinions as the Academy's Preferred Practice Patterns.

The BCSC faculty and staff are continuously striving to improve the educational usefulness of the course; you, the reader, can contribute to this ongoing process. If you have any suggestions or questions about the series, please do not hesitate to contact the faculty or the editors.

The authors, editors, and reviewers hope that your study of the BCSC will be of lasting value and that each Section will serve as a practical resource for quality patient care.

Objectives

Upon completion of BCSC Section 11, *Lens and Cataract,* the reader should be able to

- describe the normal anatomy, embryologic development, physiology, and biochemistry of the crystalline lens
- identify congenital anomalies of the lens
- distinguish types of congenital and acquired cataracts
- describe the association of cataracts with aging, trauma, medications, and systemic and ocular diseases
- appropriately evaluate and manage patients with cataract and other lens abnormalities
- explain the principles of cataract surgery techniques and associated surgical technology
- develop an appropriate differential diagnosis and management plan for intraoperative and postoperative complications of cataract surgery
- identify special circumstances in which cataract surgery techniques should be modified and develop appropriate treatment plans

Introduction

The ancient Greeks and Romans believed that the lens was the part of the eye responsible for the faculty of seeing. They theorized that the optic nerves were hollow channels through which "visual spirits" traveled from the brain to meet visual rays from the outside world at the lens, which they thought was located in the center of the globe. The visual information would then flow back to the brain. This concept was known as the *emanation theory of vision*. Celsus (25 BC–AD 50) drew the lens in the center of the globe, with an empty space called the *locus vacuus* anterior to it, in AD 30 (Fig I-1).

These erroneous ideas about lens position and function persisted through the Middle Ages and into the Renaissance, as shown by the drawings of the Belgian anatomist Andreas Vesalius in 1543 (Fig I-2). However, the true position of the crystalline lens was illustrated by the Italian anatomist Fabricius ab Aquapendente in 1600 (Fig I-3); and the Swiss physician Felix Plater (1536–1614) first postulated that the retina, and not the lens, was the part of the eye responsible for sight.

Today, many areas of lens physiology and biochemistry are still subjects of active research. No medical treatment, for example, can yet prevent the formation or progression of cataract in the lens of the otherwise healthy adult eye, and theories about cataract formation and innovative forms of management continue to be controversial. Although various risk factors for cataract development (UV-B radiation, diabetes mellitus, drug use, smoking, alcohol use, severe malnutrition, and oxidative damage) have been identified, data to develop guidelines for reducing the risk of cataract remain inconclusive.

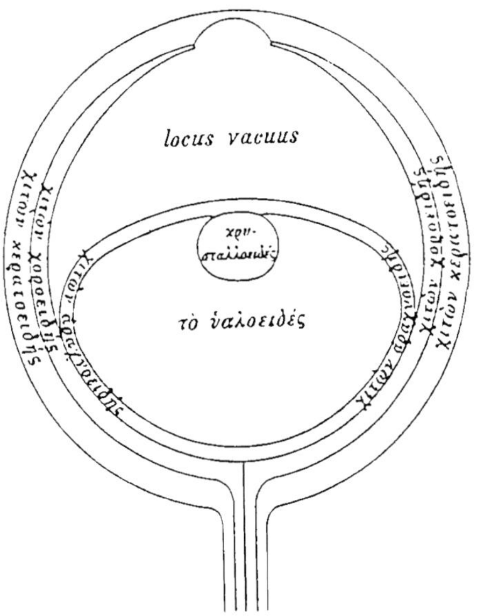

Figure I-1 The eye, after Celsus. *(From Gorin G.* History of Ophthalmology. *Wilmington: Publish or Perish, Inc; 1982.)*

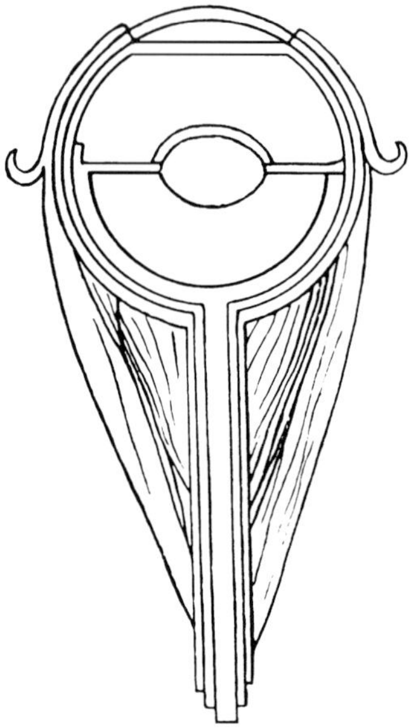

Figure I-2 Schematic eye from *De fabrica corporis humani* of Andreas Vesalius (1514–1564). *(Reproduced by permission from the Ophthalmic Publishing Company. Feigenbaum A. Early history of cataract and the ancient operation for cataract.* Am J Ophthalmol. *1960;49:307.)*

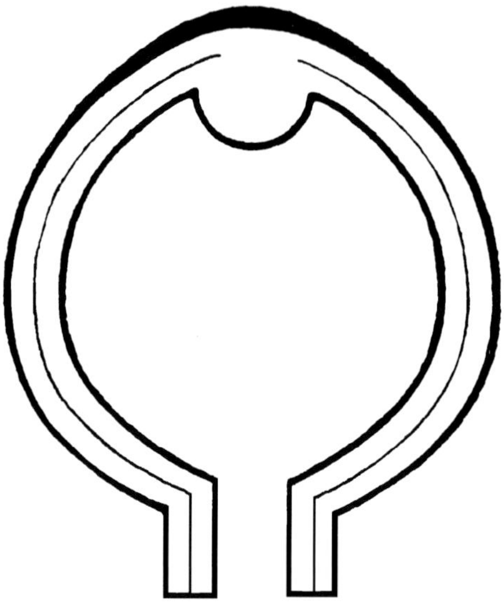

Figure I-3 Sketch from *De oculo* of Fabricius ab Aquapendente (1537–1619), showing correct position of the lens within the eyeball. *(Reproduced by permission from the Ophthalmic Publishing Company. Feigenbaum A. Early history of cataract and the ancient operation for cataract.* Am J Ophthalmol. *1960;49:307.)*

Cataract is the leading cause of preventable blindness in the world, whereas cataract extraction with intraocular lens (IOL) implantation is perhaps the most effective surgical procedure in all of medicine. More than 1.8 million cataract procedures are performed on the population older than age 65 in the United States each year, and the visual disability associated with cataract formation accounts for more than 8 million physician office visits each year.

The prevalence of lens disorders and continuing developments in their management make the basic and clinical science of the lens an important subject in ophthalmology training. The goal of Section 11 is to provide a curriculum for the study of all aspects of the lens, including the structure and function of the normal lens, the features of diseases involving the lens, and the surgical management of lens abnormalities, such as recent developments in phacoemulsification and laser capsulotomy. Because the specifics of surgical techniques and instrumentation are constantly changing, the authors of this volume have chosen to provide a balanced presentation of the general principles of cataract management, emphasizing the major prevailing approaches.

In addition, to help put today's techniques into perspective, historical vignettes describing the evolution of cataract surgery and IOL implantation appear at the beginning of Chapter 8 and in the discussion of IOLs later in that chapter.

CHAPTER 1

Anatomy

Normal Crystalline Lens

The crystalline lens is a transparent, biconvex structure whose functions are

- to maintain its own clarity
- to refract light
- to provide accommodation

The lens has no blood supply or innervation after fetal development, and it depends entirely on the aqueous humor to meet its metabolic requirements and to carry off its wastes. It lies posterior to the iris and anterior to the vitreous body (Fig 1-1). The lens is suspended in position by the zonules of Zinn, which consist of delicate yet strong fibers that support and attach it to the ciliary body. The lens is composed of the capsule, lens epithelium, cortex, and nucleus (Fig 1-2).

The anterior and posterior poles of the lens are joined by an imaginary line called the *optic axis,* which passes through them. Lines on the surface passing from one pole to the other are referred to as *meridians.* The *equator* of the lens is its greatest circumference.

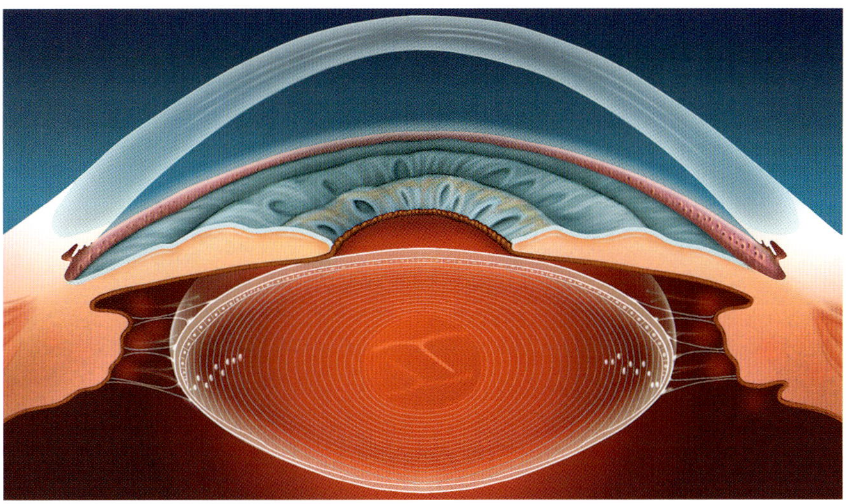

Figure 1-1 Cross section of the human crystalline lens, showing the relationship of the lens to surrounding ocular structures. *(Illustration by Christine Gralapp.)*

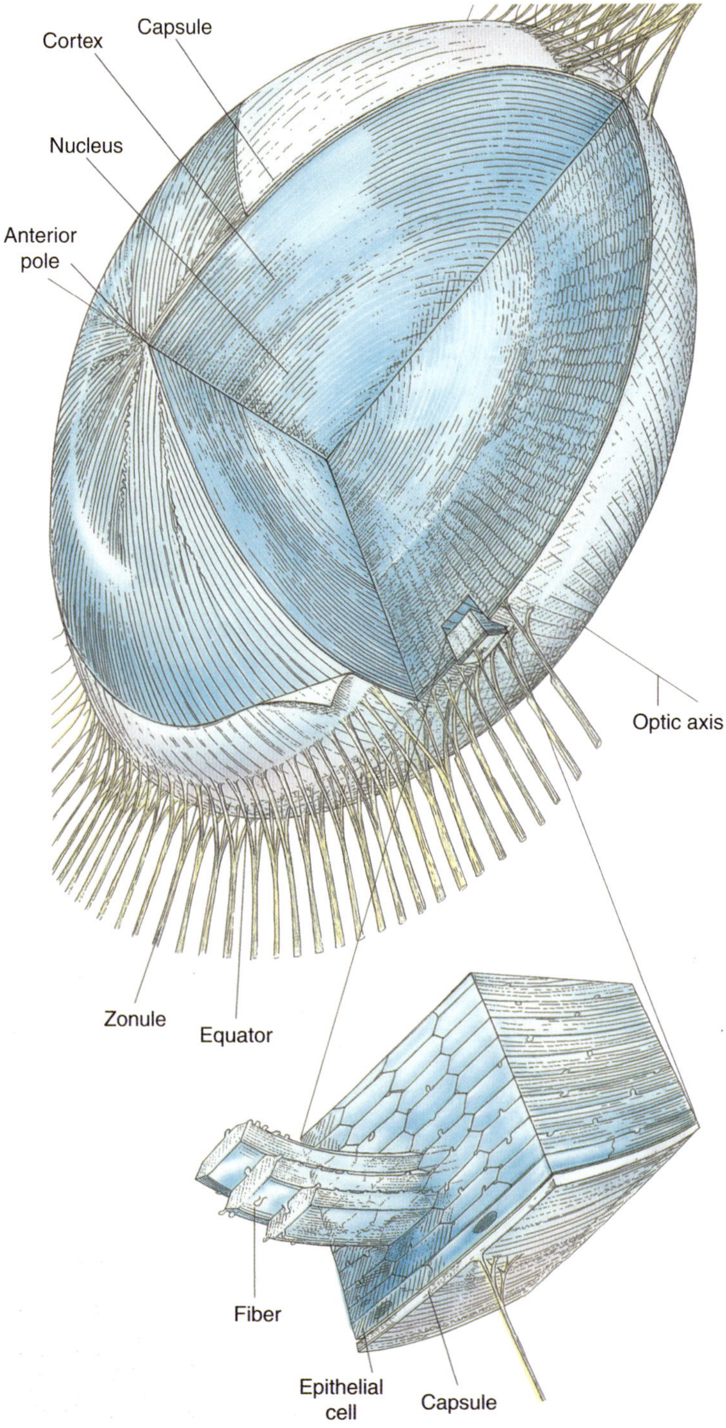

Figure 1-2 Structure of the normal human lens. *(Illustration by Carol Donner. Reproduced with permission from Koretz JF, Handelman GH. How the human eye focuses.* Scientific American. *July 1988:94.)*

The lens is able to refract light because its index of refraction—normally about 1.4 centrally and 1.36 peripherally—is different from that of the aqueous and vitreous that surround it. In its nonaccommodative state, the lens contributes about 15–20 diopters (D) of the approximately 60 D of convergent refractive power of the average human eye. The remaining 40 or so diopters of convergent refractive power occur at the air–cornea interface.

The lens continues to grow throughout life. At birth, it measures about 6.4 mm equatorially and 3.5 mm anteroposteriorly and weighs approximately 90 mg. The adult lens typically measures 9 mm equatorially and 5 mm anteroposteriorly and weighs approximately 255 mg. The relative thickness of the cortex increases with age. At the same time, the lens adopts an increasingly curved shape so that older lenses have more refractive power. However, the index of refraction decreases with age, probably as a result of the increasing presence of insoluble protein particles. Thus, the eye may become either more hyperopic or more myopic with age, depending on the balance of these opposing changes.

Capsule

The lens capsule is an elastic, transparent basement membrane composed of type IV collagen laid down by the epithelial cells. The capsule contains the lens substance and is capable of molding it during accommodative changes. The outer layer of the lens capsule, the *zonular lamella,* also serves as the point of attachment for the zonular fibers. The lens capsule is thickest in the anterior and posterior preequatorial zones and thinnest in the region of the central posterior pole, where it may be as thin as 2–4 µm. The anterior lens capsule is considerably thicker than the posterior capsule at birth and increases in thickness throughout life (Fig 1-3).

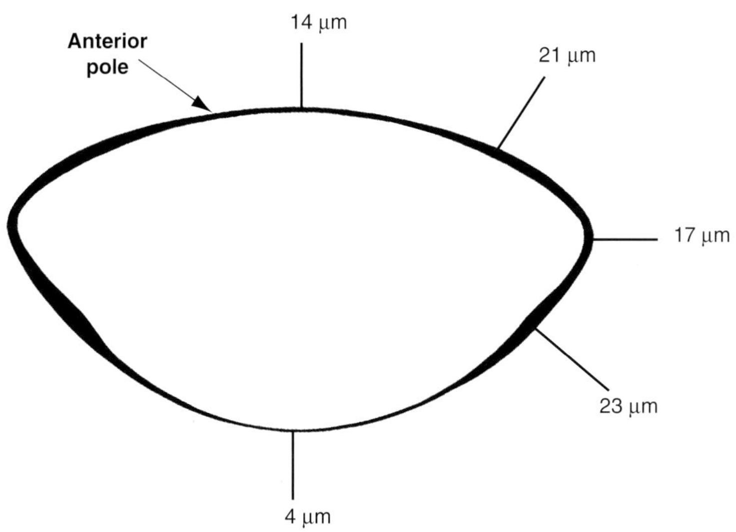

Figure 1-3 Schematic of adult human lens capsule showing relative thickness of capsule in different zones. *(Illustration by Christine Gralapp.)*

Zonular Fibers

The lens is supported by zonular fibers that originate from basal laminae of the nonpigmented epithelium of the pars plana and pars plicata of the ciliary body. These zonular fibers insert, in a continuous fashion, on the lens capsule in the equatorial region, anteriorly 1.5 mm onto the anterior lens capsule and posteriorly 1.25 mm onto the posterior lens capsule. With age, the equatorial zonular fibers regress, leaving separate anterior and posterior layers that appear in a triangular shape on cross section of the zonular ring. The fibers are 5–30 μm in diameter; light microscopy shows them to be eosinophilic structures that have a positive periodic acid–Schiff (PAS) reaction. Ultrastructurally, the fibers are composed of strands, or fibrils, 8–10 nm in diameter with 12–14 nm of banding.

Lens Epithelium

Immediately behind the anterior lens capsule is a single layer of epithelial cells. These cells are metabolically active and carry out all normal cell activities, including the biosynthesis of DNA, RNA, protein, and lipid; they also generate adenosine triphosphate to meet the energy demands of the lens. The epithelial cells are mitotic, with the greatest activity of premitotic (replicative, or S-phase) DNA synthesis occurring in a ring around the anterior lens known as the *germinative zone.* These newly formed cells migrate toward the equator, where they differentiate into fibers. As the epithelial cells migrate toward the bow region of the lens, they begin the process of terminal differentiation into lens fibers (Fig 1-4).

Perhaps the most dramatic morphologic change occurs when the epithelial cells elongate to form lens fiber cells. This change is associated with a tremendous increase in the mass of cellular proteins in the membranes of each fiber cell. At the same time, the cells lose organelles, including cell nuclei, mitochondria, and ribosomes. The loss of these organelles is optically advantageous because light passing through the lens is no longer absorbed or scattered by these structures. However, because these new lens fiber cells lack

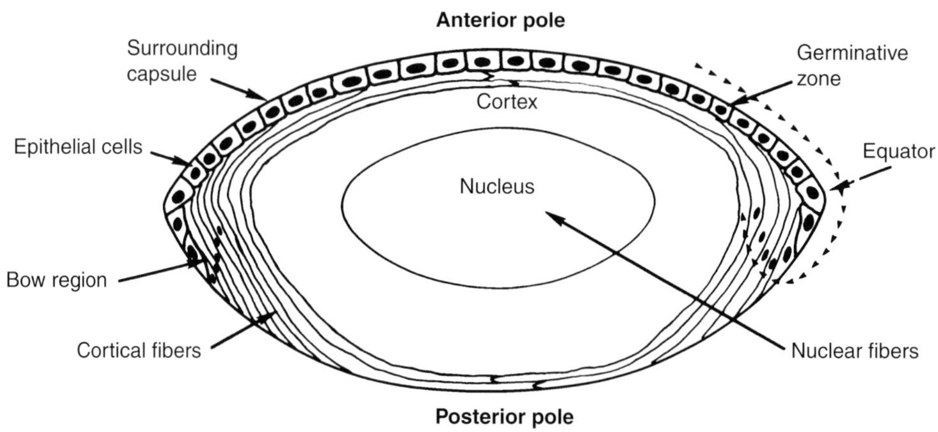

Figure 1-4 Schematic of the mammalian lens in cross section. Arrowheads indicate direction of cell migration from the epithelium to the cortex. *(From Anderson RE, ed.* Biochemistry of the Eye. *San Francisco: American Academy of Ophthalmology; 1983;6:112.)*

the metabolic functions previously carried out by the organelles, they are now dependent on glycolysis for energy production (see Chapter 2).

Nucleus and Cortex

No cells are lost from the lens; as new fibers are laid down, they crowd and compact the previously formed fibers, with the oldest layers being the most central. The oldest of these, the *embryonic* and *fetal lens nuclei,* were produced in embryonic life and persist in the center of the lens (see Fig 4-1 in Chapter 4). The outermost fibers are the most recently formed and make up the cortex of the lens.

Lens sutures are formed by the arrangement of interdigitations of apical cell processes *(anterior sutures)* and basal cell processes *(posterior sutures).* In addition to the Y-sutures located within the lens nucleus, multiple optical zones are visible by slit-lamp biomicroscopy. These zones of demarcation occur because strata of epithelial cells with differing optical densities are laid down throughout life. There is no morphologic distinction between the cortex and the nucleus; rather, the transition between these regions is gradual. Although some surgical texts make distinctions among the nucleus, epinucleus, and cortex, these terms relate only to potential differences in the behavior and appearance of the material during surgical procedures.

Kuszak JR, Clark JI, Cooper KE, et al. Biology of the lens: lens transparency as a function of embryology, anatomy and physiology. In: Albert DM, Jakobiec FA, eds. *Principles and Practice of Ophthalmology*. 2nd ed. Philadelphia: Saunders; 2000:1355–1408.

Snell RS, Lemp MA. *Clinical Anatomy of the Eye*. 2nd ed. Boston: Blackwell; 1998:197–204.

CHAPTER 2

Biochemistry

Molecular Biology

Crystallin Proteins

The human lens has a protein concentration of 33% of its wet weight, which is at least twice that of most other tissues. Lens proteins are often divided into 2 groups based on water solubility (Fig 2-1). The water-soluble fraction of the young lens accounts for approximately 80% of lens proteins and consists mainly of a group of proteins called *crystallins.* The crystallins have been subdivided into 2 major groups: the alpha and betagamma crystallins.

Alpha crystallins represent about one-third of the lens proteins by mass. In their native state, they are the largest of the crystallins, with an average molecular weight of approximately 600 kilodaltons (kDa). However, they may associate with other crystallins, yielding complexes greater than 2 megadaltons. There are 2 alpha crystallin subunits, alphaA and alphaB, each approximately 20 kDa, which form heteromeric complexes containing approximately 30 subunits. The sequence of the alpha crystallins identifies them as members of the family of small heat shock proteins. Alpha-crystallin complexes bind to partially denatured proteins and protect them from aggregating. Their primary function in lens

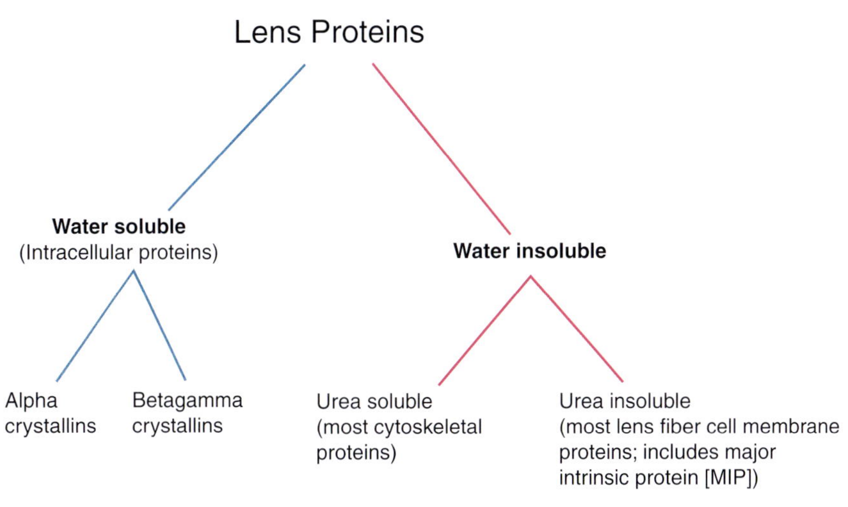

Figure 2-1 Overview of lens proteins.

fiber cells appears to be to prevent the complete denaturation and insolubilization of the other crystallins.

Betagamma crystallins are divided into 2 groups, based on molecular weight and isoelectric points. The *beta crystallins* account for 55% (by weight) of the water-soluble proteins in the lens and are encoded by 7 genes. The individual polypeptides associate with other betas, forming dimers and higher-order complexes in their native state. By gel chromatography, the betas can be separated into beta H (beta high molecular weight) and beta L (beta low molecular weight) fractions.

The *gamma crystallins* are the smallest of the crystallins, with a molecular weight in the range of 20 kDa or less. The native gamma crystallins do not associate with each other or with other proteins and, therefore, have the lowest molecular weight of the crystallin fractions. They make up approximately 15% of adult mammal lens protein. In humans, the gamma family is encoded by 4 genes. X-ray crystallographic studies have determined the 3-dimensional structure of the gamma crystallins to high resolution. Fourfold repetition of a core 3-dimensional structural motif suggests that the betagamma crystallins might have arisen from double duplication and fusion of a gene for a 40-residue polypeptide. The basic structure of the betagamma crystallins has been maintained through hundreds of millions of years of vertebrate evolution.

Membrane Structural Proteins and Cytoskeletal Proteins

The water-insoluble fraction of lens proteins can be further separated into 2 fractions, 1 soluble and 1 insoluble in 8 molar urea. The *urea-soluble fraction* of the young lens contains cytoskeletal proteins that provide the structural framework of the lens cells. Microfilaments and microtubules found in lens cells are similar to those found in other cell types. However, the lens contains 2 types of intermediate filaments that are unusual: one class is made from the protein *vimentin,* which is not usually found in epithelial cells; the other class, the *beaded filaments,* is made from the proteins phakinin and filensin, which are specific to the lens. Genetic disruption of the structure of the beaded filaments leads to disruption of the structure of the fiber cells and cataract formation.

The *urea-insoluble fraction* of the young lens contains the plasma membranes of the lens fiber cells. Several proteins are associated with these fiber cell plasma membranes. One makes up nearly 50% of the membrane proteins and has come to be known as the *major intrinsic protein (MIP).* MIP first appears in the lens just as the fibers begin to elongate. With age, this protein, which has a molecular weight of 28 kDa, undergoes proteolytic cleavage, forming a 22-kDa protein fragment. The relative proportions of these two proteins become about equal at 20–30 years of age. As expected, the 22-kDa protein predominates in the nucleus.

MIP is the founding member of a class of proteins called *aquaporins;* its other name is *aquaporin 0.* Other members of the aquaporin family are found throughout the body, where they serve predominantly as water channels. In the lens, it is not yet certain whether MIP serves primarily as a water channel, as an adhesion molecule that minimizes the extracellular space between fiber cells, or as both. Minimizing the extracellular space between fiber cells is important to reduce the scattering of light as it passes through the lens.

Increase of Water-Insoluble Proteins With Age

Over time, lens proteins aggregate to form very large particles that become water insoluble and that scatter light, thus increasing the opacity of the lens. However, it should be noted that the water-insoluble protein fraction increases with age, even if the lens remains relatively transparent. Conversion of the water-soluble proteins into water-insoluble proteins appears to be a natural process in lens fiber maturation, but it may occur to excess in cataractous lenses.

In cataracts with significant browning of the lens nucleus *(brunescent cataracts),* the increase in the amount of water-insoluble protein correlates well with the degree of opacification. In markedly brunescent cataracts, as much as 90% of the nuclear proteins may be in the insoluble fraction. Associated oxidative changes occur, including protein-to-protein and protein-to-glutathione disulfide bond formation. These changes produce decreased levels of the reduced form of glutathione and increased levels of glutathione disulfide (oxidized glutathione) in the cytoplasm of the nuclear fiber cells. It is the general view that glutathione is essential to maintain a reducing environment in the lens cytoplasm. Depletion of the reduced form of glutathione accelerates protein cross-linking, protein aggregation, and light scattering.

With age and, more notably, with brunescent nuclear cataract formation, the nuclear proteins become increasingly insoluble in urea. In addition to the increased formation of disulfide bonds, these nuclear proteins are highly cross-linked by nondisulfide bonds. This insoluble protein fraction contains yellow-to-brown pigments that are found in higher concentration in nuclear cataracts. Increased fluorescence is generated by the nondisulfide cross-links that form in brunescent nuclear cataracts.

Hejtmancik JF, Piatigorsky J. Lens proteins and their molecular biology. In: Albert DM, Jakobiec FA, eds. *Principles and Practice of Ophthalmology.* 2nd ed. Philadelphia: Saunders; 2000:1409–1428.

Carbohydrate Metabolism

The goal of lens metabolism is the maintenance of transparency. In the lens, energy production largely depends on glucose metabolism. Glucose enters the lens from the aqueous both by *simple diffusion* and by a mediated transfer process called *facilitated diffusion.* Most of the glucose transported into the lens is phosphorylated to a glucose-6-phosphate (G6P) by the enzyme hexokinase. This reaction is 70–1000 times slower than that of other enzymes involved in lens glycolysis and is, therefore, rate limited in the lens. Once formed, G6P enters one of two metabolic pathways: anaerobic glycolysis or the hexose monophosphate (HMP) shunt (Fig 2-2).

The more active of these two pathways is anaerobic glycolysis, which provides most of the high-energy phosphate bonds required for lens metabolism. Substrate-linked phosphorylation of ADP to ATP occurs at 2 steps along the way to lactate. The rate-limiting step in the glycolytic pathway itself is at the level of the enzyme phosphofructokinase, which is regulated through feedback control by metabolic products of the glycolytic pathway. This pathway is much less efficient than aerobic glycolysis because only 2 net molecules of ATP are produced for each glucose molecule utilized, whereas aerobic glycolysis produces an

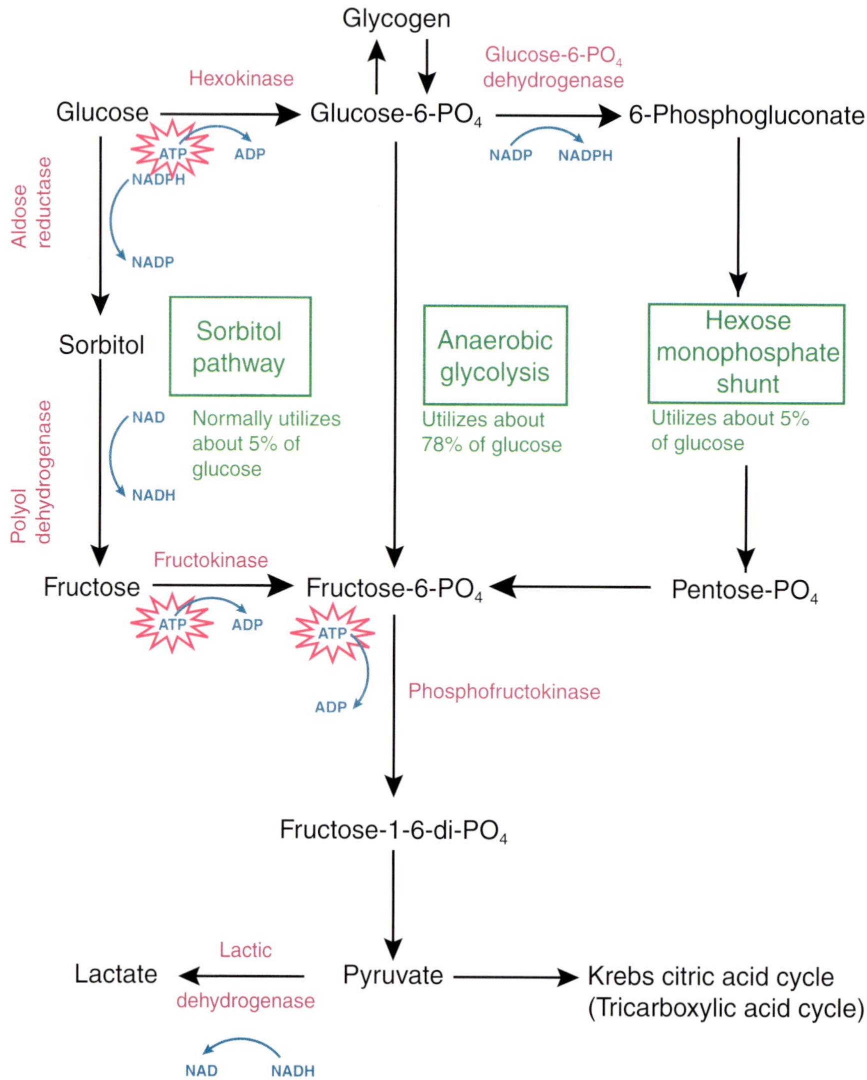

Figure 2-2 Simplified scheme of glucose metabolism in the lens. *(Adapted with permission from Hart WM Jr, ed.* Adler's Physiology of the Eye: Clinical Application. *9th ed. St Louis: Mosby; 1992:362.)*

additional 36 molecules of ATP from each glucose molecule metabolized in the citric acid cycle (oxidative metabolism). Because of the low oxygen tension in the lens, only about 3% of the lens glucose passes through the Krebs citric acid cycle to produce ATP; however, even this low level of aerobic metabolism produces approximately 25% of the lens ATP.

That the lens is not dependent on oxygen is demonstrated by its ability to sustain normal metabolism in a nitrogen environment. Provided with ample glucose, the anoxic in vitro lens remains completely transparent, has normal levels of ATP, and maintains its ion and amino acid pump activities. However, when deprived of glucose, the lens cannot maintain these functions and becomes hazy after several hours, even in the presence of oxygen.

The less active pathway for utilization of G6P in the lens is the HMP shunt, also known as the *pentose phosphate pathway.* Approximately 5% of lens glucose is metabolized by this route, although the pathway is stimulated in the presence of elevated levels of glucose. HMP shunt activity is higher in the lens than in most tissues, but the role of the HMP shunt is far from established. As in other tissues, the HMP shunt may provide NADPH (the reduced form of nicotinamide-adenine dinucleotide phosphate [NADP]) for fatty acid biosynthesis and ribose for nucleotide biosynthesis. It does provide the NADPH necessary for glutathione reductase and aldose reductase activities in the lens. The carbohydrate products of the HMP shunt enter the glycolytic pathway and are metabolized to lactate.

Aldose reductase is the key enzyme in yet another pathway for lens sugar metabolism, the *sorbitol pathway.* This enzyme has been found to play a pivotal role in the development of "sugar" cataracts. (See also the biochemistry chapters [Part IV] in BCSC Section 2, *Fundamentals and Principles of Ophthalmology.*) The Michaelis constant (K_m) of aldose reductase for glucose is about 700 times that for hexokinase. Because the affinity is actually the inverse of K_m, aldose reductase has a very low affinity for glucose compared to hexokinase. Less than 4% of lens glucose is normally converted to sorbitol.

As previously noted, the hexokinase reaction is rate limited in phosphorylating glucose in the lens and is inhibited by the feedback mechanisms of the products of glycolysis. Therefore, when glucose increases in the lens, as occurs in hyperglycemic states, the sorbitol pathway is activated relatively more than glycolysis, and sorbitol accumulates. Sorbitol is metabolized to fructose by the enzyme polyol dehydrogenase. Unfortunately, this enzyme has a relatively low affinity (high K_m), meaning that considerable sorbitol will accumulate before being further metabolized. This characteristic, combined with the poor permeability of the lens to sorbitol, results in retention of sorbitol in the lens.

A high NADPH/NADH ratio drives the reaction in the forward direction. The accumulation of NADP that occurs as a consequence of activation of the sorbitol pathway may cause the HMP shunt stimulation that is observed in the presence of elevated lens glucose. In addition to sorbitol, fructose levels increase in a lens incubated in a high-glucose environment. Together, the 2 sugars increase the osmotic pressure within the lens, drawing in water. At first, the energy-dependent pumps of the lens are able to compensate, but ultimately they are overwhelmed. The result is swelling of the fibers, disruption of the normal cytoskeletal architecture, and opacification of the lens.

Galactose is also a substrate for aldose reductase, producing the alcohol galactitol (dulcitol). Galactitol, however, is not a substrate for sugar alcohol dehydrogenase and thus accumulates rapidly, producing the same osmotic effects—and the same consequences—as sorbitol. Excess production of galactitol occurs in patients with inborn disorders of galactose metabolism. The patient with an inborn error of galactose metabolism is unable to utilize galactose properly and accumulates galactitol and other galactose metabolites. Galactose cataracts can be induced experimentally in animals maintained on diets extremely rich in galactose.

The pivotal role of aldose reductase in cataractogenesis in animals is apparent from studies of the development of sugar-induced cataract in various animal species. Those species that have high aldose reductase activities develop lens opacities, whereas those lacking aldose reductase do not. In addition, specific inhibitors of this enzymatic activity, applied either systemically or topically to 1 eye, decrease the rate of onset and the severity of sugar cataracts in experimental studies.

Oxidative Damage and Protective Mechanisms

Free radicals are generated in the course of normal cellular metabolic activities and may also be produced by external agents such as radiant energy. These highly reactive free radicals can lead to the damage of lens fibers. Peroxidation of lens fiber plasma or lens fiber plasma membrane lipids has been suggested as a factor contributing to lens opacification. In the process of lipid peroxidation, the oxidizing agent removes a hydrogen atom from the polyunsaturated fatty acid, forming a fatty acid radical, which, in turn, attacks molecular oxygen, forming a lipid peroxy radical. This reaction may propagate the chain, leading to the formation of lipid peroxide (LOOH), which eventually can react further to yield malondialdehyde (MDA), a potent cross-linking agent. It has been hypothesized that MDA cross-reacts with membrane lipids and proteins, rendering them incapable of performing their normal functions.

Because oxygen tension in and around the lens is normally low, free radical reactions may not involve molecular oxygen; instead, the free radicals may react directly with molecules. DNA is easily damaged by free radicals. Some of the damage to the lens is reparable, but some may be permanent. Free radicals can also attack the proteins or membrane lipids in the cortex. No repair mechanisms are known to ameliorate such damage, which increases with time. In lens fibers, where protein synthesis no longer takes place, free radical damage may lead to polymerization and cross-linking of lipids and proteins, resulting in an increase in the water-insoluble protein content.

The lens is equipped with several enzymes that protect against free radical or oxygen damage. These include glutathione peroxidase, catalase, and superoxide dismutase. Superoxide dismutase catalyzes the destruction of the superoxide anion, O_2^-, and produces hydrogen peroxide: $2O_2^- + 2H^+ \rightarrow H_2O_2 + O_2$. Catalase may break down the peroxide by the reaction: $2H_2O_2 \rightarrow 2H_2O + O_2$. Glutathione peroxidase catalyzes the reaction: $2GSH + LOOH \rightarrow GSSG + LOH + H_2O$. The glutathione disulfide (GSSG) is then reconverted to glutathione (GSH) by glutathione reductase, using the pyridine nucleotide NADPH provided by the HMP shunt as the reducing agent: $GSSG + NADPH + H^+ \rightarrow 2GSH + NADP^+$. Thus, glutathione acts indirectly as a major free radical scavenger in the lens. In addition, both vitamin E and ascorbic acid are present in the lens. Each of these substances can act as a free radical scavenger and thus protect against oxidative damage.

Exposure of the lens to an increased level of oxygen during long-term hyperbaric oxygen therapy leads to a myopic shift, increased opacification of the lens nucleus and, in many cases, the formation of nuclear cataracts. The lens is also exposed to increased levels of oxygen during retinal surgery and for months following vitrectomy. Because vitrectomy is associated with very high rates of nuclear cataract formation, it has been suggested that the low oxygen level existing around the lens protects it from oxidative damage and that loss of the gel structure of the vitreous body increases exposure of the lens to oxygen and the risk of nuclear cataracts.

Andley UP, Liang JJN, Lou MF. Biochemical mechanisms of age-related cataract. In: Albert DM, Jakobiec FA, eds. *Principles and Practice of Ophthalmology*. 2nd ed. Philadelphia: Saunders; 2000:1428–1449.

Beebe DC. Lens. In: Kaufman PL, Alm A, eds. *Adler's Physiology of the Eye: Clinical Application*. 10th ed. St Louis: Mosby; 2003:117–158.

Bloemendal H, de Jong W, Jaenicke R, Lubsen NH, Slingsby C, Tardieu A. Aging and vision: structure, stability and function of lens crystallins. *Prog Biophys Mol Biol*. 2004;86(3):407–485.

Jaffe NS, Horwitz J. Evolution and molecular biology of lens proteins. In: Podos SM, Yanoff M, eds. *Textbook of Ophthalmology, vol 3, Lens and Cataract*. New York: Gower Medical Publishing; 1992.

CHAPTER 3

Physiology

Throughout life, lens epithelial cells at the equator continue to divide and develop into lens fibers, resulting in continual growth of the lens. The lens cells with the highest metabolic rate are in the epithelium and the outer cortex. These superficial cells utilize oxygen and glucose for the active transport of electrolytes, carbohydrates, and amino acids into the lens. Because the lens is avascular, several challenges are involved in the task of maintaining transparency. The older cells, toward the center of the lens, must be able to communicate with the superficial cells and the environment outside the lens. This communication is accomplished through low-resistance gap junctions that facilitate the exchange of small molecules from cell to cell. Lens fiber cells also have abundant water channels in their membranes, made from the major intrinsic protein (MIP—also known as *aquaporin 0*). Whether the function of MIP is primarily as a water channel, as a contributor to cell–cell adhesion, or both is not yet certain.

Maintenance of Lens Water and Cation Balance

Perhaps the most important aspect of lens physiology is the mechanism that controls water and electrolyte balance, which is critical to lens transparency. Because transparency is highly dependent on the structural and macromolecular components of the lens, perturbation of cellular hydration can readily lead to opacification. It is noteworthy that disruption of water and electrolyte balance is not a feature of nuclear cataracts. In cortical cataracts, however, the water content rises significantly.

The normal human lens contains approximately 66% water and 33% protein, and this amount changes very little with aging. The lens cortex is more hydrated than the lens nucleus. About 5% of the lens volume is the water found between the lens fibers in the extracellular spaces. Within the lens, sodium and potassium concentrations are maintained at 20 millimolars (mM) and 120 mM, respectively. Aqueous and vitreous levels are markedly different, with the sodium concentration maintained at 150 mM and potassium at 5 mM.

Lens Epithelium: Site of Active Transport

The lens is dehydrated and has higher levels of potassium ions (K^+) and amino acids than the surrounding aqueous and vitreous. Conversely, the lens contains lower levels of sodium ions (Na^+), chloride ions (Cl^-), and water than the surrounding environment.

The cation balance between the inside and outside of the lens is the result both of the permeability properties of the lens cell membranes and of the activity of the sodium pumps that reside within the cell membranes of the lens epithelium and each lens fiber. The sodium pumps function by pumping sodium ions out while taking potassium ions in. This mechanism depends on the breakdown of adenosine triphosphate (ATP) and is regulated by the enzyme Na^+,K^+-ATPase. This balance is easily disrupted by the specific ATPase inhibitor ouabain. Inhibition of Na^+,K^+-ATPase leads to loss of cation balance and elevated water content in the lens. Whether Na^+,K^+-ATPase is depressed in the development of cortical cataract is uncertain; some studies have shown reduced Na^+,K^+-ATPase activity, whereas others have shown no change. Still other studies have suggested that the passive membrane permeability to cations is increased with aging and cataract development.

Pump-Leak Theory

The combination of active transport and membrane permeability is often referred to as the pump-leak system of the lens (Fig 3-1). According to the *pump-leak theory,* potas-

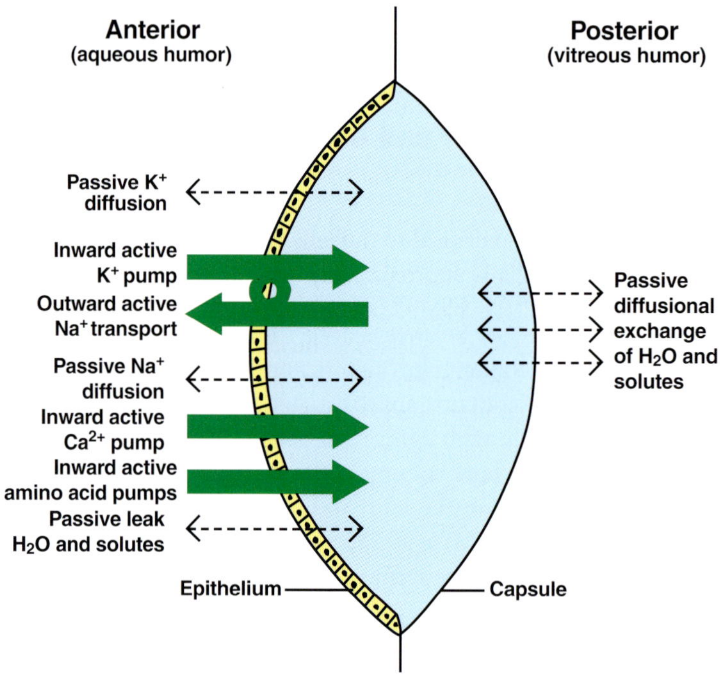

Figure 3-1 The pump-leak hypothesis of pathways of solute movement in the lens. The major site of active transport mechanisms is in the anterior epithelium, whereas passive diffusion occurs over both surfaces of the lens. *(Modified with permission from Paterson CA, Delamere NA. The lens. In: Hart WM Jr, ed.* Adler's Physiology of the Eye. *9th ed. St Louis: Mosby; 1992:365.)*

sium and various other molecules such as amino acids are actively transported into the anterior lens via the epithelium anteriorly. They then diffuse out with the concentration gradient through the back of the lens, where there are no active transport mechanisms. Conversely, sodium flows in through the back of the lens with the concentration gradient and then is actively exchanged for potassium by the epithelium. In support of this theory, an anteroposterior gradient was found for both ions: potassium was concentrated in the anterior lens; sodium, in the posterior lens. Conditions such as refrigeration that inactivate the energy-dependent enzyme pumps also abolish these gradients. Most of the Na^+,K^+-ATPase activity is found in the lens epithelium and the superficial cortical fiber cells. The active transport mechanisms are lost if the capsule and attached epithelium are removed from the lens but not if the capsule alone is removed by enzymatic degradation with collagenase. These findings support the hypothesis that the epithelium is the primary site for active transport in the lens. This asymmetric arrangement results in sodium and potassium gradients across the lens, with the concentration of potassium being higher at the front of the lens and lower at the back. Conversely, sodium concentration is higher at the back of the lens and lower at the front. Much of the diffusion throughout the lens occurs from cell to cell through the low-resistance gap junctions.

The membrane transport processes that establish the ion gradients across lens cell membranes generate extracellular currents around the outside of the lens. Sodium preferentially enters the lens at the poles, and potassium preferentially exits from the equator.

The unequal distribution of electrolytes across the lens cell membranes results in an electrical potential difference between the inside and outside of the lens. The inside of the lens is electronegative, measuring approximately –70 millivolts (mV). There is even a –23-mV potential difference between the anterior and posterior surfaces of the lens. The normal potential difference of about 70 mV is readily altered by changes in pump activity or membrane permeability.

Calcium homeostasis is also critical to the lens. The normal intracellular level of calcium in the lens epithelial cells is approximately 100 nanomolars, whereas the exterior calcium level is close to 1 mM. This large transmembrane calcium gradient is maintained primarily by the calcium pump (Ca^{2+}-ATPase). The lens cell membranes are also relatively impermeable to calcium. Free calcium levels in lens fiber cells are much higher, averaging 10 micromolars. Loss of calcium homeostasis can be highly disruptive of lens metabolism. Increased levels of calcium can result in many deleterious changes, including depressed glucose metabolism, formation of high-molecular-weight protein aggregates, and activation of destructive proteases.

Membrane transport and permeability are also important considerations in lens nutrition. Active amino acid transport takes place at the lens epithelium by a mechanism dependent on the sodium gradient, which is brought about by the sodium pump. Glucose enters the lens by a process of facilitated diffusion not directly linked to an active transport system. The waste products of lens metabolism leave the lens by simple diffusion. A variety of substances, including ascorbic acid, *myo*-inositol, and choline, have specialized transport mechanisms in the lens.

Accommodation

Accommodation, the mechanism by which the eye changes focus from distant to near images, is produced by a change in lens shape resulting from the action of the ciliary muscle on the zonular fibers. The lens substance is most malleable during childhood and the young adult years, progressively losing its ability to change shape with age. After approximately 40 years, the rigidity of the lens nucleus clinically reduces accommodation because the sclerotic nucleus cannot bulge anteriorly and change its anterior curvature as it could before. Recent studies have shown that, throughout life, the hardness or stiffness of the human lens increases more than 1000-fold.

According to the classic theory of von Helmholtz, most of the accommodative change in lens shape occurs at the central anterior lens surface. The central anterior capsule is thinner than the peripheral capsule (see Fig 1-3 in Chapter 1), and the anterior zonular fibers insert slightly closer to the visual axis than do the posterior zonular fibers, resulting in a central anterior bulge with accommodation. The posterior lens surface curvature changes minimally with accommodation. The central posterior capsule, which is the thinnest area of the capsule, tends to bulge posteriorly to the same extent regardless of zonular tension.

The ciliary muscle is a ring that, upon contraction, has the opposite effect from that intuitively expected of a sphincter. When a sphincter muscle contracts, it usually tightens its grip. However, when the ciliary muscle contracts, the diameter of the muscle ring is reduced, thereby relaxing the tension on the zonular fibers and allowing the lens to become more spherical. Thus, when the ciliary muscle contracts, the axial thickness of the lens increases, its diameter decreases, and its dioptric power increases, producing accommodation. When the ciliary muscle relaxes, the zonular tension increases, the lens flattens, and the dioptric power of the lens decreases (Table 3-1).

The accommodative response may be stimulated by the known or apparent size and distance of an object or by blur, chromatic aberration, or a continual oscillation of ciliary tone. Accommodation is mediated by the parasympathetic fibers of cranial nerve III (oculomotor). Parasympathomimetic drugs (eg, pilocarpine) induce accommodation, whereas parasympatholytic medications (eg, atropine) block accommodation. Drugs that relax the ciliary muscle are called *cycloplegics.*

Table 3-1 Changes With Accommodation

	With Accommodation	Without Accommodation
Ciliary muscle action	Contraction	Relaxation
Ciliary ring diameter	Decreases	Increases
Zonular tension	Decreases	Increases
Lens shape	More spherical	Flatter
Lens equatorial diameter	Decreases	Increases
Axial lens thickness	Increases	Decreases
Central anterior lens capsule curvature	Steepens	Flattens
Central posterior lens capsule curvature	Minimal change	Minimal change
Lens dioptric power	Increases	Decreases

The *amplitude of accommodation* is the amount of change in the eye's refractive power that is produced by accommodation. It diminishes with age and may be affected by some medications and diseases. Adolescents generally have 12–16 D of accommodation, whereas adults at age 40 have 4–8 D. After age 50, accommodation decreases to less than 2 D. It is thought that hardening of the lens with age is the principal cause of this loss of accommodation, which is called *presbyopia*. Research is under way into other possible contributing factors in presbyopia, such as changes in lens dimensions, in the elasticity of the lens capsule, and in the geometry of zonular attachments with age.

Glasser A, Kaufman PL. Accommodation and presbyopia. In: Kaufman PL, Alm A, eds. *Adler's Physiology of the Eye: Clinical Application*. 10th ed. St Louis: Mosby; 2003:197–233.

Presbyopia

Presbyopia is the loss of accommodation due to aging. According to the theory of von Helmholtz, as the crystalline lens ages, it becomes firmer and more sclerotic and resists deformation when the ciliary muscle contracts. Hence, it cannot bulge enough anteriorly to increase the lens curvature and dioptric power to focus at near. Most studies have supported this explanation of the cause of presbyopia, including measurements of lens position and curvature in the intact eye, and of increasing lens rigidity and sclerosis with age.

Glasser A, Kaufman PL. The mechanism of accommodation in primates. *Ophthalmology.* 1999;106(5):863–872.

Heys KR, Cram SL, Truscott RJ. Massive increase in the stiffness of the human lens nucleus with age: the basis for presbyopia? *Mol Vis.* 2004;10:956–963.

Winkler J, Wirbelauer C, Frank V, Laqua H. Quantitative distribution of glycosaminoglycans in young and senile (cataractous) anterior lens capsules. *Exp Eye Res.* 2001;72(3):311–318.

This chapter was prepared with the assistance of David Beebe, PhD.

CHAPTER 4

Embryology

Normal Development

The formation of the human crystalline lens begins very early in embryogenesis (Fig 4-1). At approximately 25 days of gestation, 2 lateral evaginations, called the *optic vesicles,* form from the forebrain, or diencephalon. As the optic vesicles enlarge and extend laterally, they become closely apposed and adherent to the *surface ectoderm,* a single layer of cuboidal cells, in 2 patches on either side of the head.

Lens Placode

The ectoderm cells that overlie the optic vesicles become columnar at approximately 27 days of gestation. This area of thickened cells is called the *lens placode.* Growth factors of the *bone morphogenetic protein (BMP)* family are required for the formation of the lens placode and for subsequent lens formation.

Lens Pit

The lens pit appears at 29 days of gestation as an indentation (infolding) of the lens placode. The lens pit deepens and invaginates to form the lens vesicle.

Lens Vesicle

As the lens pit continues to invaginate, the stalk of cells that connects it to the surface ectoderm degenerates by programmed cell death (apoptosis), thereby separating the lens cells from the surface ectoderm. The resultant sphere, a single layer of cuboidal cells encased in a basement membrane (the *lens capsule*), is called the *lens vesicle.* At the time of its formation at 30 days' gestation, the lens vesicle is approximately 0.2 mm in diameter.

Because the lens vesicle was formed through a process of invagination of the surface ectoderm, the apices of the single layer of cells are oriented toward the lumen of the lens vesicle, with the base of each cell attached to the capsule around the periphery of the vesicle. At the same time that the lens vesicle is forming, the optic vesicle is invaginating to form the 2-layered *optic cup.*

Primary Lens Fibers and the Embryonic Nucleus

The cells in the posterior layer of the lens vesicle stop dividing and begin to elongate. As they elongate, they begin to fill the lumen of the lens vesicle. At approximately 40 days of

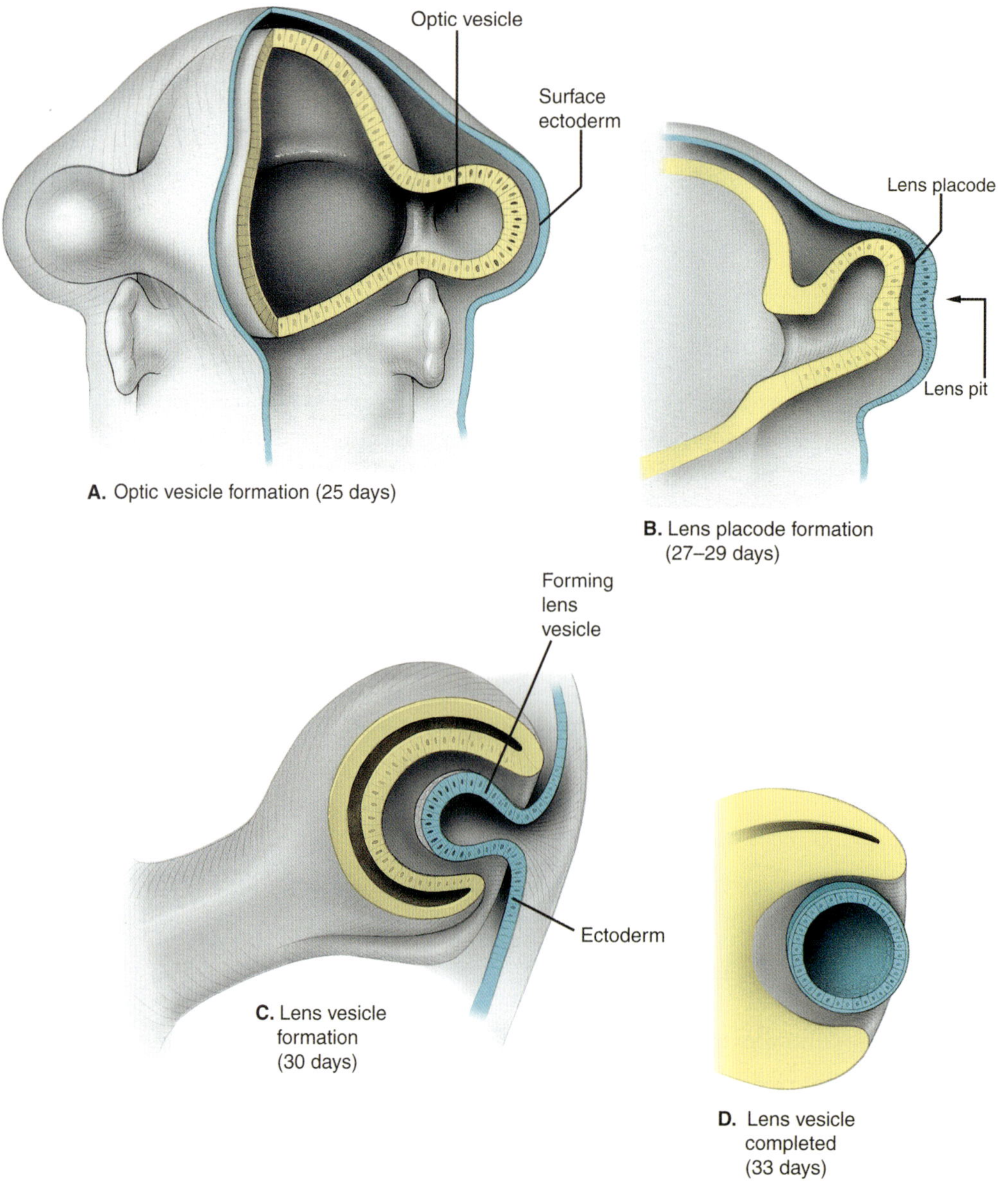

Figure 4-1 Embryologic development of the lens. See text for detailed description of artwork. *(Illustration by Christine Gralapp.)* *(continued)*

gestation, the lumen of the lens vesicle is obliterated. The elongated cells are called the *primary lens fibers.* As the fiber cells mature, their nuclei and other membrane-bound organelles undergo degradation, a process that reduces light scattering. The primary lens fibers make up the embryonic nucleus that will ultimately occupy the central area of the lens in adult life.

The cells of the anterior lens vesicle remain as a monolayer of cuboidal cells, the *lens epithelium.* Subsequent growth of the lens is due to proliferation within the epithelium.

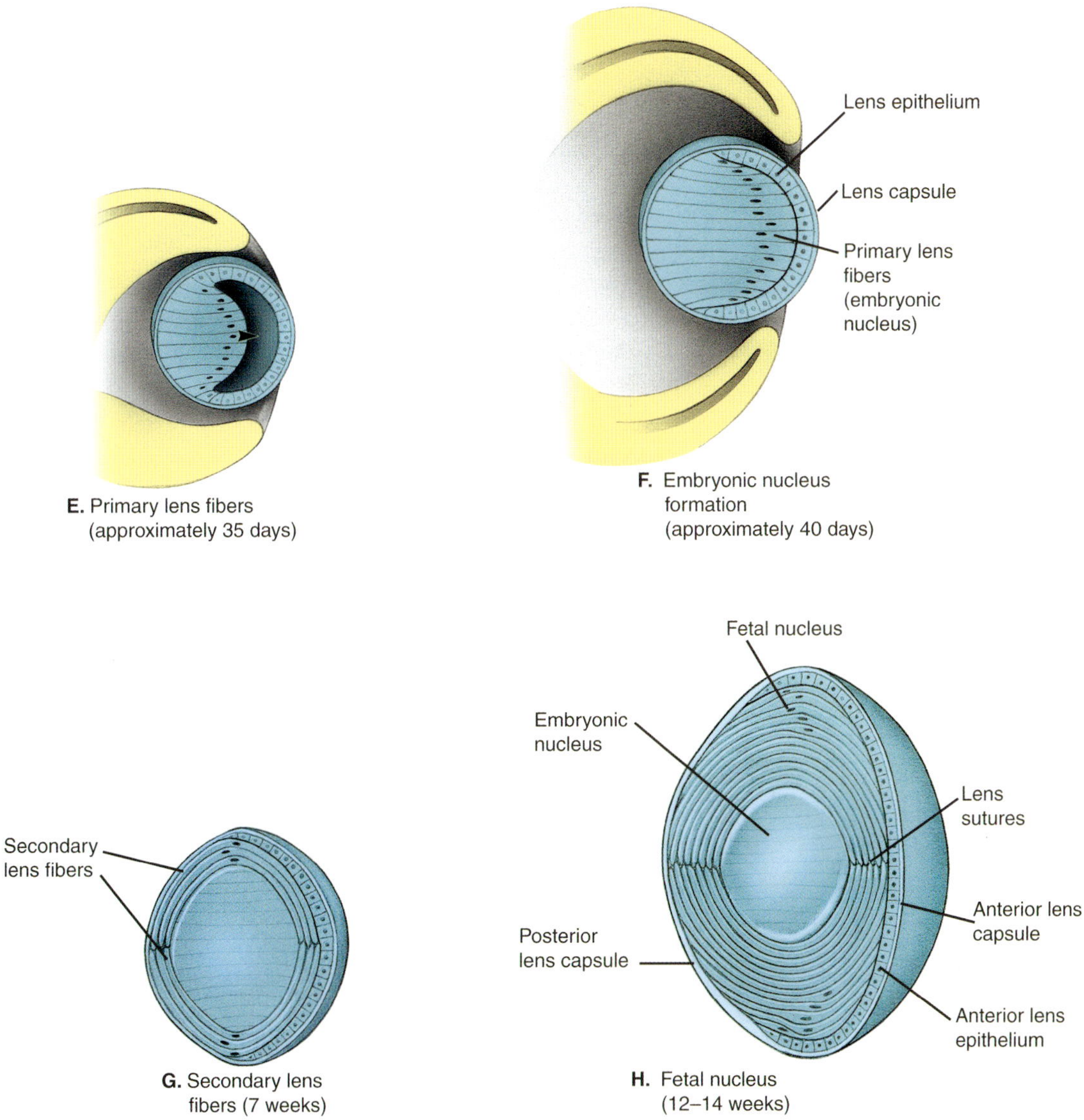

Figure 4-1 *(continued from previous page)*

The *lens capsule* develops as a basement membrane elaborated by the lens epithelium anteriorly and by lens fibers posteriorly.

Secondary Lens Fibers

After they proliferate, the epithelial cells near the lens equator elongate to form secondary lens fibers. The anterior aspect of each developing lens fiber extends anteriorly beneath the lens epithelium, toward the anterior pole of the lens. The posterior aspect of each developing lens fiber extends posteriorly along the capsule toward the posterior pole of the lens. In this manner, new lens fibers are continually formed, layer upon layer. As each secondary fiber cell detaches from the capsule, it loses its nucleus and membrane-bound organelles. The secondary lens fibers formed between 2 and 8 months of gestation make up the *fetal nucleus.*

Lens Sutures and the Fetal Nucleus

As lens fibers grow anteriorly and posteriorly, a pattern emerges where the ends of the fibers meet and interdigitate with the ends of fibers arising on the opposite side of the lens, near the anterior and posterior poles. These patterns of cell association are known as *sutures.* Y-shaped sutures are recognizable at about 8 weeks of gestation, with an erect Y-suture appearing anteriorly and an inverted Y-suture posteriorly (Fig 4-2). As the lens fibers continue to form and the lens continues to grow, the pattern of lens sutures becomes increasingly complex, resulting in 12 or more suture branches in the adult eye. The influences responsible for the precise formation and changing organization of the suture pattern remain a mystery.

The human lens weighs approximately 90 mg at birth, and it increases in mass at the rate of about 2 mg per year as new fibers form throughout life. The central, or oldest, lens

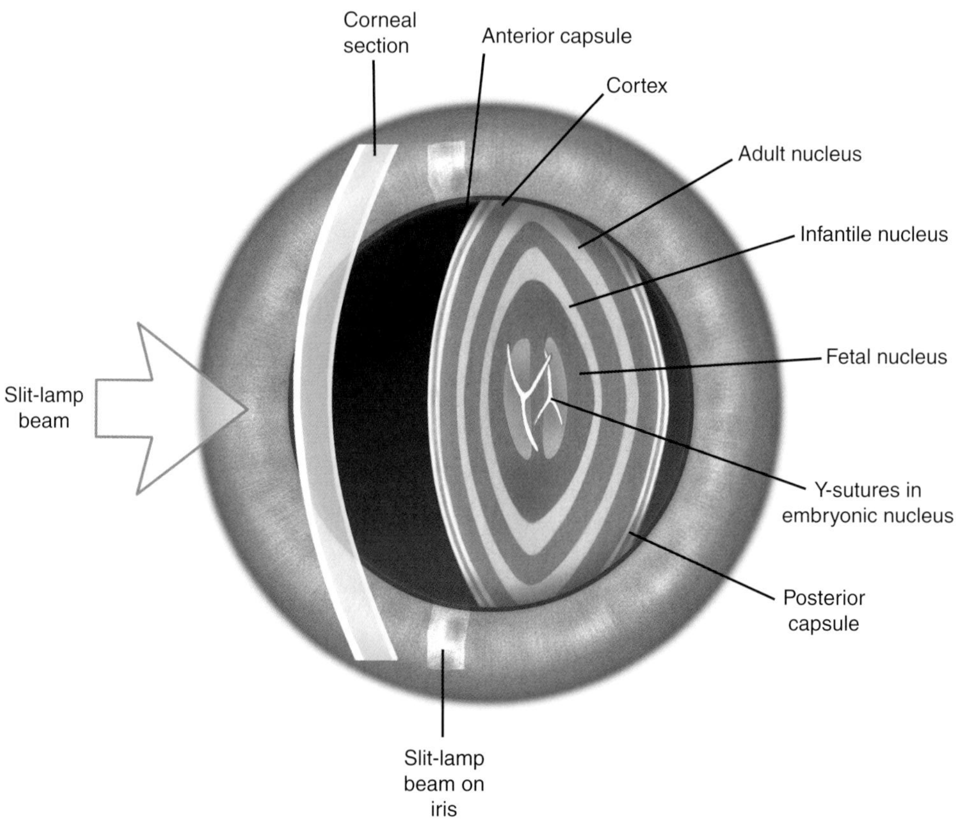

Figure 4-2 Y-shaped sutures, formed during embryogenesis, are visible within the adult lens with the use of the slit lamp. *(Illustration by Christine Gralapp.)*

fibers gradually become less malleable and the lens nucleus becomes more rigid. This process progressively reduces the amplitude of accommodation.

Tunica Vasculosa Lentis

At about 1 month of gestation, the hyaloid artery, which enters the eye at the optic disc, branches to form a network of capillaries, the tunica vasculosa lentis, on the posterior surface of the lens capsule (Fig 4-3). These capillaries grow toward the equator of the lens, where they anastomose with a second network of capillaries, called the *anterior pupillary membrane,* which derives from the ciliary veins and which covers the anterior surface of the lens. At approximately 9 weeks of gestation, the capillary network surrounding the lens is fully developed; it disappears by an orderly process of programmed cell death shortly before birth. Sometimes a remnant of the tunica vasculosa lentis persists as a small opacity or strand, called a *Mittendorf dot,* on the posterior aspect of the lens. In other eyes, remnants of the pupillary membrane are often visible as pupillary strands.

Zonules of Zinn

Experimental evidence suggests that the zonular fibers are secreted by the ciliary epithelium, although how these fibers insert into the lens capsule is not known. The zonular fibers begin to develop at the end of the third month of gestation.

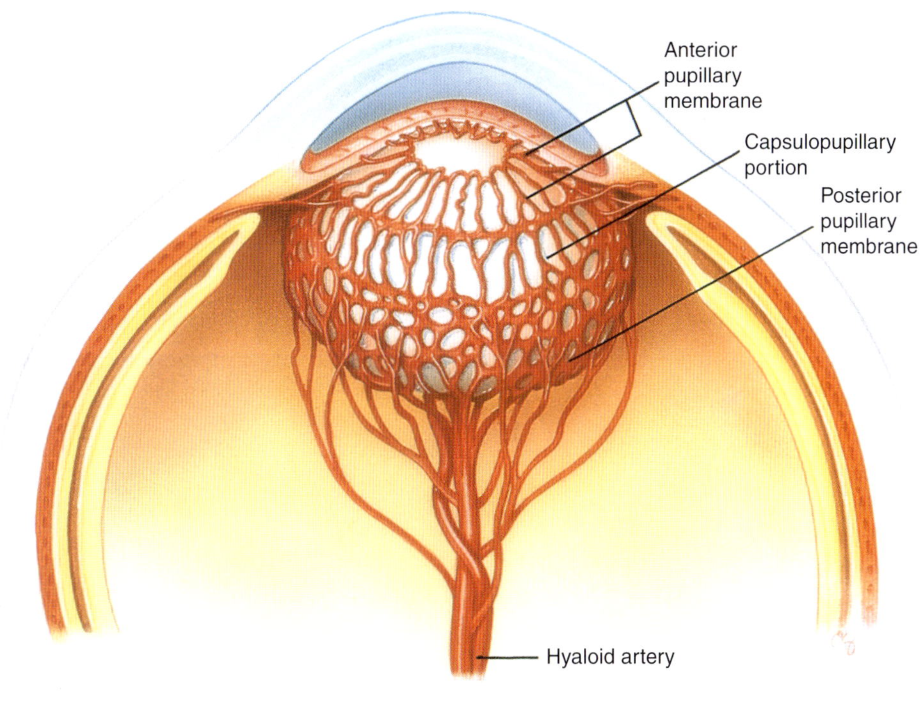

Figure 4-3 Components of the tunica vasculosa lentis. *(Illustration by Christine Gralapp.)*

Duke-Elder S, ed. *System of Ophthalmology*. St Louis: Mosby; 1973:chap 4, pp 127–137.

Kuszak JR, Clark JI, Cooper KE, et al. Biology of the lens: lens transparency as a function of embryology, anatomy, and physiology. In: Albert DM, Jakobiec FA, eds. *Principles and Practice of Ophthalmology*. 2nd ed. Philadelphia: Saunders; 2000:1355–1408.

Kuszak JR, Costello MJ. Embryology and anatomy of human lenses. In: Tasman W, Jaeger EA, eds. *Duane's Clinical Ophthalmology*. Vol 1. Philadelphia: Lippincott; 2002:chap 71A, pp 1–20.

Streeten BW. Zonular apparatus; Worgul BV. The lens. In: Jakobiec FA, ed. *Ocular Anatomy, Embryology, and Teratology*. Philadelphia: Harper & Row; 1982:331–353.

Congenital Anomalies and Abnormalities

Congenital Aphakia

The lens is absent in congenital aphakia, a very rare anomaly. Two forms of congenital aphakia have been described. In *primary aphakia,* the lens placode fails to form from the surface ectoderm in the developing embryo. In *secondary aphakia,* the more common type, the developing lens is spontaneously absorbed. Both forms of aphakia are usually associated with other malformations of the eye.

Lenticonus and Lentiglobus

Lenticonus is a localized, cone-shaped deformation of the anterior or posterior lens surface (Fig 4-4). Posterior lenticonus is more common than anterior lenticonus and is usually unilateral and axial in location. Anterior lenticonus, which is often bilateral, may be associated with Alport syndrome.

In lentiglobus, the localized deformation of the lens surface is spherical. Posterior lentiglobus is more common than anterior lentiglobus and is often associated with posterior pole opacities that vary in density.

Retinoscopy through the center of the lens reveals a distorted and myopic reflex in both lenticonus and lentiglobus. These deformations can also be seen in the red reflex, where, by retroillumination, they appear as an "oil droplet." (This condition should not be

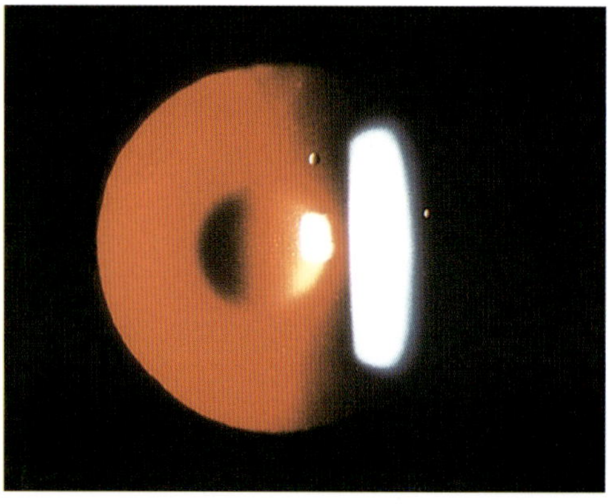

Figure 4-4 Posterior lenticonus as viewed by retroillumination.

confused with the "oil droplet" cataract of galactosemia, which is discussed in Chapter 5.) The posterior bulging may progress with initial worsening of the myopia, followed by opacification of the defect. Surrounding cortical lamellae may also opacify.

Lens Coloboma

A lens coloboma is an anomaly of lens shape (Fig 4-5). Lens colobomas may be classified into 2 types: *primary coloboma,* a wedge-shaped defect or indentation of the lens periphery that occurs as an isolated anomaly; and *secondary coloboma,* a flattening or indentation of the lens periphery caused by the lack of ciliary body or zonular development. Lens colobomas are typically located inferiorly and may be associated with colobomas of the uvea. Cortical lens opacification or thickening of the lens capsule may appear adjacent to the coloboma. The zonular attachments in the region of the coloboma usually are weakened or absent.

Mittendorf Dot

Mittendorf dot, mentioned earlier in this chapter, is a common anomaly observed in many healthy eyes. A small, dense white spot generally located inferonasal to the posterior pole of the lens, a Mittendorf dot is a remnant of the posterior pupillary membrane of the tunica vasculosa lentis. It marks the place where the hyaloid artery came into contact with the posterior surface of the lens in utero. Sometimes a Mittendorf dot is associated with a fibrous tail or remnant of the hyaloid artery projecting into the vitreous body.

Epicapsular Star

Another very common remnant of the tunica vasculosa lentis is an epicapsular star (Fig 4-6). As its name suggests, it consists of a star-shaped distribution of tiny brown or golden flecks on the central anterior lens capsule. It may be unilateral or bilateral.

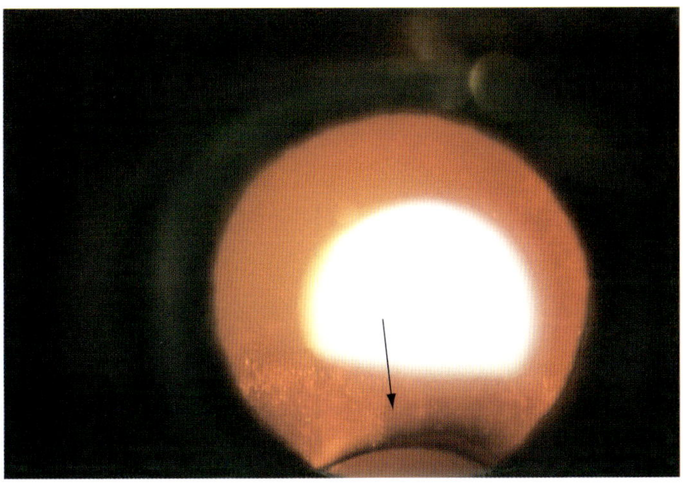

Figure 4-5 Coloboma of the lens *(arrow)* as viewed by retroillumination.

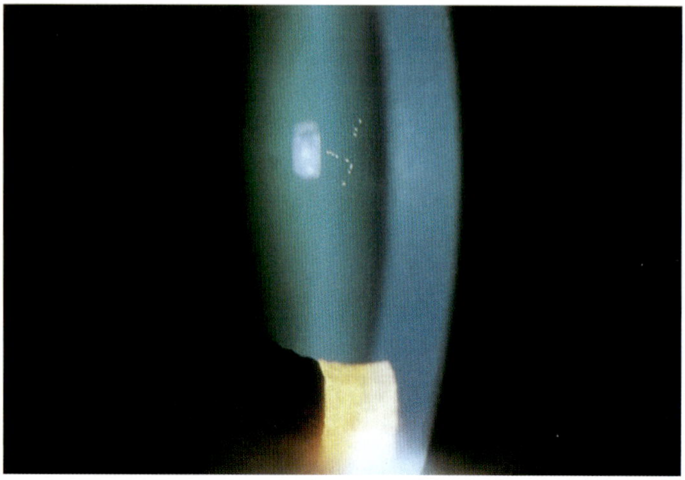

Figure 4-6 Epicapsular star.

Peters Anomaly

Peters anomaly, historically called *posterior corneal defect,* is part of a spectrum of disorders known as *anterior segment dysgenesis syndrome,* also known as *neurocristopathy* or *mesodermal dysgenesis.* Peters anomaly is characterized by a central or paracentral corneal opacity (leukoma) associated with the thinning or absence of adjacent endothelium and Descemet's membrane. In normal ocular development, the lens vesicle separates from the surface ectoderm (the future corneal epithelium) at about 33 days' gestation. Peters anomaly is typically linked with the absence of this separation. It is often associated with mutations in or deletion of one allele of the genes normally involved in anterior segment development, including the transcription factors *PAX6, PITX2,* and *FOXC1.* Patients with Peters anomaly may also display the following lens anomalies:

- adhesions between lens and cornea
- anterior cortical or polar cataract
- a misshapen lens displaced anteriorly into the pupillary space and the anterior chamber
- microspherophakia

Microspherophakia

Microspherophakia is a developmental abnormality in which the lens is small in diameter and spherical. The entire lens equator can be visualized at the slit lamp when the pupil is widely dilated (Fig 4-7). The spherical shape of the lens results in increased refractive power, which causes the eye to be highly myopic.

Faulty development of the secondary lens fibers during embryogenesis is believed to be the cause of microspherophakia. Microspherophakia is most often seen as a part of Weill-Marchesani syndrome. This condition may also occur as an isolated hereditary abnormality or, occasionally, in association with Peters anomaly, Marfan syndrome, Alport syndrome, Lowe syndrome, or congenital rubella. People with Weill-Marchesani syndrome commonly

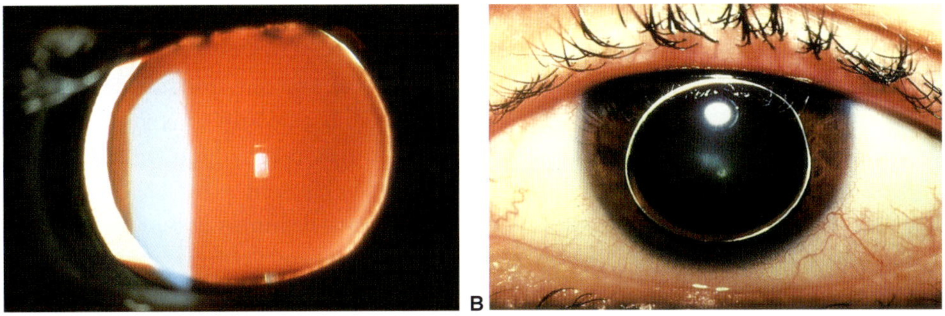

Figure 4-7 Microspherophakia. **A,** When the pupil is dilated, the entire lens equator can be seen at the slit lamp. **B,** Anterior dislocation of a microspherophakic lens. *(Part A courtesy of Karla J. Johns, MD.)*

have small stature, short and stubby fingers, and broad hands with reduced joint mobility. Weill-Marchesani syndrome is usually inherited as an autosomal recessive trait.

The spherical lens can block the pupil, causing secondary angle-closure glaucoma. Miotics aggravate this condition by increasing pupillary block and allowing further forward lens displacement. Cycloplegics are the medical treatment of choice to break an attack of angle-closure glaucoma in patients with microspherophakia because they decrease pupillary block by tightening the zonular fibers, decreasing the anteroposterior lens diameter, and pulling the lens posteriorly. A laser iridotomy may also be useful in relieving angle closure in patients with microspherophakia. (See also BCSC Section 10, *Glaucoma*.)

Aniridia

Aniridia is an uncommon panocular syndrome in which the most dramatic manifestation is partial or nearly complete absence of the iris (Fig 4-8). Aniridia has been linked to the loss of one allele of the *PAX6* gene, a transcription factor that is important for the development

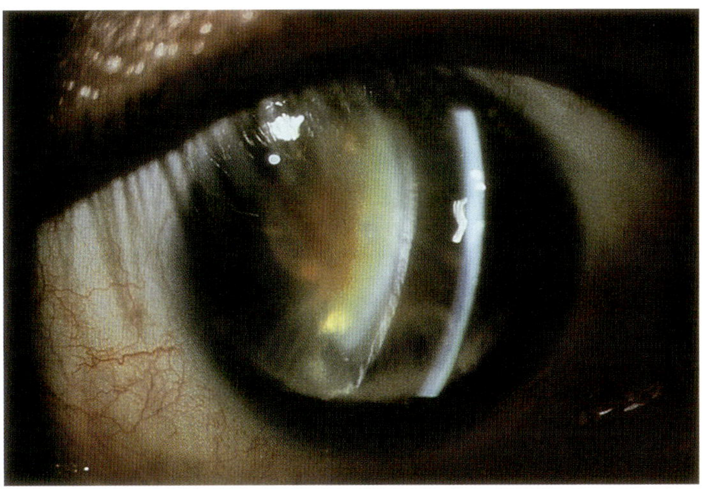

Figure 4-8 Cataract in aniridic patient.

and function of the cornea, lens, and retina. Associated findings include corneal pannus and epitheliopathy, glaucoma, foveal and optic nerve hypoplasia, and nystagmus. Aniridia is almost always bilateral. Two-thirds of cases are familial, and one-third are sporadic. Sporadic cases of aniridia are associated with a high incidence of Wilms tumor and the WAGR complex (*W*ilms tumor, *a*niridia, *g*enitourinary malformations, and mental *r*etardation).

Anterior and posterior polar lens opacities may be present at birth in patients with aniridia. Cortical, subcapsular, and lamellar opacities develop in 50%–85% of patients within the first 2 decades. The lens opacities may progress and further impair vision. Poor zonular integrity and ectopia lentis have also been reported in patients with aniridia.

Congenital and Infantile Cataract

The term *congenital cataract* refers to a lens opacity present at birth. Lens opacities that develop during the first year of life are called *infantile cataracts.* Because some lens opacities escape detection at birth and are noted only on later examination, these terms are used interchangeably by many physicians. Congenital and infantile cataracts are fairly common, occurring in 1 of every 2000 live births. Congenital and infantile cataracts cover a broad spectrum of severity: whereas some lens opacities do not progress and are visually insignificant, others can produce profound visual impairment.

Congenital and infantile cataracts may be unilateral or bilateral. They can be classified by morphology, presumed or defined genetic etiology, presence of specific metabolic disorders, or associated ocular anomalies or systemic findings (Table 4-1). In general, approximately one-third of congenital or infantile cataracts are a component of a more extensive syndrome or disease (eg, cataract resulting from congenital rubella syndrome), one-third occur as an isolated inherited trait, and one-third result from undetermined causes. Metabolic diseases tend to be more commonly associated with bilateral cataracts. (For a discussion of the systemic evaluation of patients with congenital cataracts, see BCSC Section 6, *Pediatric Ophthalmology and Strabismus.*) Congenital cataracts occur in a variety of morphologic configurations, including lamellar, polar, sutural, coronary, cerulean, nuclear, capsular, complete, and membranous. Each of these categories encompasses a range of severity.

Lamellar

Of the congenital and infantile cataracts, lamellar, or zonular, cataracts are the most common type (Fig 4-9). They are characteristically bilateral and symmetric, and their effect on visual acuity varies with the size and density of the opacity. Lamellar cataracts may be inherited as an autosomal dominant trait. In some cases, they may be the result of a transient toxic influence during embryonic lens development. The earlier this toxic influence occurs, the smaller and deeper is the resulting lamellar cataract.

Lamellar cataracts are opacifications of specific layers or zones of the lens. Clinically, the cataract is visible as an opacified layer that surrounds a clearer center and is itself surrounded by a layer of clear cortex. Viewed from the front, the lamellar cataract has a disk-shaped configuration. Often, additional arcuate opacities within the cortex straddle the equator of the lamellar cataract; these horseshoe-shaped opacities are called *riders.*

Table 4-1 Etiology of Pediatric Cataracts

Bilateral cataracts
Idiopathic
Hereditary cataracts (autosomal dominant most common; also autosomal recessive or X-linked)
Genetic and metabolic diseases
Down syndrome
Hallermann-Streiff syndrome
Lowe syndrome
Galactosemia
Marfan syndrome
Trisomy 13–15
Hypoglycemia
Alport syndrome
Myotonic dystrophy
Fabry disease
Hypoparathyroidism
Conradi syndrome
Maternal infection
Rubella
Cytomegalovirus
Varicella
Syphilis
Toxoplasmosis
Ocular anomalies
Aniridia
Anterior segment dysgenesis syndrome
Toxic
Corticosteroids
Radiation (may also be unilateral)
Unilateral cataracts
Idiopathic
Ocular anomalies
Persistent fetal vasculature (PFV)
Anterior segment dysgenesis
Posterior lenticonus
Posterior pole tumors
Traumatic (rule out child abuse)
Rubella
Masked bilateral cataract

Polar

Polar cataracts are lens opacities that involve the subcapsular cortex and capsule of the anterior or posterior pole of the lens (Fig 4-10). *Anterior polar cataracts* are usually small, bilateral, symmetric, nonprogressive opacities that do not impair vision. They are frequently inherited in an autosomal dominant pattern. Anterior polar cataracts are sometimes seen in association with other ocular abnormalities, including microphthalmos, persistent pupillary membrane, and anterior lenticonus. They do not require treatment but often cause anisometropia.

Posterior polar cataracts generally produce more visual impairment than do anterior polar cataracts because they tend to be larger and are positioned closer to the nodal point

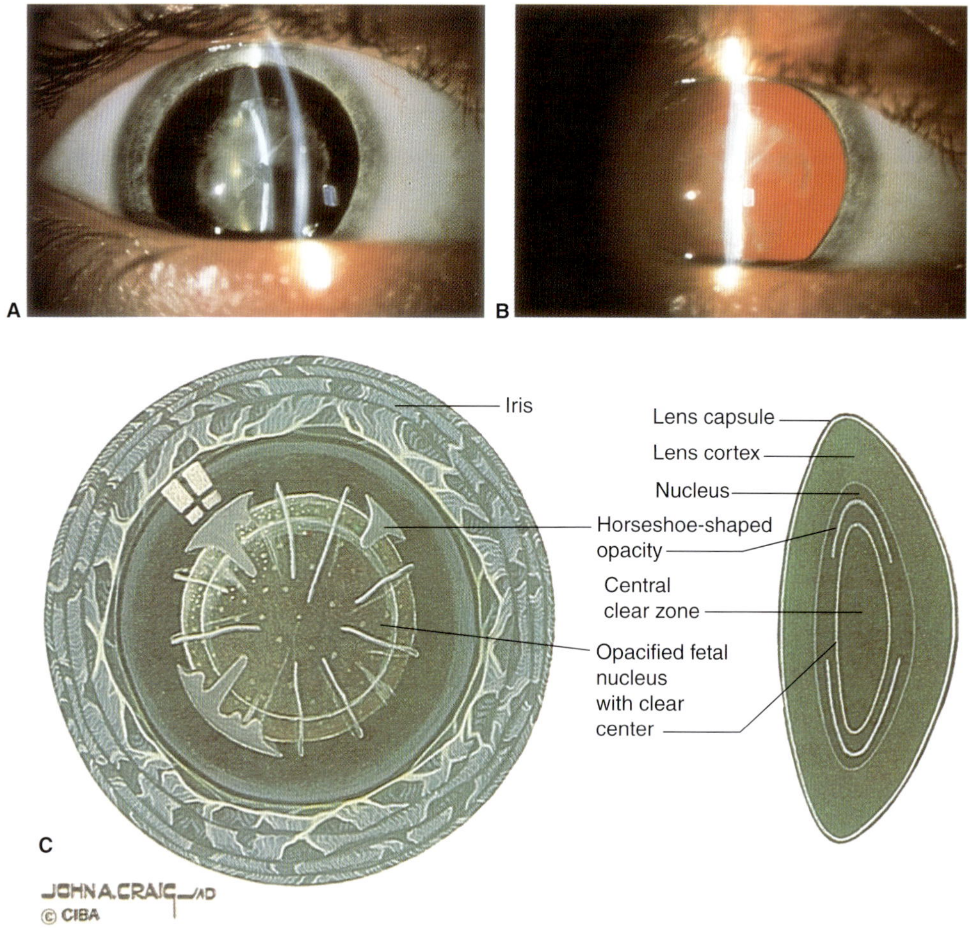

Figure 4-9 **A,** Lamellar cataract. **B,** Lamellar cataract viewed by retroillumination. **C,** Schematic of lamellar cataract. *(Courtesy of CIBA Pharmaceutical Co., division of CIBA-GEIGY Corp. Reproduced with permission from* Clinical Symposia. *Illustration by John A. Craig.)*

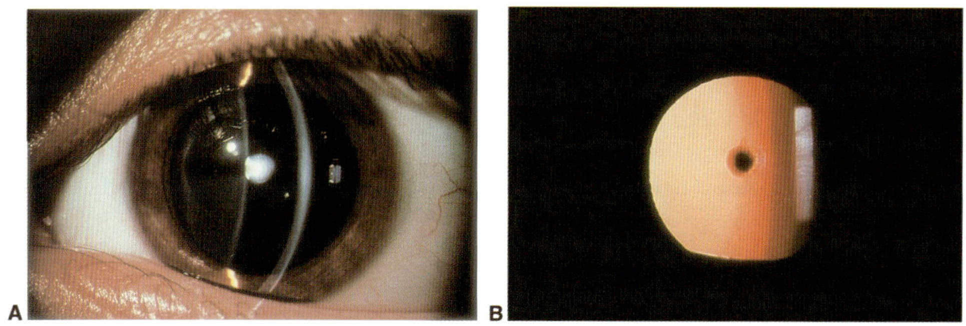

Figure 4-10 **A,** Anterior polar cataract. **B,** Anterior polar cataract viewed by retroillumination.

of the eye. Capsular fragility has been reported. Posterior polar cataracts are usually stable but occasionally progress. They may be familial or sporadic. Familial posterior polar cataracts are usually bilateral and inherited in an autosomal dominant pattern. Sporadic posterior polar cataracts are often unilateral and may be associated with remnants of the tunica vasculosa lentis or with an abnormality of the posterior capsule such as lenticonus or lentiglobus.

Sutural

The sutural, or stellate, cataract is an opacification of the Y-sutures of the fetal nucleus. It usually does not impair vision (Fig 4-11). These opacities often have branches or knobs projecting from them. Bilateral and symmetric, sutural cataracts are frequently inherited in an autosomal dominant pattern.

Coronary

Coronary cataracts are so named because they consist of a group of club-shaped opacities in the cortex that are arranged around the equator of the lens like a crown, or corona. They cannot be seen unless the pupil is dilated, and they usually do not affect visual acuity. Coronary cataracts are often inherited in an autosomal dominant pattern.

Cerulean

Cerulean cataracts are small bluish opacities located in the lens cortex (Fig 4-12); hence, they are also known as *blue-dot cataracts*. They are nonprogressive and usually do not cause visual symptoms.

Nuclear

Congenital nuclear cataracts are opacities of the embryonic nucleus alone or of both embryonic and fetal nuclei (Fig 4-13). They are usually bilateral, with a wide spectrum

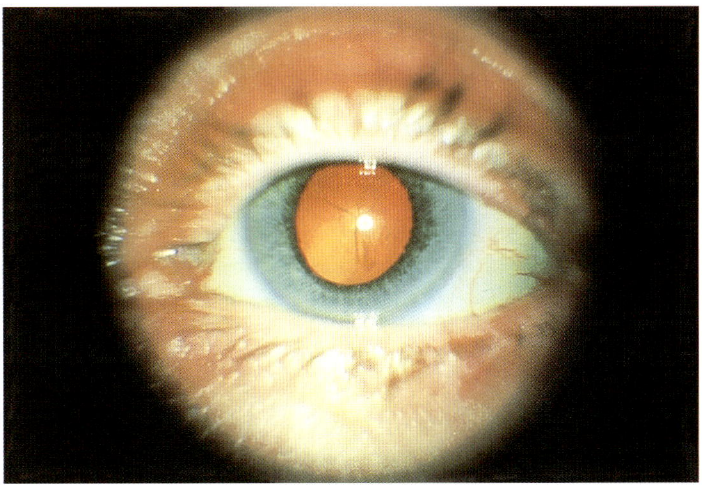

Figure 4-11 Sutural cataract.

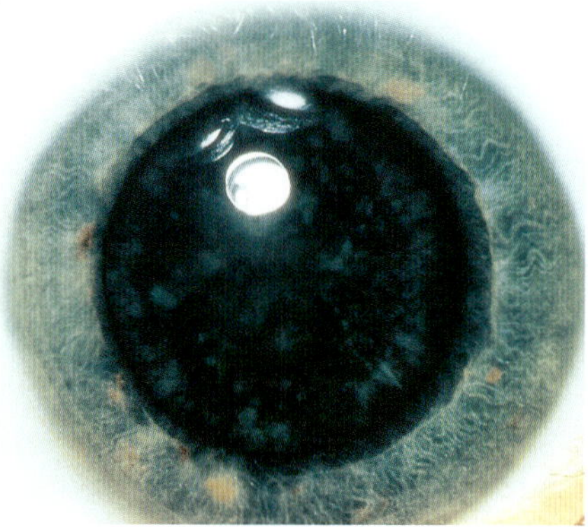

Figure 4-12 A cerulean cataract consists of small bluish opacities in the cortex. *(Courtesy of Karla J. Johns, MD.)*

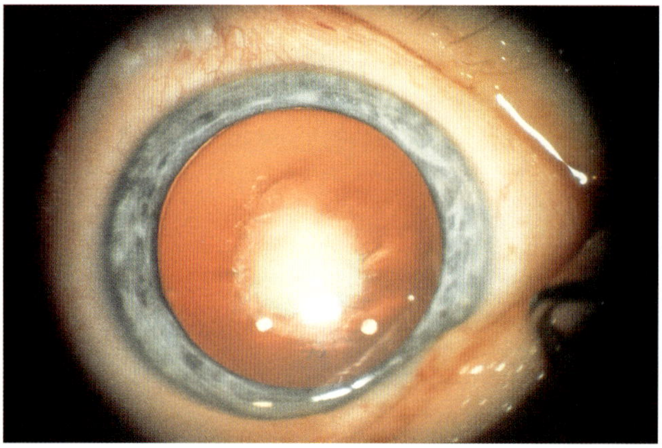

Figure 4-13 Congenital nuclear cataract. *(Reproduced from Day SH.* Understanding and Preventing Amblyopia. *Eye Care Skills for the Primary Care Physician Series [slidescript]. San Francisco: American Academy of Ophthalmology; 1987.)*

of severity. Lens opacification may involve the complete nucleus or be limited to discrete layers within the nucleus. Eyes with congenital nuclear cataracts tend to be microphthalmic.

Capsular

Capsular cataracts are small opacifications of the lens epithelium and anterior lens capsule that spare the cortex. They are differentiated from anterior polar cataracts by their protrusion into the anterior chamber. Capsular cataracts generally do not adversely affect vision.

Complete

With complete, or total, cataract, all of the lens fibers are opacified. The red reflex is completely obscured, and the retina cannot be seen with either direct or indirect ophthalmoscopy. Some cataracts may be subtotal at birth and progress rapidly to become complete cataracts. Complete cataracts may be unilateral or bilateral, and they produce profound visual impairment.

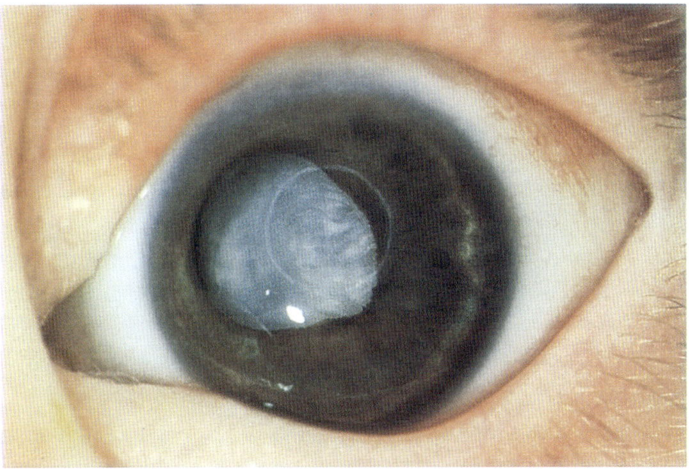

Figure 4-14 Membranous cataract.

Membranous

Membranous cataracts occur when lens proteins are resorbed from either an intact or a traumatized lens, allowing the anterior and posterior lens capsules to fuse into a dense white membrane (Fig 4-14). The resulting opacity and lens distortion generally cause significant visual disability.

Rubella

Maternal infection with the rubella virus, an RNA togavirus, can cause fetal damage, especially if the infection occurs during the first trimester of pregnancy. Systemic manifestations of congenital rubella infection include cardiac defects, deafness, and mental retardation.

Cataracts resulting from *congenital rubella syndrome* are characterized by pearly white nuclear opacifications. Sometimes the entire lens is opacified (complete cataract), and the cortex may liquefy. Histopathologically, lens fiber nuclei are retained deep within the lens substance. Live virus particles may be recovered from the lens as late as 3 years after the patient's birth. Cataract removal may be complicated by excessive postoperative inflammation caused by release of these live virus particles.

Other ocular manifestations of congenital rubella syndrome include diffuse pigmentary retinopathy, microphthalmos, glaucoma, and transient or permanent corneal clouding. Although congenital rubella syndrome may cause cataract or glaucoma, both conditions are usually not present simultaneously in the same eye.

Developmental Defects

Ectopia Lentis

Ectopia lentis is a displacement of the lens that may be congenital, developmental, or acquired. A *subluxated* lens is partially displaced from its normal position but remains in the pupillary area. A *luxated,* or *dislocated,* lens is completely displaced from the pupil, implying separation of all zonular attachments. Findings associated with lens subluxation include decreased vision, marked astigmatism, monocular diplopia, and iridodonesis (tremulous iris). Potential complications of ectopia lentis include cataract and displacement of the lens into the anterior chamber or into the vitreous. Dislocation into the anterior chamber or pupil may cause pupillary block and angle-closure glaucoma. Dislocation of the lens posteriorly into the vitreous cavity often has no adverse sequelae.

Trauma is the most common cause of acquired lens displacement. Nontraumatic ectopia lentis is commonly associated with Marfan syndrome, homocystinuria, aniridia, and congenital glaucoma. Less frequently, it appears with Ehlers-Danlos syndrome, hyperlysinemia, and sulfite oxidase deficiency. Ectopia lentis may occur as an isolated anomaly (simple ectopia lentis), usually inherited as an autosomal dominant trait. Ectopia lentis can also be associated with pupillary abnormalities in the ocular syndrome ectopia lentis et pupillae (see Developmental Defects, Ectopia Lentis et Pupillae, later in this chapter).

Marfan Syndrome

Marfan syndrome is a heritable disorder with ocular, cardiac, and skeletal manifestations. Though usually inherited as an autosomal dominant trait, the disorder appears with no family history in approximately 15% of cases. Marfan syndrome is believed to result from an abnormality of fibrillin, a connective tissue component. Affected individuals are tall, with arachnodactyly (Fig 4-15A) and chest wall deformities. Associated cardiac abnormalities include dilated aortic root and mitral valve prolapse.

From 50% to 80% of patients with Marfan syndrome exhibit ectopia lentis (Fig 4-15B). The lens subluxation tends to be bilateral and symmetric (usually superior and temporal), but variations do occur. The zonular attachments commonly remain intact but become stretched and elongated. Ectopia lentis in Marfan syndrome is probably congenital in most cases. Progression of lens subluxation is observed in some patients over time, whereas in many patients the lens position remains stable.

Ocular abnormalities associated with Marfan syndrome include axial myopia and an increased risk of retinal detachment. Patients with Marfan syndrome may develop pupil-

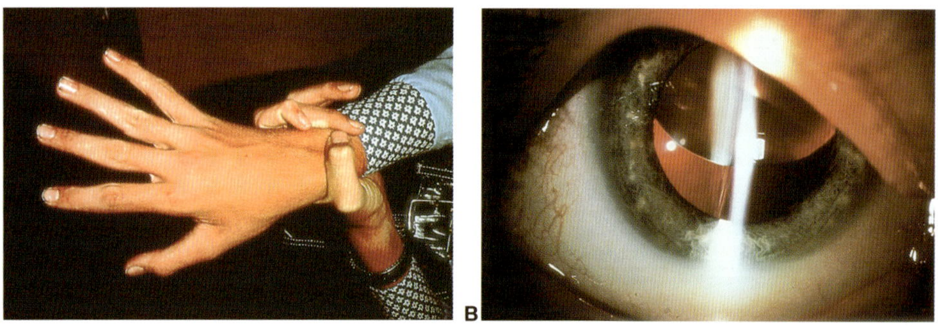

A B

Figure 4-15 Marfan syndrome. **A,** Arachnodactyly in a patient with Marfan syndrome. **B,** Subluxated lens in Marfan syndrome. *(Part A courtesy of Karla J. Johns, MD.)*

lary block glaucoma if the lens dislocates into the pupil or anterior chamber. Open-angle glaucoma may also occur. In addition, children with lens subluxation may develop amblyopia if their refractive error shows significant asymmetry or remains uncorrected in early childhood.

Spectacle or contact lens correction of the refractive error provides satisfactory visual acuity in most cases. Pupillary dilation is sometimes helpful. The clinician may refract both the phakic and the aphakic portions of the pupil to determine the optimum visual acuity. A reading add is often necessary because the subluxated lens lacks sufficient accommodation.

In some cases, adequate visual acuity cannot be obtained with spectacle or contact lens correction, and removal of the lens may be indicated. Lens extraction—either extracapsular or intracapsular—in patients with Marfan syndrome is associated with a high rate of complications such as vitreous loss and complex retinal detachment. (Intracapsular and extracapsular cataract extraction are discussed in detail in Chapter 8.) Improved results have been reported with lensectomy using vitrectomy instrumentation, although the long-term results are not yet known.

Homocystinuria

Homocystinuria is an autosomal recessive disorder, an inborn error of methionine metabolism. Serum levels of homocystine and methionine are elevated. Affected individuals are healthy at birth but develop seizures and osteoporosis and soon display mental retardation. They are usually tall and have light-colored hair. Patients with homocystinuria are also prone to thromboembolic episodes, and surgery and general anesthesia are thought to increase the risk of thromboembolism.

Lens dislocation in homocystinuria tends to be bilateral and symmetric. The dislocation appears in infancy in approximately 30% of affected individuals, and by the age of 15 years, it appears in 80% of those affected. The lenses are usually subluxated inferiorly and nasally, but variations have been reported. Because zonular fibers of the lens are known to have a high concentration of cysteine, deficiency of cysteine is thought to disturb normal zonular development; affected fibers tend to be brittle and easily disrupted. Studies of infants with homocystinuria treated with a low-methionine, high-cysteine diet and vitamin supplementation with the coenzyme pyridoxine (vitamin B_6) have shown that this therapy holds promise in reducing the incidence of ectopia lentis.

Hyperlysinemia

Hyperlysinemia, an inborn error of metabolism of the amino acid lysine, is associated with ectopia lentis. Affected individuals also show mental retardation and muscular hypotony.

Sulfite Oxidase Deficiency

Sulfite oxidase deficiency is a very rare autosomal recessive metabolic disorder of sulfur metabolism. In addition to ectopia lentis, other manifestations include severe mental retardation and seizures.

Ectopia Lentis et Pupillae

In the autosomal recessive disorder ectopia lentis et pupillae, the lens and the pupil are displaced in opposite directions. The pupil is irregular, usually slit shaped, and displaced from the normal position. The dislocated lens may bisect the pupil or may be completely luxated from the pupillary space. This disorder is usually bilateral but not symmetric. Characteristically, the iris dilates poorly. Associated ocular anomalies include severe axial myopia, retinal detachment, enlarged corneal diameter, cataract, and abnormal iris transillumination.

Persistent Fetal Vasculature

Persistent fetal vasculature (PFV), also known as *persistent hyperplastic primary vitreous (PHPV),* is a congenital, nonhereditary ocular malformation that frequently involves the lens. In 90% of patients, it is unilateral. A white, fibrous, retrolental tissue is present, often in association with posterior cortical opacification. Progressive cataract formation often occurs, sometimes leading to a complete cataract. Other abnormalities associated with PFV include elongation of the ciliary processes, prominent radial iris vessels, and persistent hyaloid artery. (See also BCSC Section 6, *Pediatric Ophthalmology and Strabismus;* and Section 12, *Retina and Vitreous.*)

Beebe DC. The lens. In: *Adler's Physiology of the Eye: Clinical Application.* Kaufman PL, Alm A, eds. 10th ed. St Louis: Mosby; 2003:117–158.

Gold DH, Weingeist TA, eds. *The Eye in Systemic Disease.* Philadelphia: Lippincott; 1990:309–414, 513–580.

Goldberg MF. Persistent fetal vasculature (PFV): an integrated interpretation of signs and symptoms associated with persistent hyperplastic primary vitreous (PHPV). LIV Edward Jackson Memorial Lecture. *Am J Ophthalmol.* 1997;124:587–626.

Hiles DA, Kilty LA. Disorders of the lens. In: Isenberg SJ, ed. *The Eye in Infancy.* 2nd ed. St Louis: Mosby; 1994:336–373.

Jaffe NS, Horwitz J. Lens alterations. In: Podos SM, Yanoff M, eds. *Textbook of Ophthalmology.* Vol 3. New York: Gower; 1992:chap 8, pp 8.1–8.16.

Lambert S. Lens. In: Taylor D, ed. *Paediatric Ophthalmology.* 2nd ed. Boston: Blackwell Science; 1997:445–476.

Shortt AJ, Lanigan B, O'Keefe M. Pars plana lensectomy for the management of ectopia lentis in children. *J Pediatr Ophthalmol Strabismus.* 2004;41(5):289–294.

Streeten BW. Pathology of the lens. In: Albert DM, Jakobiec FA, eds. *Principles and Practice of Ophthalmology.* 2nd ed. Philadelphia: Saunders; 2000:chap 4, pp 3685–3749.

CHAPTER 5

Pathology

Aging Changes

As the lens ages, it increases in weight and thickness and decreases in accommodative power. As new layers of cortical fibers are formed concentrically, the lens nucleus undergoes compression and hardening (nuclear sclerosis). Chemical modification and proteolytic cleavage of crystallins (lens proteins) result in the formation of high-molecular-weight protein aggregates. These aggregates may become large enough to cause abrupt fluctuations in the local refractive index of the lens, thereby scattering light and reducing transparency. Chemical modification of lens nuclear proteins also increases pigmentation, such that the lens increasingly takes on a yellow or brownish hue with advancing age (Fig 5-1). Other age-related changes include decreased concentrations of glutathione and potassium and increased concentrations of sodium and calcium in the lens cell cytoplasm.

A very common cause of visual impairment in older adults is *age-related cataract,* the pathogenesis of which is multifactorial and not completely understood. There are 3 main types of age-related cataracts: nuclear, cortical, and posterior subcapsular. In many patients, components of more than one type are present. (See also BCSC Section 4, *Ophthalmic Pathology and Intraocular Tumors.*)

Nuclear Cataracts

Some degree of nuclear sclerosis and yellowing is normal in adult patients past middle age. In general, this condition interferes only minimally with visual function. An excessive amount of light scattering and yellowing is called a *nuclear cataract,* which causes a central opacity (Fig 5-2). The ophthalmologist can evaluate the degree of increased color and of opacification by using a slit-lamp biomicroscope and by examining the red reflex with the pupil dilated.

Nuclear cataracts tend to progress slowly. Although they are usually bilateral, they may be asymmetric. Nuclear cataracts typically cause greater impairment of distance vision than of near vision. In the early stages, the progressive hardening of the lens nucleus frequently causes an increase in the refractive index of the lens and thus a myopic shift in refraction *(lenticular myopia).* In hyperopic eyes, the myopic shift enables otherwise presbyopic individuals to read without spectacles, a condition referred to as *second sight.* Occasionally, the abrupt change in refractive index between the sclerotic nucleus (or other

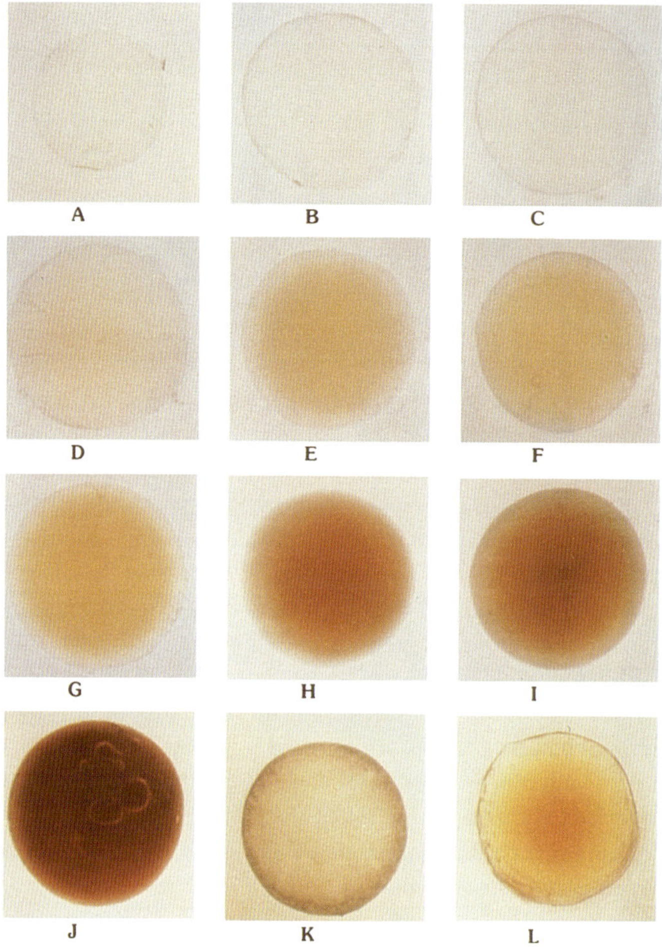

Figure 5-1 Increasing yellow-to-brown coloration of the human lens from 6 months *(A)* through 8 years *(B)*, 12 years *(C)*, 25 years *(D)*, 47 years *(E)*, 60 years *(F)*, 70 years *(G)*, 82 years *(H)*, and 91 years *(I)*. Brown nuclear cataract in 70-year-old patient *(J)*, cortical cataract in 68-year-old *(K)*, and mixed nuclear and cortical cataract in 74-year-old *(L)*. *(Reproduced with permission from Lerman S. Phototoxicity: clinical considerations.* Focal Points: Clinical Modules for Ophthalmologists. *San Francisco: American Academy of Ophthalmology; 1987, module 8.)*

lens opacities) and the lens cortex can cause monocular diplopia. Progressive yellowing or browning of the lens causes poor hue discrimination, especially at the blue end of the visible light spectrum. Photopic retinal function may decrease with advanced nuclear cataract. In very advanced cases, the lens nucleus becomes opaque and brown and is called a *brunescent* nuclear cataract.

Histopathologically, the nucleus in nuclear cataract is difficult to distinguish from the nucleus of normal, aged lenses. Investigations by electron microscopy have identified an increased number of lamellar membrane whorls in some nuclear cataracts. The degree to which protein aggregates or these membrane modifications contribute to the increased light scattering of nuclear cataracts is unclear.

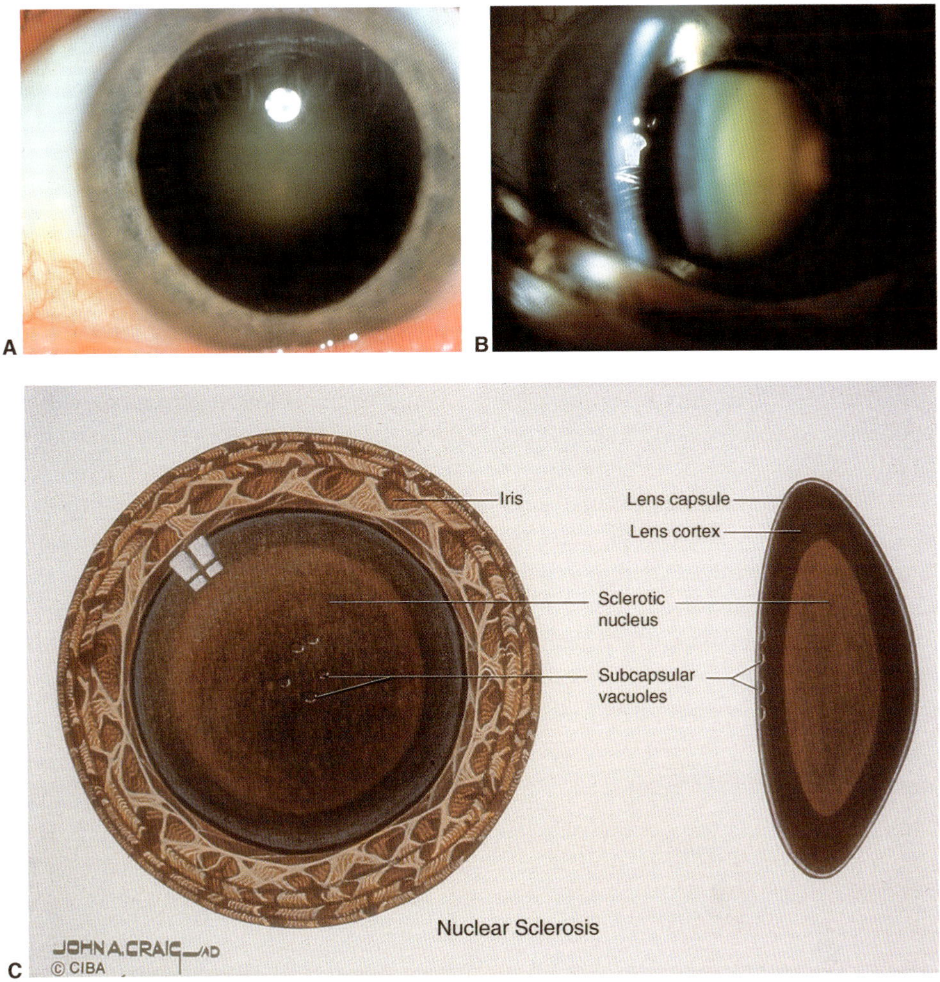

Figure 5-2 Nuclear cataract viewed with diffuse illumination **(A)** and with a slit beam **(B)**. **C,** Schematic of nuclear cataract. *(Courtesy of CIBA Pharmaceutical Co., division of CIBA-GEIGY Corp. Reproduced with permission from* Clinical Symposia. *Illustration by John A. Craig.)*

Cortical Cataracts

In contrast to nuclear cataracts, cortical cataracts are associated with the local disruption of the structure of mature fiber cells. Once membrane integrity is compromised, essential metabolites are lost from the affected cells. This loss leads to extensive protein oxidation and precipitation. Cortical cataracts are usually bilateral but are often asymmetric. Their effect on visual function varies greatly, depending on the location of the opacification relative to the visual axis. A common symptom of cortical cataracts is glare from intense focal light sources, such as car headlights. Monocular diplopia may also result. Cortical cataracts vary greatly in their rate of progression; some cortical opacities remain unchanged for prolonged periods, whereas others progress rapidly.

The first signs of cortical cataract formation visible with the slit-lamp biomicroscope are vacuoles and water clefts in the anterior or posterior cortex (Fig 5-3). The cortical lamellae may be separated by fluid. Wedge-shaped opacities (often called *cortical spokes* or cuneiform opacities) form near the periphery of the lens, with the pointed end of the opacities oriented toward the center (Fig 5-4). Since these peripheral opacities occur in fiber cells that extend from the posterior to the anterior sutures, they affect only the central regions of the fiber cells. In the initial stages of the cataract, affected fiber cells remain clear at their anterior and posterior ends. The cortical spokes appear as white opacities when viewed with the slit-lamp biomicroscope and as dark shadows when viewed on retroillumination. The wedge-shaped opacities may spread to adjacent fiber cells and along the length of affected fibers, causing the degree of opacity to increase and extend toward the visual axis. When the entire cortex from the capsule to the nucleus becomes white and opaque, the cataract is said to be *mature* (Fig 5-5). In mature opacities, the lens takes up water, swelling to become an *intumescent* cortical cataract.

A *hypermature* cataract occurs when degenerated cortical material leaks through the lens capsule, leaving the capsule wrinkled and shrunken (Fig 5-6). A *morgagnian* cataract occurs when further liquefaction of the cortex allows free movement of the nucleus within the capsular bag (Fig 5-7).

Histopathologically, cortical cataracts are characterized by local swelling and disruption of the lens fiber cells. Globules of eosinophilic material (morgagnian globules) are observed in slitlike spaces between lens fibers.

Posterior Subcapsular Cataracts

Posterior subcapsular cataracts (PSCs) are often seen in patients younger than those presenting with nuclear or cortical cataracts. PSCs are located in the posterior cortical layer

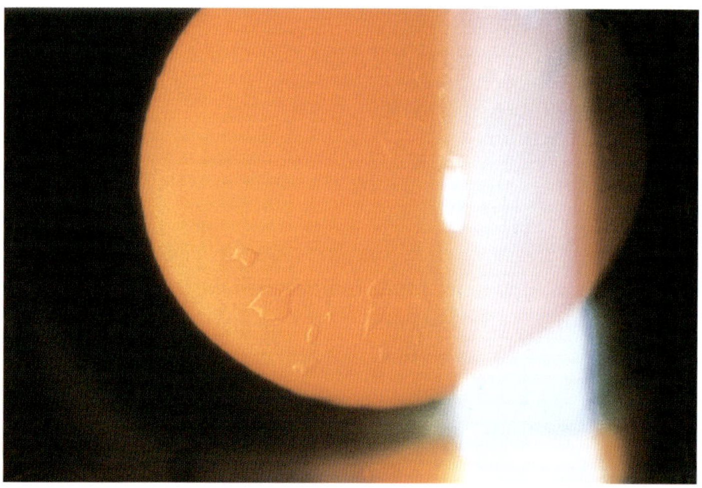

Figure 5-3 Vacuoles in early cortical cataract development.

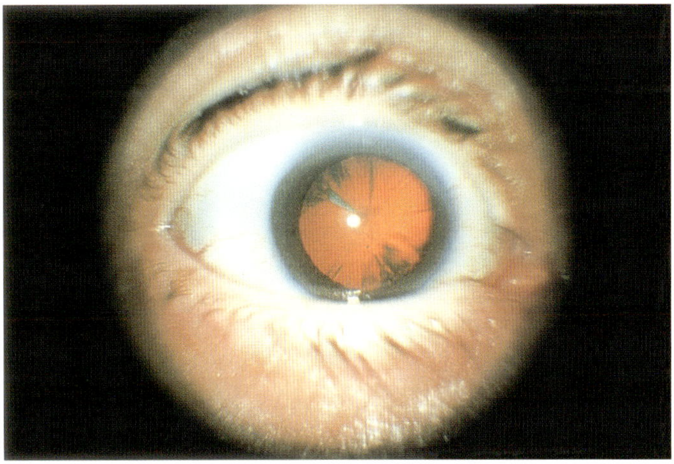

A

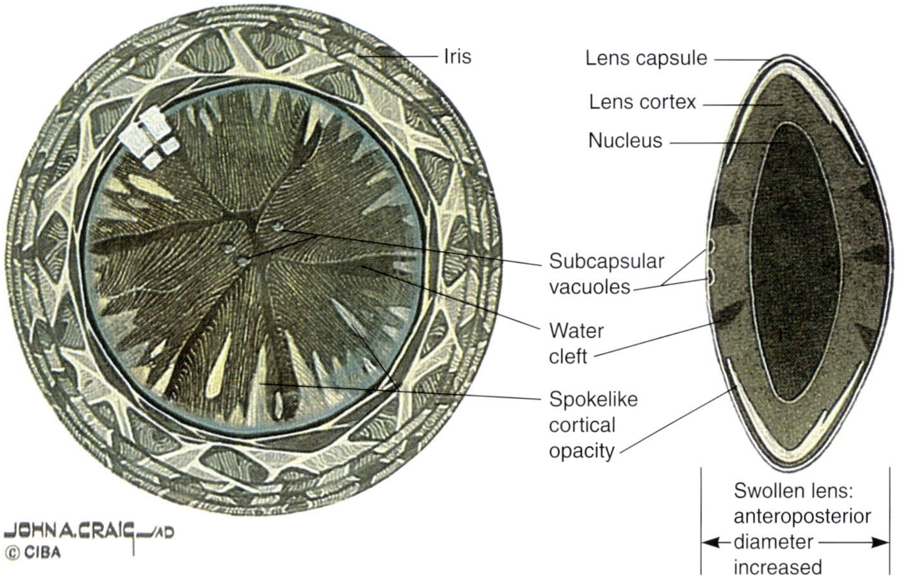

B

Figure 5-4 **A,** Cortical cataract viewed by retroillumination. **B,** Schematic of immature cortical cataract. *(Courtesy of CIBA Pharmaceutical Co., division of CIBA-GEIGY Corp. Reproduced with permission from* Clinical Symposia. *Illustration by John A. Craig.)*

and are usually axial (Fig 5-8). The first indication of PSC formation is a subtle iridescent sheen in the posterior cortical layers visible with the slit lamp. In later stages, granular opacities and a plaquelike opacity of the posterior subcapsular cortex appear.

The patient often complains of glare and poor vision under bright lighting conditions because the PSC obscures more of the pupillary aperture when miosis is induced by bright lights, accommodation, or miotics. Near visual acuity tends to be reduced more than distance visual acuity. Some patients experience monocular diplopia.

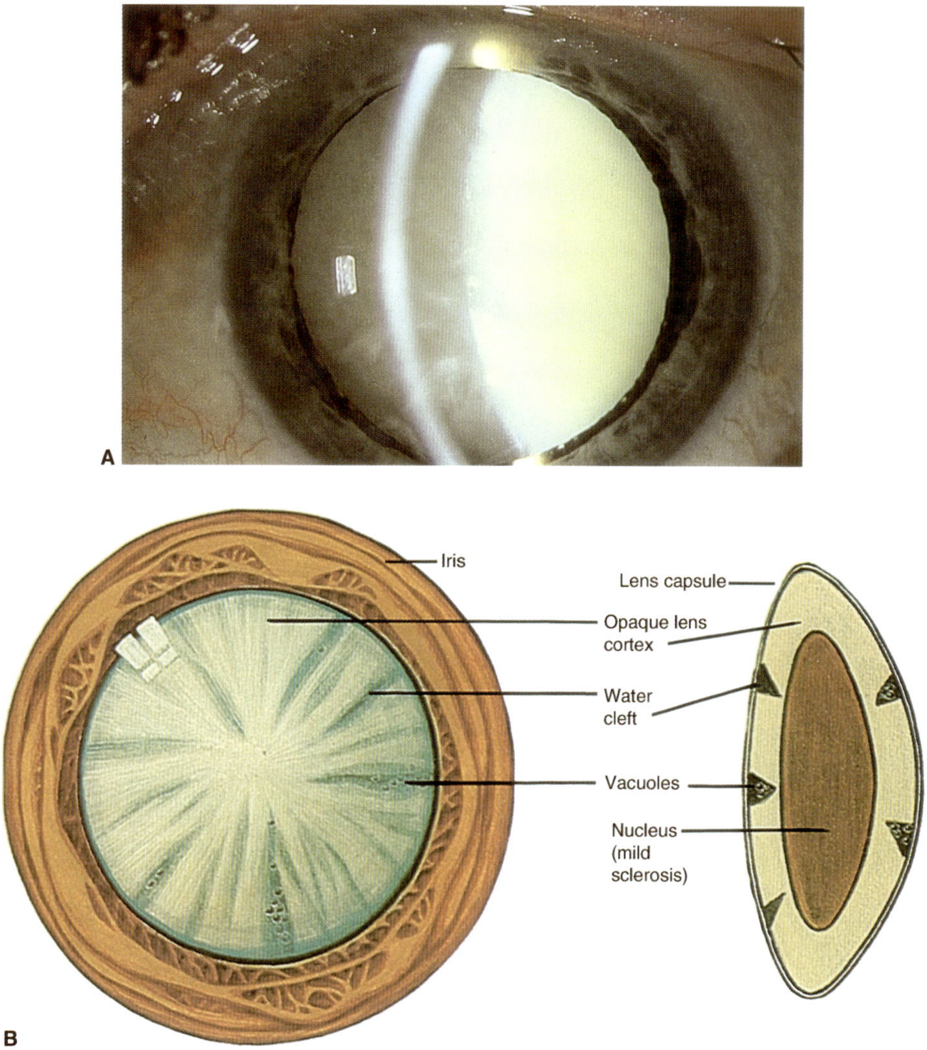

Figure 5-5 **A,** Mature cortical cataract. **B,** Schematic of mature cortical cataract. *(Courtesy of CIBA Pharmaceutical Co., division of CIBA-GEIGY Corp. Reproduced with permission from* Clinical Symposia. *Illustration by John A. Craig.)*

Slit-lamp detection of PSCs can best be accomplished through a dilated pupil. Retro-illumination is also helpful.

As stated earlier, PSCs are one of the main types of cataract related to aging. However, they can also occur as a result of trauma; systemic, topical, or intraocular corticosteroid use; inflammation; exposure to ionizing radiation; and alcoholism.

Histopathologically, PSC is associated with posterior migration of the lens epithelial cells from the lens equator to the axis on the inner surface of the posterior capsule. Dur-

A

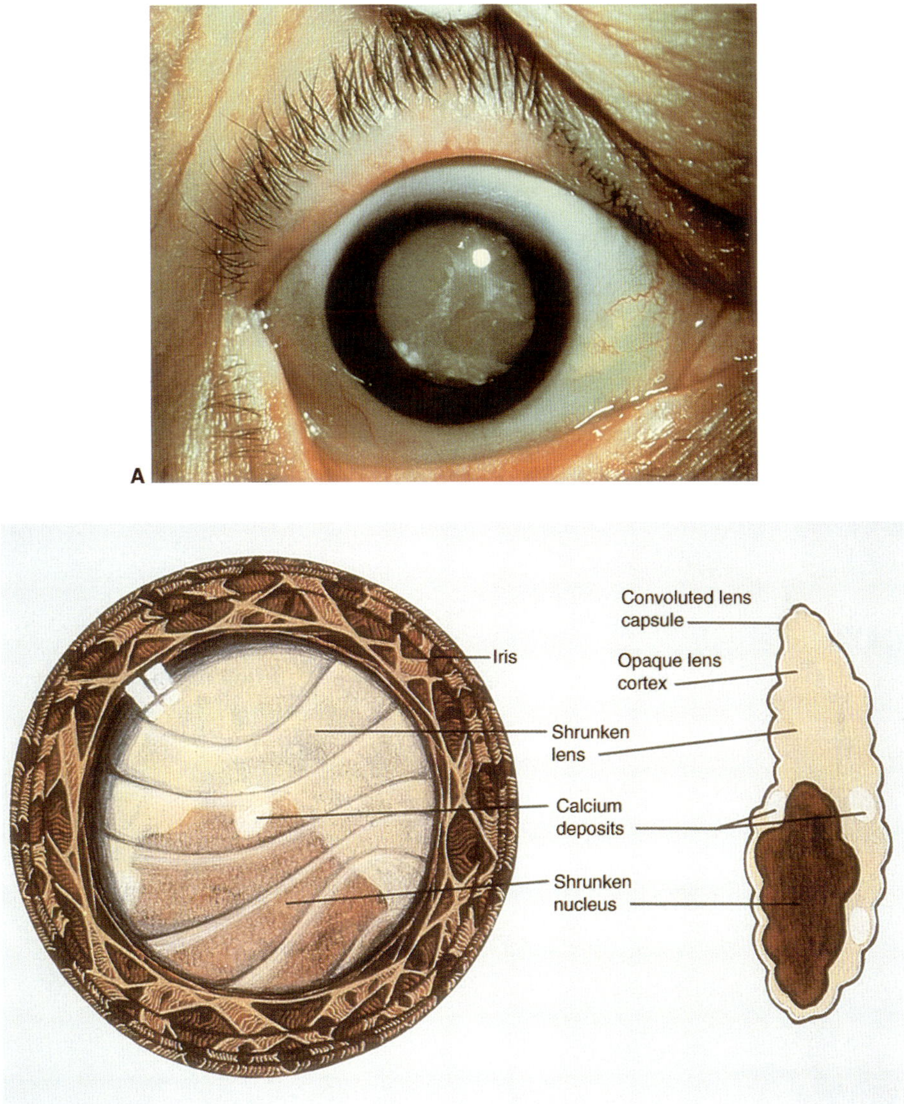

B

Figure 5-6 **A,** Hypermature cortical cataract. **B,** Schematic of hypermature cortical cataract. *(Courtesy of CIBA Pharmaceutical Co., division of CIBA-GEIGY Corp. Reproduced with permission from* Clinical Symposia. *Illustration by John A. Craig.)*

ing their migration to or after their arrival at the posterior axis, the cells undergo aberrant enlargement. These swollen cells are called *Wedl,* or *bladder,* cells.

Kuszak JR, Deutsch TA, Brown HG. Anatomy of aged and senile cataractous lenses. In: Albert DM, Jakobiec FA, eds. *Principles and Practice of Ophthalmology*. Philadelphia: Saunders; 1994:564–575.

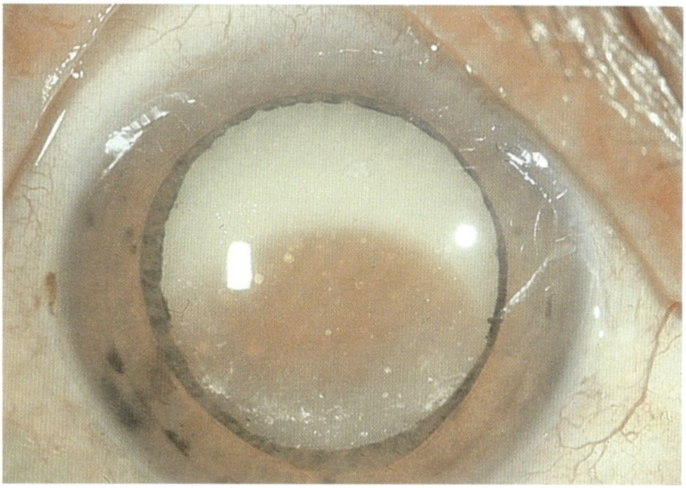
A

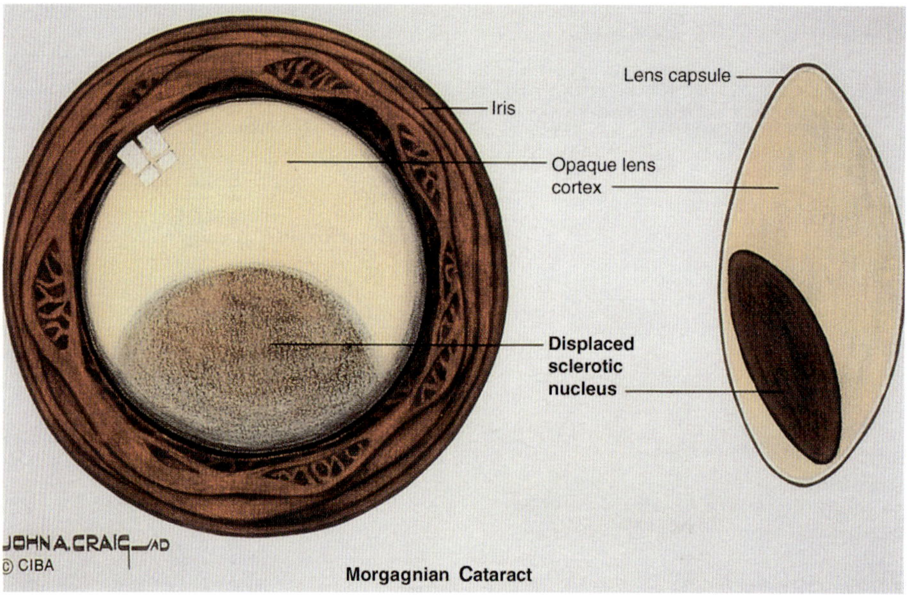

B

Figure 5-7 **A,** Morgagnian cataract. **B,** Schematic of morgagnian cataract. *(Courtesy of CIBA Pharmaceutical Co., division of CIBA-GEIGY Corp. Reproduced with permission from* Clinical Symposia. *Illustration by John A. Craig.)*

Genetic Contributions to Age-Related Cataracts

Studies of identical and fraternal twins and of familial associations suggest that a large proportion of the risk of age-related cataracts is inherited. It is estimated that inheritance accounts for more than 50% of the risk of cortical cataracts. Strikingly, most of this risk is associated with variations at a single locus. The gene responsible has not yet been identified. Similarly, 35%–50% of the risk of nuclear cataracts can be traced to inheritance.

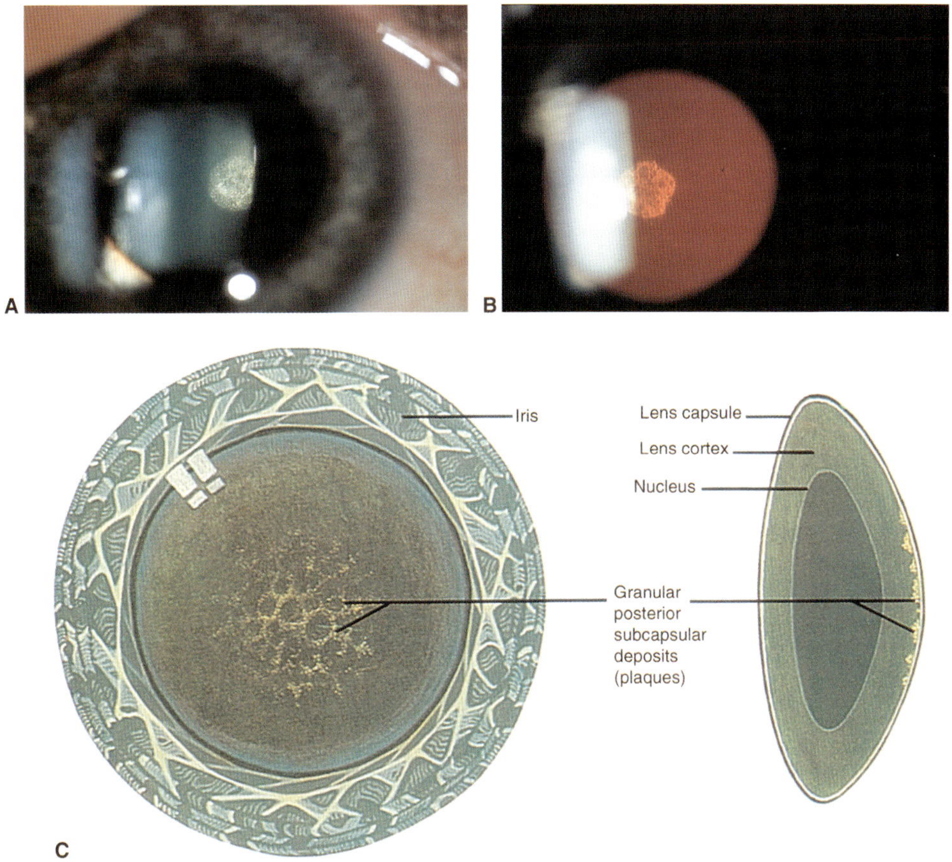

Figure 5-8 Posterior subcapsular cataract (PSC) viewed at the slit lamp **(A)** and with indirect illumination **(B)**. **C,** Schematic of PSC. *(Courtesy of CIBA Pharmaceutical Co., division of CIBA-GEIGY Corp. Reproduced with permission from* Clinical Symposia. *Illustration by John A. Craig.)*

Again, much of this risk seems to be accounted for by a single dominant gene. Identification of these genes will be important, because understanding the biochemical pathways in which they function may suggest ways to slow the progression or prevent the development of age-related cataracts in a large number of cases.

Hammond CJ, Duncan DD, Snieder H, et al. The heritability of age-related cortical cataract: the twin eye study. *Invest Ophthalmol Vis Sci.* 2001;42(3):601–605.

Hammond CJ, Snieder H, Spector TD, Gilbert CE. Genetic and environmental factors in age-related nuclear cataracts in monozygotic and dizygotic twins. *N Engl J Med.* 2000;342(24):1786–1790.

Heiba IM, Elston RC, Klein BE, Klein R. Genetic etiology of nuclear cataract: evidence for a major gene. *Am J Med Genet.* 1993;47(8):1208–1214.

Iyengar SK, Klein BE, Klein R, et al. Identification of a major locus for age-related cortical cataract on chromosome 6p12-q12 in the Beaver Dam Eye Study. *Proc Natl Acad Sci USA.* 2004;101(40):14485–14490.

Drug-Induced Lens Changes

Corticosteroids

Long-term use of corticosteroids may cause PSCs. The incidence of corticosteroid-induced PSCs is related to dose and duration of treatment. Cataract formation has been reported following administration of corticosteroids by several routes: systemic, topical, subconjunctival, and inhaled. The increasing use of high-dose intraocular steroids to treat retinal neovascularization and inflammation has resulted in a substantial rise in the incidence of PSCs and of steroid-induced ocular hypertension. Coincidentally, the patients who are susceptible to steroid-induced increases in intraocular pressure are frequently those who develop PSCs after intravitreal injection of triamcinolone acetonide.

Histopathologically and clinically, PSC formation occurring subsequent to corticosteroid use cannot be distinguished from senescent PSC formation. Some steroid-induced PSCs in children may resolve with cessation of the drug.

Gillies MC, Kuzniarz M, Craig J, Ball M, Luo W, Simpson JM. Intravitreal triamcinolone-induced elevated intraocular pressure is associated with the development of posterior subcapsular cataract. *Ophthalmology.* 2005;112(1):139–143.

Phenothiazines

Phenothiazines, a major group of psychotropic medications, can cause pigmented deposits in the anterior lens epithelium in an axial configuration (Fig 5-9). These deposits appear to be dependent on both drug dose and treatment duration. In addition, they are more likely to be seen with the use of some phenothiazines, notably chlorpromazine and thioridazine, than with others. The visual changes associated with phenothiazine use are generally insignificant.

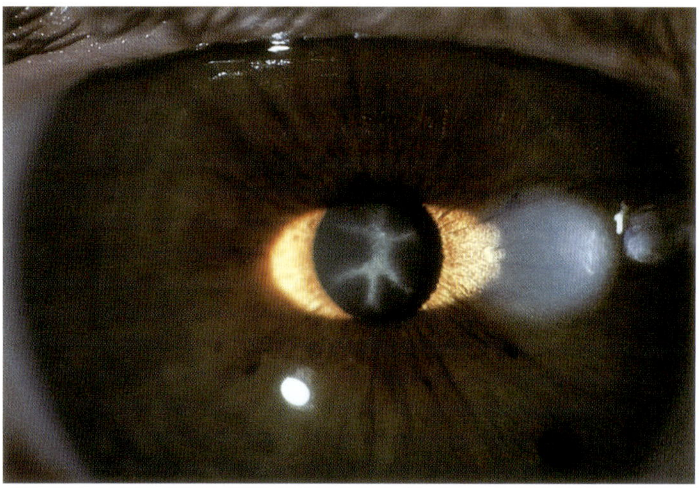

Figure 5-9 Pigmented deposits on anterior lens capsule in patient treated with phenothiazines.

Miotics

The use of anticholinesterases can cause cataracts. The incidence of cataracts has been reported as high as 20% in patients after 55 months of pilocarpine use and 60% in patients after echothiophate iodide (Phospholine Iodide) use. Usually, this type of cataract first appears as small vacuoles within and posterior to the anterior lens capsule and epithelium. These vacuoles are best appreciated on retroillumination. The cataract may progress to posterior cortical and nuclear lens changes as well. Cataract formation is more likely in patients receiving anticholinesterase therapy over a long period and in those receiving more frequent dosage. Although visually significant cataracts are common in elderly patients using topical anticholinesterases, progressive cataract formation has not been reported in children given echothiophate for the treatment of accommodative esotropia.

Amiodarone

The use of amiodarone, an antiarrhythmia medication, has been reported to cause stellate anterior axial pigment deposition. Only very rarely is this condition visually significant. Amiodarone is also deposited in the corneal epithelium and is the cause of a rare optic neuropathy.

Statins

Studies in dogs demonstrated that some 3-hydroxy-3-methylglutaryl coenzyme A (HMG-CoA) reductase inhibitors (statins) are associated with cataract when given in excessive doses. Long-term use of statins in humans has been shown not to be associated with an increased cataract risk, and a longitudinal study reported a 50% reduction in the 5-year incidence of nuclear cataracts in patients treated with statins. However, concomitant use of simvastatin and erythromycin, which increases circulating statin levels, may be associated with approximately a twofold increased risk of cataract.

Klein BE, Klein R, Lee KE, Grady LM. Statin use and incident nuclear cataract. *JAMA.* 2006;295(23):2752–2758.

Schlienger RG, Haefeli WE, Jick H, Meier CR. Risk of cataract in patients treated with statins. *Arch Intern Med.* 2001;161:2021–2026.

Trauma

Traumatic lens damage may be caused by mechanical injury and by physical forces (radiation, chemicals, electrical current).

Contusion

Vossius ring

Blunt injury to the eye can sometimes cause pigment from the pupillary ruff to be imprinted onto the anterior surface of the lens in a Vossius ring. Although a Vossius ring is visually insignificant and gradually resolves with time, it serves as an indicator of prior blunt trauma.

Traumatic cataract

A blunt, nonperforating injury may cause lens opacification either as an acute event or as a late sequela. A contusion cataract may involve only a portion of the lens or the entire lens. Often, the initial manifestation of a contusion cataract is a stellate or rosette-shaped opacification *(rosette cataract),* usually axial in location, that involves the posterior lens capsule (Fig 5-10). In some cases, blunt trauma causes both dislocation and cataract formation (Fig 5-11). Mild contusion cataracts can improve spontaneously in rare cases.

Dislocation and subluxation

During a blunt injury to the eye, rapid expansion of the globe in an equatorial plane can follow compression. This rapid equatorial expansion can disrupt the zonular fibers, causing dislocation or subluxation of the lens. The lens may be dislocated in

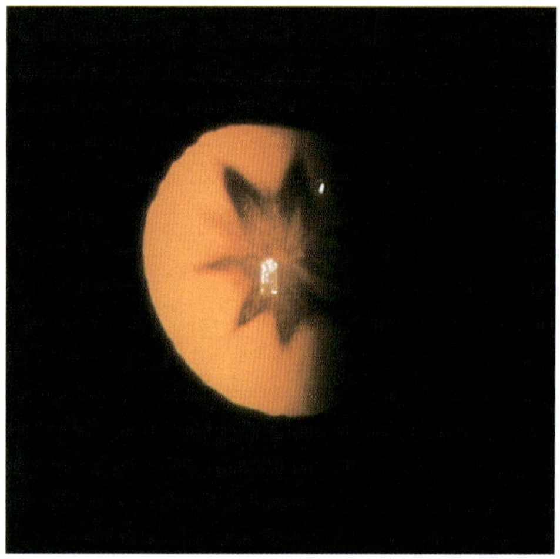

Figure 5-10 Stellate lens opacity following contusion.

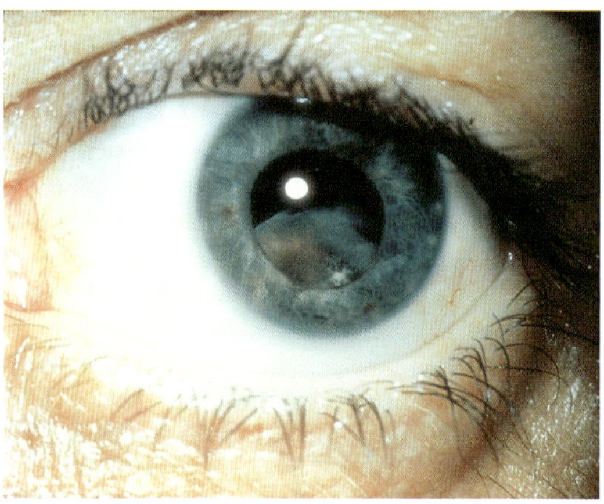

Figure 5-11 Dislocated cataractous lens following blunt trauma. *(Courtesy of Karla J. Johns, MD.)*

any direction, including posteriorly into the vitreous cavity or anteriorly into the anterior chamber.

Symptoms and signs of traumatic lens subluxation include fluctuation of vision, impaired accommodation, monocular diplopia, and high astigmatism. Often, iridodonesis or phacodonesis is present. Retroillumination of the lens at the slit lamp through a dilated pupil may reveal the zonular disruption. In some cases, blunt trauma causes both dislocation and cataract formation.

Perforating and Penetrating Injury

A perforating or penetrating injury of the lens often results in opacification of the cortex at the site of the rupture, usually progressing rapidly to complete opacification (Fig 5-12). Occasionally, a small perforating injury of the lens capsule may heal, resulting in a stationary focal cortical cataract (Fig 5-13).

Radiation

Ionizing radiation

The lens is extremely sensitive to ionizing radiation; however, as much as 20 years may pass after exposure before a cataract becomes clinically apparent. This period of latency is related to the dose of radiation and to the patient's age; younger patients are more susceptible because they have more actively growing lens cells. Ionizing radiation in the x-ray range (0.001–10.0 nm wavelength) can cause cataracts in some individuals in doses as low as 200 rads in one fraction. (A routine chest x-ray equals 0.1 rad exposure to the thorax.)

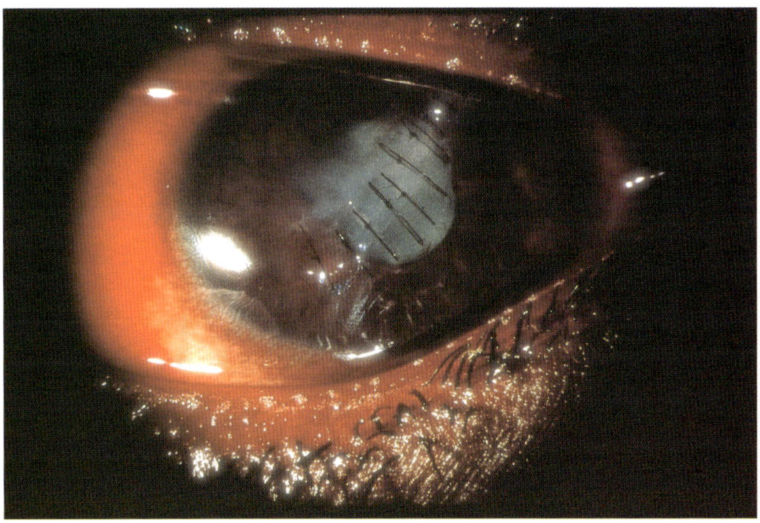

Figure 5-12 Complete cortical opacification after perforating injury, with disruption of the lens capsule.

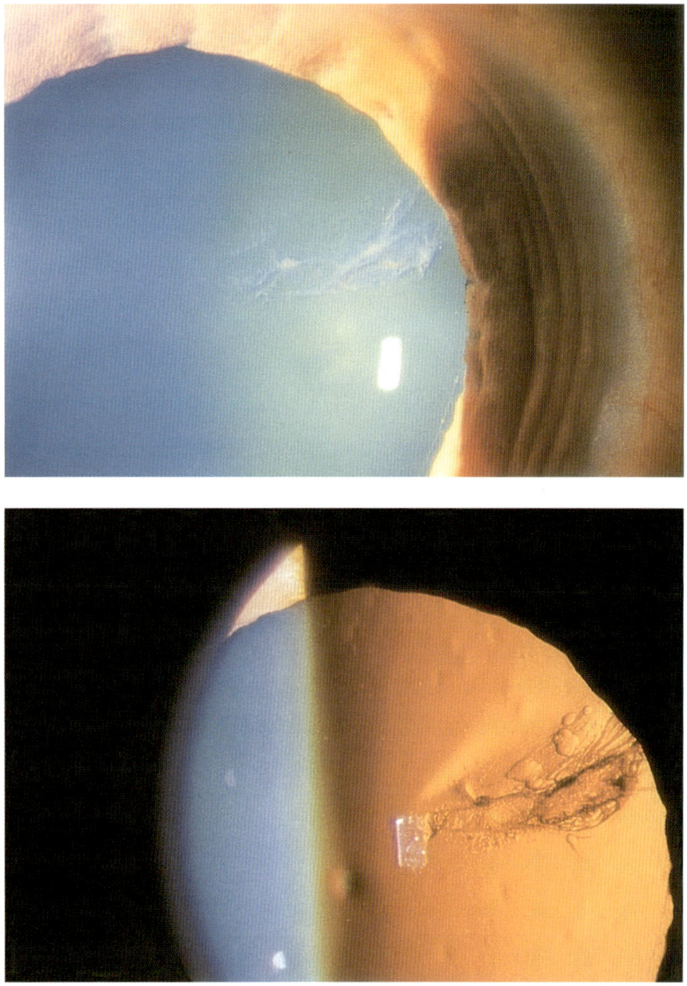

A

B

Figure 5-13 **A,** Focal cortical cataract from a small perforating injury to the lens capsule. **B,** Focal cortical cataract viewed by retroillumination.

The first clinical signs of radiation-induced cataract are often punctate opacities within the posterior capsule and feathery anterior subcapsular opacities that radiate toward the equator of the lens. These opacities may progress to complete opacification of the lens.

Infrared radiation (glassblowers' cataract)

Exposure of the eye to infrared radiation and intense heat over time can cause the outer layers of the anterior lens capsule to peel off as a single layer. Such true exfoliation of the lens capsule, in which the exfoliated outer lamella tends to scroll up on itself, is rarely seen today. Cortical cataract may be associated. (See the section Pseudoexfoliation Syndrome.)

Ultraviolet radiation

Experimental evidence suggests that the lens is susceptible to damage from ultraviolet (UV) radiation. Epidemiologic evidence indicates that long-term exposure to sunlight is associated with increased risk of cortical cataracts. Although sunlight exposure accounts for only about 10% of the total risk of cortical cataract in the general population, this risk is avoidable. Since exposure to UV radiation can produce other morbidity, avoiding excessive sunlight exposure should be encouraged. UV-absorbing corrective lenses and nonprescription sunglasses decrease UV transmission by more than 80%, and wearing a hat with a brim decreases ocular sun exposure by 30%–50%.

Microwave radiation

Microwave radiation has been shown to cause cataracts in laboratory animals. Human case reports and epidemiologic studies are more controversial and less conclusive than experimental studies. Cataracts caused by microwave radiation are likely to be anterior and/or posterior subcapsular opacities.

Chemical Injuries

Alkali injuries to the ocular surface often result in cataract, in addition to damaging the cornea, conjunctiva, and iris. Alkali compounds penetrate the eye readily, causing an increase in aqueous pH and a decrease in the level of aqueous glucose and ascorbate. Cortical cataract formation may occur acutely or as a delayed effect of chemical injury. Because acid tends to penetrate the eye less easily than alkali, acid injuries are less likely to result in cataract formation.

Intralenticular Foreign Bodies

Rarely, a small foreign body can perforate the cornea and the anterior lens capsule and become lodged within the lens. If the foreign body is not composed of a ferric or cupric material and the anterior lens capsule seals the perforation site, the foreign body may be retained within the lens without significant complication. Intralenticular foreign bodies may cause cataract formation in some cases but do not always lead to lens opacification.

Metallosis

Siderosis bulbi

Iron intraocular foreign bodies can result in siderosis bulbi, a condition characterized by deposition of iron molecules in the trabecular meshwork, lens epithelium, iris, and retina (Fig 5-14A). The epithelium and cortical fibers of the affected lens at first show a yellowish tinge, followed later by a rusty brown discoloration (Fig 5-14B). Lens involvement occurs more rapidly if the retained foreign body is embedded close to the lens. Later manifestations of siderosis bulbi are complete cortical cataract formation and retinal dysfunction. See also BCSC Section 12, *Retina and Vitreous.*

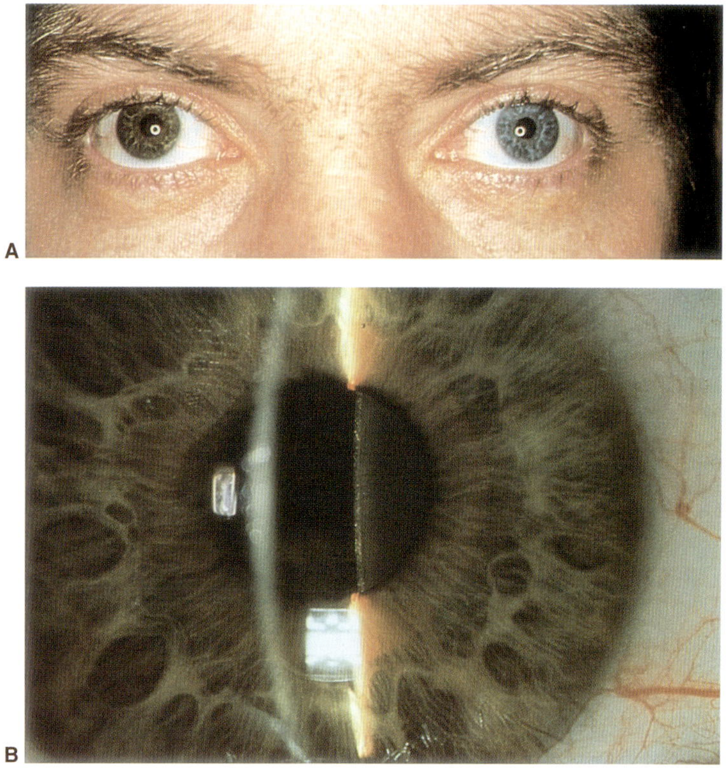

Figure 5-14 Siderosis bulbi. **A,** Heterochromia iridis caused by siderosis bulbi. **B,** Discoloration of lens capsule and cortex.

Chalcosis

Chalcosis occurs when an intraocular copper-containing foreign body deposits copper in Descemet's membrane, the anterior lens capsule, or other intraocular basement membranes. A *sunflower cataract* is a petal-shaped deposition of yellow or brown pigmentation in the lens capsule that radiates from the anterior axial pole of the lens to the equator. Usually, the sunflower cataract causes no significant loss of visual acuity. However, intraocular foreign bodies containing almost pure copper (more than 90%) can cause a severe inflammatory reaction and intraocular necrosis.

Electrical Injury

Electrical shock can cause protein coagulation and cataract formation. Lens manifestations are more likely when the transmission of current involves the patient's head. Initially, lens vacuoles appear in the anterior midperiphery of the lens, followed by linear opacities in the anterior subcapsular cortex. A cataract induced by an electrical injury may regress, remain stationary, or mature to complete cataract over months or years (Fig 5-15).

Portellos M, Orlin SE, Kozart DM. Electric cataracts [photo essay]. *Arch Ophthalmol.* 1996;114:1022–1023.

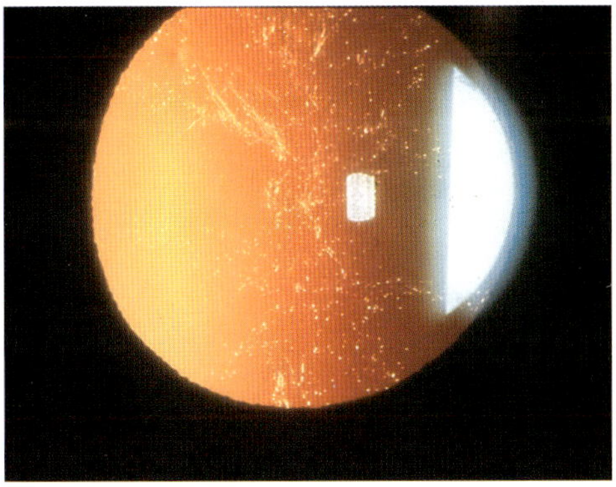

Figure 5-15 Electrical injury. *(Courtesy of Karla J. Johns, MD.)*

Metabolic Cataract

Diabetes Mellitus

Diabetes mellitus can affect lens clarity, as well as the refractive index and accommodative amplitude of the lens. As the blood glucose level increases, so also does the glucose content in the aqueous humor. Because glucose from the aqueous enters the lens by diffusion, glucose content in the lens will likewise be increased. Some of the glucose is converted to sorbitol, the sugar alcohol of glucose, by the enzyme aldose reductase. Sorbitol is metabolized slowly by the lens and accumulates in the lens cell cytoplasm. The resulting increase in osmotic pressure may cause an influx of water, which leads to swelling of the lens fibers. The state of lenticular hydration can affect the refractive power of the lens. Patients with uncontrolled diabetes may show transient refractive changes owing to large changes in their blood glucose level. Acute myopic shifts may indicate undiagnosed or poorly controlled diabetes. People with diabetes have a decreased amplitude of accommodation compared to age-matched controls, and presbyopia may present at a younger age in patients with diabetes than in those without.

Cataract is a common cause of visual impairment in patients with diabetes. Acute *diabetic cataract,* or *snowflake cataract,* consists of bilateral, widespread subcapsular lens changes of abrupt onset, typically in young people with uncontrolled diabetes mellitus (Fig 5-16). Multiple gray-white subcapsular opacities that have a snowflake appearance are seen initially in the superficial anterior and posterior lens cortex. Vacuoles and clefts form in the underlying cortex. Intumescence and maturity of the cortical cataract follow shortly thereafter. Researchers believe that the underlying metabolic changes associated with the acute diabetic cataract in humans are closely allied to the sorbitol cataract studied in experimental animals. Although acute diabetic cataracts are rarely encountered in clinical practice today, any rapidly maturing bilateral cortical cataracts in a child or young adult should alert the clinician to the possibility of diabetes mellitus.

Diabetic patients develop age-related lens changes that are indistinguishable from nondiabetic age-related cataracts, except that these lens changes tend to occur at a younger age in patients with diabetes than in those without the disease. The increased risk or earlier onset of age-related cataracts in diabetic patients may be a result of the accumulation

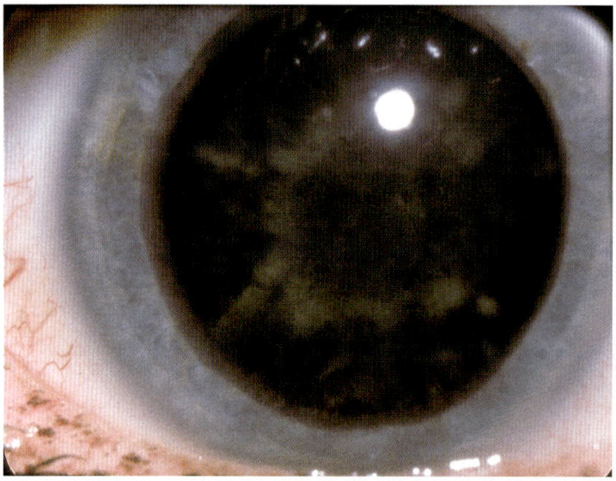

Figure 5-16 Diabetic cataract, also called *snowflake cataract,* consists of gray-white subcapsular opacities. This type of cataract is seen, in rare cases, in patients with uncontrolled diabetes mellitus. *(Courtesy of Karla J. Johns, MD.)*

of sorbitol within the lens and accompanying changes in hydration, increased nonenzymatic glycosylation (glycation) of lens proteins, or greater oxidative stress from alterations in lens metabolism.

Flynn HW Jr, Smiddy WE, eds. *Diabetes and Ocular Disease: Past, Present, and Future Therapies.* Ophthalmology Monograph 14. San Francisco: American Academy of Ophthalmology; 2000:49–53, 226.

Galactosemia

Galactosemia is an inherited autosomal recessive inability to convert galactose to glucose. As a consequence of this inability, excessive galactose accumulates in body tissues, with further metabolic conversion of galactose to galactitol (dulcitol), the sugar alcohol of galactose. Galactosemia can result from defects in 1 of 3 enzymes involved in the metabolism of galactose: galactose 1-phosphate uridyltransferase (Gal-1-PUT), galactokinase, or UDP galactose 4-epimerase. The most common and the severest form, known as *classic galactosemia,* is caused by a defect in Gal-1-PUT.

In classic galactosemia, symptoms of malnutrition, hepatomegaly, jaundice, and mental deficiency present within the first few weeks of life. The disease is fatal if undiagnosed and untreated. The diagnosis of classic galactosemia can be confirmed by demonstration of the non–glucose-reducing substance galactose in the urine.

Of patients with classic galactosemia, 75% will develop bilateral cataracts, usually within the first few weeks of life. Accumulation of galactose and galactitol within the lens cells leads to an increase in intracellular osmotic pressure and an influx of fluid in the lens. Typically, the nucleus and deep cortex become increasingly opacified, causing an "oil droplet" appearance on retroillumination (Fig 5-17). If the disease remains untreated, the cataracts progress to total opacification of the lenses. Treatment of galactosemia includes elimination of milk and milk products from the diet. In some cases, early cataract formation can be reversed by timely diagnosis and dietary intervention.

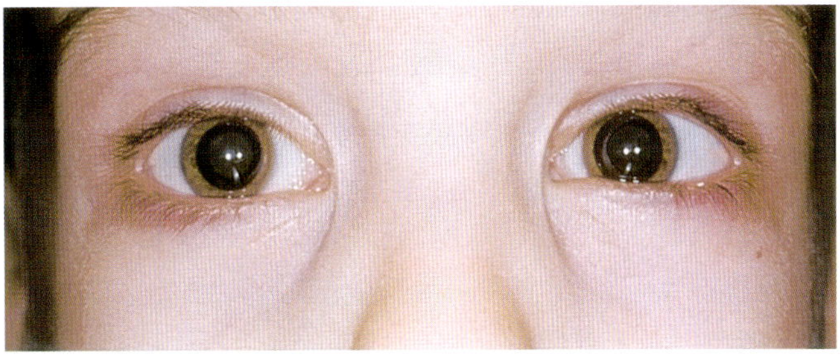

Figure 5-17 "Oil droplet" bilateral cataracts in galactosemia.

Deficiencies of the 2 other enzymes, galactokinase and epimerase, can also cause galactosemia. These deficiencies are less common, however, and cause less severe systemic abnormalities. Cataracts caused by deficiencies in these enzymes tend to present later in life than those seen in classic galactosemia.

Hypocalcemia

Cataracts may occur in association with any condition that results in hypocalcemia. *Hypocalcemia* may be idiopathic, or it may appear as a result of unintended destruction of the parathyroid glands during thyroid surgery. Usually bilateral, hypocalcemic (tetanic) cataracts are punctate iridescent opacities in the anterior and posterior cortex. They lie beneath the lens capsule and are usually separated from it by a zone of clear lens. These discrete opacities may either remain stable or mature into complete cortical cataracts.

Wilson Disease

Wilson disease (hepatolenticular degeneration) is an inherited autosomal recessive disorder of copper metabolism. The characteristic ocular manifestation of Wilson disease is the Kayser-Fleischer ring, a golden brown discoloration of Descemet's membrane around the periphery of the cornea. In addition, a characteristic sunflower cataract often develops. Reddish brown pigment (cuprous oxide) is deposited in the anterior lens capsule and subcapsular cortex in a stellate shape that resembles the petals of a sunflower. In most cases, the sunflower cataract does not produce serious visual impairment.

Myotonic Dystrophy

Myotonic dystrophy is an inherited autosomal dominant condition characterized by delayed relaxation of contracted muscles, ptosis, weakness of the facial musculature, cardiac conduction defects, and prominent frontal balding in affected male patients. Patients with this disorder typically develop polychromatic iridescent crystals in the lens cortex (Fig 5-18), with sequential PSC progressing to complete cortical opacification. Ultrastructurally, these crystals are composed of whorls of plasmalemma from the lens fibers. Polychromatic iridescent crystals are occasionally seen in the lens cortex of patients who do not have myotonic dystrophy; these crystals are thought to be caused by cholesterol crystal deposition in the lens.

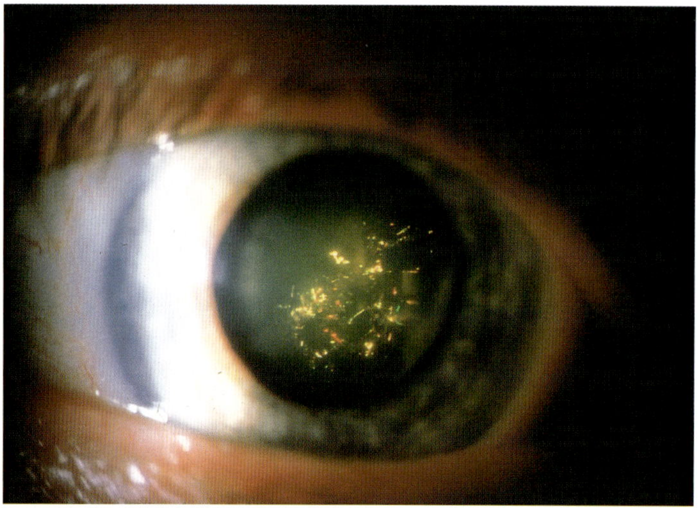

Figure 5-18 Myotonic dystrophy. *(Courtesy of Karla J. Johns, MD.)*

Effects of Nutrition and Smoking

Although nutritional deficiencies have been demonstrated to cause cataracts in animal models, this etiology has been difficult to confirm in humans. Numerous population-based studies have found that lower socioeconomic status, lower education level, and poorer overall nutrition are associated with increased prevalence of age-related cataracts. The identification of specific dietary deficiencies that lead to cataract and of supplements that protect against cataract has been more difficult. Some studies have suggested that taking multivitamin supplements, vitamin A, vitamin C, vitamin E, niacin, thiamine, riboflavin, beta carotene, or increased protein may have a protective effect on cataract development. Other studies have found that vitamins C and E have little or no effect on cataract development. Most recently, the Age-Related Eye Disease Study (AREDS) showed that over 7 years, increased intake of vitamins C and E and beta carotene did not decrease the development or progression of cataract. Use of the multivitamin supplement offered to all AREDS participants (Centrum) was moderately protective against the development of nuclear opacities. It is important to remember that high-dose vitamin use may pose risks. Smokers taking high doses of beta carotene have been shown to have an increased risk of lung cancer, of death from lung cancer, and of death from cardiovascular disease. In addition, women taking supplemental doses of vitamin A have been shown to be at increased risk of hip fracture.

Lutein and zeaxanthin are the only carotenoids found in human lenses, and recent studies have shown a moderate decrease in the risk of cataract with the increased frequency of intake of food high in lutein (eg, spinach, kale, and broccoli). Eating cooked spinach more than twice a week decreased the risk of cataract. This decreased risk was unrelated to healthy lifestyle. In contrast to the effects of such dietary supplements, severe episodes of diarrhea associated with severe dehydration may be linked to an increased risk of cataract formation.

Smoking or the use of smokeless tobacco products is the most significant, avoidable risk factor for cataracts. In numerous studies worldwide, smoking has consistently been associated with an increase in the frequency of nuclear opacities. Although the general health risks of smoking are well known, specific ocular risks such as macular degeneration and cataract may not be. The ophthalmologist can inform patients about these risks and is in a strong position to encourage individuals to stop smoking.

Age-Related Eye Disease Study Research Group. A randomized, placebo-controlled, clinical trial of high-dose supplementation with vitamins C and E and beta carotene for age-related cataract and vision loss: AREDS report no. 9. *Arch Ophthalmol.* 2001;119:1439–1452.

Berendschot TT, Broekmans WM, Klöpping-Ketalaars IA, Kardinaal AF, Van Poppel G, Van Norren D. Lens aging in relation to nutritional determinants and possible risk factors for age-related cataract. *Arch Ophthalmol.* 2002;120:1732–1737.

Chasan-Taber L, Willett WC, Seddon JM, et al. A prospective study of carotenoid and vitamin A intakes and risk of cataract extraction in US women. *Am J Clin Nutr.* 1999;70:509–516.

Christen WG, Manson JE, Seddon JM, et al. A prospective study of cigarette smoking and risk of cataract in men. *JAMA.* 1992;268:989–993.

Cumming RG, Mitchell P, Smith W. Diet and cataract: the Blue Mountains Eye Study. *Ophthalmology.* 2000;107:450–456.

Goodman GE, Thornquist MD, Balmes J, et al. The Beta-Carotene and Retinol Efficacy Trial: incidence of lung cancer and cardiovascular disease mortality during 6-year follow-up after stopping beta-carotene and retinol supplements. *J Natl Cancer Inst.* 2004;96(23):1743–1750.

Hankinson SE, Willett WC, Colditz GA, et al. A prospective study of cigarette smoking and risk of cataract surgery in women. *JAMA.* 1992;268:994–998.

Leske MC, Chylack LT Jr, He Q, et al. Antioxidant vitamins and nuclear opacities: the longitudinal study of cataract. *Ophthalmology.* 1998;105:831–836.

Lyle BJ, Mares-Perlman JA, Klein BE, Klein R, Greger JL. Antioxidant intake and risk of incident age-related nuclear cataracts in the Beaver Dam Eye Study. *Am J Epidemiol.* 1999;149:801–809.

Milton RC, Sperduto RD, Clemons TE, Ferris FL 3rd; Age-Related Eye Disease Study Research Group. Centrum use and progression of age-related cataract in the Age-Related Eye Disease Study: a propensity score approach. AREDS report no. 21. *Ophthalmology.* 2006;113(8):1264–1270.

Omenn GS, Goodman GE, Thornquist MD, et al. Effects of a combination of beta carotene and vitamin A on lung cancer and cardiovascular disease. *N Engl J Med.* 1996;334:1150–1155.

Opotowsky AR, Bilezikian JP. Serum vitamin A concentration and the risk of hip fracture among women 50 to 74 years old in the United States: a prospective analysis of the NHANES I follow-up study. *Am J Med.* 2004;117(3):169–174.

Raju P, George R, Ve Ramesh S, Arvind H, Baskaran M, Vijaya L. Influence of tobacco use on cataract development. *Br J Ophthalmol.* 2006;90(11):1374–1377. Epub 2006 Jul 12.

Cataract Associated With Uveitis

Lens changes often occur as a result of chronic uveitis or associated corticosteroid therapy. Typically, a PSC appears; anterior lens changes may also occur (Fig 5-19). The formation of posterior synechiae is common in uveitis, often with thickening of the anterior lens capsule, which may have an associated fibrous pupillary membrane. Lens changes in

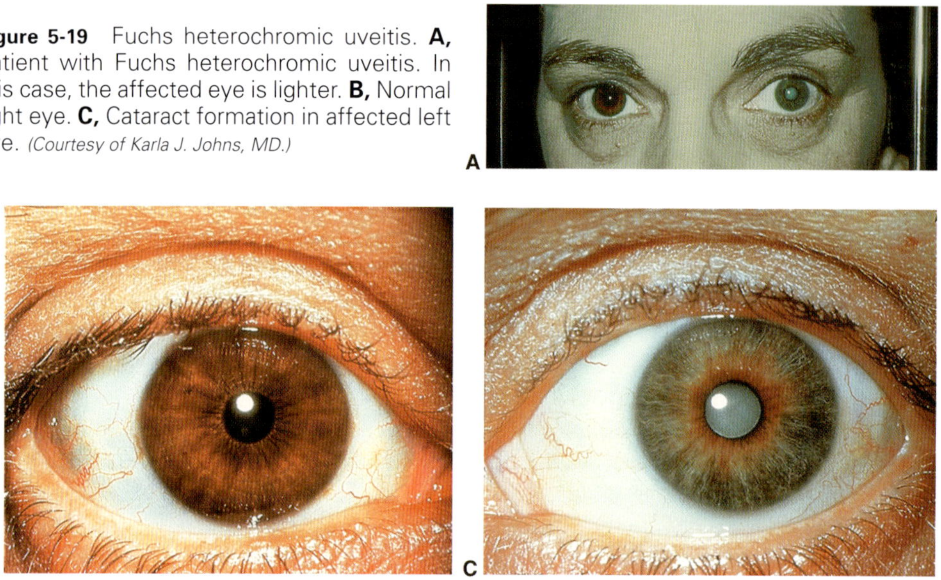

Figure 5-19 Fuchs heterochromic uveitis. **A,** Patient with Fuchs heterochromic uveitis. In this case, the affected eye is lighter. **B,** Normal right eye. **C,** Cataract formation in affected left eye. *(Courtesy of Karla J. Johns, MD.)*

cataract secondary to uveitis may progress to a mature cataract. Calcium deposits may be observed on the anterior capsule or within the lens substance.

Cortical cataract formation occurs in up to 70% of cases of Fuchs heterochromic uveitis (see Fig 5-19). Because posterior synechiae do not commonly occur in this syndrome, formation of pupillary membranes is unlikely, and long-term corticosteroid therapy is not indicated. Cataract extraction in patients with Fuchs heterochromic uveitis generally has a favorable prognosis. Intraoperative anterior chamber hemorrhages have been reported in approximately 25% of cases.

Cataracts Associated With Ocular Therapies

Posterior subcapsular cataract secondary to corticosteroid treatment is discussed in the previous section. Vitrectomy is another cause of treatment-induced cataract. Transient opacities involving the posterior sutures can occur soon after vitrectomy, but these opacities usually resolve spontaneously. However, more than 60% and up to 95% of patients who undergo vitrectomy during surgical treatment of a variety of retinal problems develop nuclear cataracts within 2 years of the surgery. Postvitrectomy cataracts are less common in patients younger than 50 years. The formation of nuclear cataracts after vitrectomy seems to be associated with disruption of the vitreous body structure and does not seem to be a consequence of the retinal disease. Retinal surgery performed without vitrectomy is not associated with increased lens opacification. In this regard, age-related degeneration of the vitreous body has also been associated with increased risk of nuclear opacification.

Lens changes may also occur after hyperbaric oxygen therapy. Several studies found a myopic shift during the course of several weeks of hyperbaric oxygen therapy for different conditions. Since no change in axial length or corneal curvature was detected, the refractive change was presumed to be due to increased nuclear sclerosis. In most cases, the myopic shift resolved after cessation of therapy. In patients exposed to hyperbaric oxygen at least 150 times during a 1-year period, nearly 50% of patients with previously clear lenses developed frank nuclear cataracts. An increase in nuclear light scatter was shown in most of the other patients in this treatment group when they were compared with older, sicker patients who were in the same clinic but not eligible for hyperbaric oxygen therapy.

Harocopos GJ, Shui YB, McKinnon M, Holekamp NM, Gordon MO, Beebe DC. Importance of vitreous liquefaction in age-related cataract. *Invest Ophthalmol Vis Sci.* 2004;45(1):77–85.

Melberg NS, Thomas MA. Nuclear sclerotic cataract after vitrectomy in patients younger than 50 years of age. *Ophthalmology.* 1995;102(10):1466–1471.

Palmquist BM, Philipson B, Barr PO. Nuclear cataract and myopia during hyperbaric oxygen therapy. *Br J Ophthalmol.* 1984;68(2):113–117.

Sawa M, Ohji M, Kusaka S, et al. Nonvitrectomizing vitreous surgery for epiretinal membrane long-term follow-up. *Ophthalmology.* 2005;112(8):1402–1408.

Pseudoexfoliation Syndrome

Pseudoexfoliation (PEX) syndrome is a systemic disease in which a matrix of fibrotic material is deposited in many bodily organs. In the eye, a basement membrane–like fibrillogranular white material is deposited on the lens, cornea, iris, anterior hyaloid face, ciliary processes, zonular fibers, and trabecular meshwork. These deposits, believed to comprise elastic microfibrils, appear as grayish white flecks that are prominent at the pupillary margin and on the lens capsule (Fig 5-20). Associated with this condition are atrophy of the iris at the pupillary margin, deposition of pigment on the anterior surface of the iris, poorly dilating pupil, increased pigmentation of the trabecular meshwork, capsular fragility, zonular weakness, and open-angle glaucoma. PEX is a unilateral or bilateral disorder that becomes more apparent with increasing age.

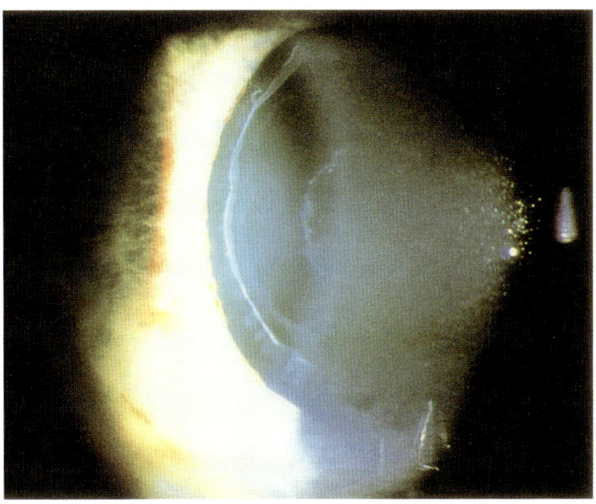

Figure 5-20 Pseudoexfoliation.

Increased oxidative stress caused by abnormalities in transforming growth factor-β (TGF-β) contributes to the formation of cataracts. Patients with this syndrome may also experience weakness of the zonular fibers and spontaneous lens subluxation and phacodonesis. Poor zonular integrity may affect cataract surgery technique and IOL implantation. The PEX material may be elaborated even after the crystalline lens is removed.

Ritch R. Exfoliation syndrome. *Focal Points: Clinical Modules for Ophthalmologists*. San Francisco: American Academy of Ophthalmology; 1994, module 9.

Schlötzer-Schrehardt U, Naumann GO. Ocular and systemic pseudoexfoliation syndrome. *Am J Ophthalmol*. 2006;141(5):921–937.

Cataract and Skin Diseases

Atopic Dermatitis

Atopic dermatitis is a chronic, itching, erythematous dermatitis, often seen in conjunction with increased levels of immunoglobulin E (IgE) and a history of multiple allergies or asthma. Cataract formation has been reported in up to 25% of patients with atopic dermatitis. The cataracts are usually bilateral, and onset occurs in the second to third decade. Typically, these cataracts are anterior subcapsular opacities in the pupillary area that resemble shieldlike plaques.

Mannis MJ, Macsai MS, Huntley AC, eds. *Eye and Skin Disease*. Philadelphia: Lippincott-Raven; 1996.

Phacoantigenic Uveitis

In the normal eye, minute amounts of lens proteins leak out through the lens capsule. The eye appears to have immunologic tolerance to these small amounts of lens antigens. However, the release of a large amount of lens protein into the anterior chamber disrupts this immunologic tolerance and may trigger a severe inflammatory reaction. Phacoantigenic uveitis, sometimes referred to as *phacoanaphylactic uveitis,* is an immune-mediated granulomatous inflammation initiated by lens proteins released through a ruptured lens capsule. Phacoantigenic uveitis usually occurs following traumatic rupture of the lens capsule or following cataract surgery when cortical material is retained within the eye. Onset is days to weeks after the injury or surgery.

The disease is characterized by a red, painful eye with chemosis and anterior chamber inflammation with cells, flare, and keratic precipitates. Occasionally, glaucoma secondary to blockage of the trabecular meshwork and formation of synechiae may occur. Late complications include cyclitic membrane, hypotony, and phthisis bulbi. Rarely, phacoantigenic uveitis can give rise to an inflammatory reaction in the fellow eye. Lens extraction is the definitive therapy for the condition. Histopathologic examination shows a zonal granulomatous inflammation surrounding a breach of the lens capsule. (See BCSC

Section 4, *Ophthalmic Pathology and Intraocular Tumors,* and BCSC Section 9, *Intraocular Inflammation and Uveitis.*)

Lens-Induced Glaucoma

Phacolytic Glaucoma

Phacolytic glaucoma is a complication of a mature or hypermature cataract. Denatured, liquefied high-molecular-weight lens proteins leak through an intact but permeable lens capsule. An immune response is not elicited; rather, macrophages ingest these lens proteins. The trabecular meshwork can become clogged with both the lens proteins and the engorged macrophages. The usual clinical presentation of phacolytic glaucoma consists of abrupt onset of pain and redness in a cataractous eye that has had poor vision for some time. The cornea may be edematous, and significant flare reaction occurs in the anterior chamber. White flocculent material appears in the anterior chamber and often adheres to the lens capsule as well. Intraocular pressure (IOP) is markedly elevated, and the anterior chamber angle is open, although the same material may be seen in the trabecular meshwork. Initial treatment of phacolytic glaucoma consists of controlling IOP with antiglaucoma medications and managing inflammation with topical corticosteroids. Surgical removal of the lens is the definitive treatment.

Lens Particle Glaucoma

Following a penetrating lens injury, extracapsular cataract extraction (ECCE) with retained cortical material, or, rarely, Nd:YAG capsulotomy, particles of lens cortex may migrate into the anterior chamber, where they cause obstruction to aqueous outflow through the trabecular meshwork. In most instances, the onset of glaucoma is delayed by days or weeks after the surgical event or lens injury. Examination reveals hydrated cortical material in the anterior chamber, sometimes in association with an anterior segment inflammatory reaction. Gonioscopy shows that the angle is open, and cortical material can often be seen deposited along the trabecular meshwork. Medical therapy to lower IOP and to reduce intraocular inflammation is indicated. If the IOP and inflammation do not respond quickly to this treatment, surgical removal of the retained lens material may be required.

Phacomorphic Glaucoma

An intumescent cataractous lens can cause pupillary block and induce secondary angle-closure glaucoma, or it can physically push the iris forward and thus cause shallowing of the anterior chamber. Typically, the patient presents with a red, painful eye and a history of decreased vision as a result of cataract formation prior to the acute event (Fig 5-21). The cornea may be edematous. The anterior chamber is shallow, and gonioscopy reveals a closed anterior chamber angle. Initial management includes medical treatment to lower the IOP. The condition responds to laser iridotomy, but definitive treatment consists of cataract extraction.

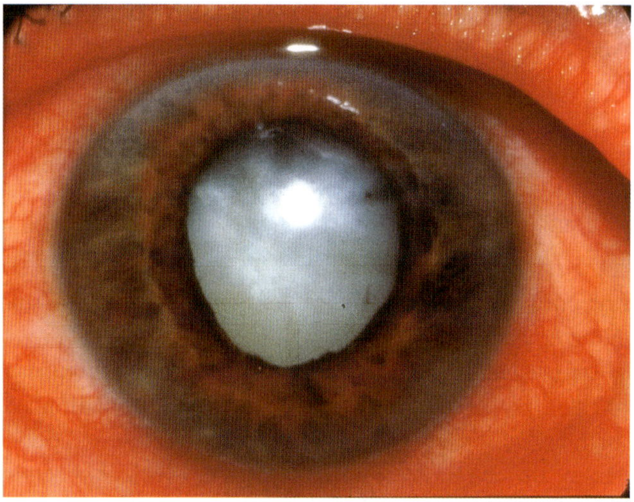

Figure 5-21 Phacomorphic glaucoma.

Glaukomflecken

Glaukomflecken are gray-white epithelial and anterior cortical lens opacities that occur following an episode of markedly elevated IOP, as in acute angle-closure glaucoma. Histopathologically, glaukomflecken are composed of necrotic lens epithelial cells and degenerated subepithelial cortex.

Ischemia

Ischemic ocular conditions, such as pulseless disease (Takayasu arteritis), thromboangiitis obliterans (Buerger disease), and anterior segment necrosis, can cause PSC. The cataract may progress rapidly to total opacification of the lens.

Cataracts Associated With Degenerative Ocular Disorders

Cataracts can occur secondary to many degenerative ocular diseases, such as retinitis pigmentosa, essential iris atrophy, chronic hypotony, and absolute glaucoma. These secondary cataracts usually begin as PSCs and may progress to total lens opacification. The mechanisms responsible for cataractogenesis in degenerative ocular disorders are not well understood.

Burke JP, O'Keefe M, Bowell R, Naughten ER. Ophthalmic findings in classical galactosemia: a screened population. *J Pediatr Ophthalmol Strabismus*. 1989;26:165–168.

Cruickshanks KF, Klein BE, Klein R. Ultraviolet light exposure and lens opacities: the Beaver Dam Eye Study. *Am J Public Health*. 1992;82:1658–1662.

Edwards MC, Johnson JL, Marriage B, et al. Isolated sulfite oxidase deficiency: review of two cases in one family. *Ophthalmology*. 1999;106:1957–1961.

Fraunfelder FT, Fraunfelder FW. *Drug-Induced Ocular Side Effects*. 5th ed. Boston: Butterworth-Heinemann; 2001.

Gold DH, Weingeist TA, eds. *The Eye in Systemic Disease.* Philadelphia: Lippincott; 1990:90, 330–331, 390, 434.

Havener WH. *Ocular Pharmacology.* 5th ed. St Louis: Mosby; 1983:366, 487–489.

Irvine JA, Smith RE. Lens injuries. In: Shingleton BJ, Hersh PS, Kenyon KR, eds. *Eye Trauma.* St Louis: Mosby; 1991:126–135.

Johns KJ. Diabetes and the lens. In: Feman SS, ed. *Ocular Problems in Diabetes Mellitus.* Boston: Blackwell; 1992:221–244.

Klein BE, Klein R, Lee KE. Incidence of age-related cataract: the Beaver Dam Eye Study. *Arch Ophthalmol.* 1998;116:219–225.

Liebman JM, Ritch R. Glaucoma secondary to lens intumescence and dislocation. In: Ritch R, Shields MB, Krupin T, eds. *The Glaucomas.* 2nd ed. St Louis: Mosby; 1996.

Lipman RM, Tripathi BJ, Tripathi RC. Cataracts induced by microwave and ionizing radiation. *Surv Ophthalmol.* 1988;33:200–210.

Nelson LB, Spaeth GL, Nowinski TS, Margo CE, Jackson L. Aniridia: a review. *Surv Ophthalmol.* 1984;28:621–642.

Richter C, Epstein DL. Lens-induced open-angle glaucoma. In: Ritch R, Shields MB, Krupin T, eds. *The Glaucomas.* 2nd ed. St Louis: Mosby; 1996.

Urban RC Jr, Cotlier E. Corticosteroid-induced cataracts. *Surv Ophthalmol.* 1986;31:102–110.

West SK, Duncan DD, Muñoz B, et al. Sunlight exposure and risk of lens opacities in a population-based study: the Salisbury Eye Evaluation Project. *JAMA*. 1998;280:714–718.

West SK, Valmadrid CT. Epidemiology of risk factors for age-related cataract. *Surv Ophthalmol.* 1995;39:323–334.

Young RW. *Age-Related Cataract*. New York: Oxford University Press; 1991.

CHAPTER 6

Epidemiology of Cataracts

According to the World Health Organization (WHO), cataract is the leading cause of blindness and visual impairment throughout the world. With the general aging of the population, the overall prevalence of visual loss as a result of lenticular opacities increases each year. In 2002, the WHO estimated that cataracts caused reversible blindness in more than 17 million (47.8%) of the 37 million blind individuals worldwide, and this number is projected to reach 40 million by 2020. The WHO proposes that between 2000 and 2020, the number of cataract surgeries performed worldwide will need to triple in order to keep pace with the needs of the population. It has been shown that visual impairment and age-related cataract may be independent risk factors for increased mortality in older persons. Cataract affects nearly 20.5 million Americans aged 40 and older, or about 1 in every 6 people in this age range. It is estimated that 2.5 million cataract surgeries were performed in the United States in 2004, of which 1.8 million were performed on Medicare beneficiaries. The rate of cataract surgery in the United States is thus greater than 8000 cataract surgeries per million population, whereas in China the number is fewer than 500 cataract surgeries per million. In parts of the developing world, the number may be as low as 50 surgeries per million.

Because surgery is the only treatment currently available for visually significant lenticular opacity, the growing need for surgical resources compounds the already significant socioeconomic impact of cataracts in particular and blindness in general. The problem is especially critical in developing countries, where 1 blind individual takes 2 individuals out of the workforce, if the blind person requires the care of an able adult.

The economic impact of cataract surgery in the United States alone is enormous. It is estimated that the federal government spends more than $3.4 billion each year treating cataract through the Medicare program. In addition to the vast number of cataract operations performed each year in the United States, an even greater number of related office visits and tests contribute to the financial impact of cataracts. Further, patients with visual loss incur significantly higher medical costs, and 90% of these costs are unrelated to the eye.

Although cataracts may be congenital, metabolic, or traumatic in origin, age-related cataracts have the greatest socioeconomic impact because of their prevalence. The lack of a widely accepted, standardized classification system for lens opacities makes it difficult to evaluate precisely the prevalence and incidence of cataracts. The size, shape, density, and location of age-related lens opacities are variable, and most definitions of cataract require a quantifiable reduction in visual acuity in addition to alterations in lens morphology visible at the slit lamp. Further, examination methods are often subjective and require patient participation. Thus, studies are easily biased. Most estimates of age-related cataract frequency are based on data from selective groups rather than from general populations. Finally, in many elderly patients, eyes may have coexisting pathology, producing visual loss that might have been incorrectly attributed to lens changes.

A number of studies on cataract have been carried out in recent years. The Age-Related Eye Disease Study (AREDS) was performed during the 1990s. The study demonstrated, among other findings, a high degree of reliability in grading the severity of lens opacities in a large study cohort with mostly early lens changes. The AREDS system for classifying cataracts from photography may be useful in future studies of cataract incidence and progression.

Age-Related Eye Disease Study Research Group. The age-related eye disease study (AREDS) system for classifying cataracts from photographs: AREDS report no. 4. *Am J Ophthalmol.* 2001;131:167–175.

Javitt JC, Zhou Z, Willke R. Association between vision loss and higher medical care costs in Medicare beneficiaries costs are greater for those with progressive vision loss. *Ophthalmology.* 2007;114:238–245.

The Beaver Dam Eye Study was a large population-based study that was performed in the late 1980s (data published in the 1990s). It reported that 38.8% of men and 45.9% of women older than 74 years had visually significant cataracts. For this study, "significance" was determined by photographic grading of lens opacities and best-corrected visual acuity of 20/32 (logMAR equivalent closest to 20/30 Snellen fraction), excluding those with severe age-related maculopathy. The prevalence of cataract in this study is shown in Table 6-1.

A follow-up to the Beaver Dam Eye Study was performed between 1993 and 1995 to estimate the incidence of nuclear, cortical, and posterior subcapsular cataract (PSC) in the study cohort. Incident nuclear cataract occurred in 13.1%, cortical cataract in 8.2%, and PSC in 3.4%. The cumulative incidence of nuclear cataract increased from 2.9% in persons aged 43–54 years at baseline to 40.0% in those aged 75 years or older. For cortical cataract and PSC, the corresponding values were 1.9% and 21.8% and 1.4% and 7.3%, respectively. Women were more likely than men to have nuclear cataracts, even after adjusting for age.

Table 6-1 Percent Prevalence of Visually Significant* Cataract in the Beaver Dam Eye Study, 1988–1990

	Women		Men	
Age	**Worse Eye (%)**	**Better Eye (%)**	**Worse Eye (%)**	**Better Eye (%)**
43–54	2.6	0.4	0.4	0.0
55–64	10.0	1.0	3.9	0.3
65–74	23.5	8.3	14.3	3.4
75+	45.9	25.4	38.8	12.6

*Visually significant indicates visual acuity in the affected eye of 20/32 or worse (Snellen fraction equivalent of 45 letters correct on logMAR chart). This excludes subjects with geographic atrophy or exudative maculopathy in the affected eye.

Adapted from Klein BK, Klein R, Linton KL. Prevalence of age-related lens opacities in a population. The Beaver Dam Eye Study. *Ophthalmology.* 1992;99:546–552.

Klein BE, Klein R, Lee KE. Incidence of age-related cataract: the Beaver Dam Eye Study. *Arch Ophthalmol.* 1998;116:219–225.

The Baltimore Eye Survey revealed that cataract was the leading cause of blindness (20/200 or worse vision) among those 40 years and older. Untreated cataract was the source of blindness in 27% of African Americans and 13% of Caucasians.

The Longitudinal Study of Cataract (LSC) was an epidemiologic study of the natural history of and risk factors for lens opacities. In this study, nuclear opacification was linked with increasing age, white race, lower education, gout medication, current smoking, family history of cataract, preexisting PSC, and early use of eyeglasses. The LSC assessed new lens opacities and the progression of lenticular opacities using a research instrument called the *Lens Opacities Classification System III (LOCS III).* The median age of study participants was 65 years, and the incidence of new opacities was 6% after 2 years and 8% after 5 years. After 5 years' follow-up, the incidence rates for developing cortical and posterior subcapsular opacities were 7.7% and 4.3%, respectively. The progression of preexisting posterior subcapsular opacities was higher, reaching 55.1% after 5 years of follow-up. Although the incidence rates for both cortical and posterior subcapsular opacities were much higher for those aged 65 years or older than for those younger than 65 years, the progression rates for these two age groups were very similar. The Barbados Eye Study provided prevalence data on lens opacities in a predominantly black population. Cortical opacities were the most frequent type of cataract, and women had a higher frequency of opacification.

In a US-based cohort of 8363 individuals older than 61 years at intake, the cumulative rate of cataract surgery was 7.4% annually over 5 years. A second study indicated that each year, 5.7% of individuals aged 49 years or older become unilaterally pseudophakic. Applied to data from the most recent US census, these percentages translate to 3.3 million cataract surgeries in patients aged 62 years or older and 5.2 million procedures when those aged 49 years or older are included, although these results seem much higher than the census data would suggest.

Leske MC, Chylack LT Jr, He Q, et al. Incidence and progression of cortical and posterior subcapsular opacities: the Longitudinal Study of Cataract. The LSC Group. *Ophthalmology.* 1997;104:1987–1993.

Leske MC, Connell AM, Wu SY, Hyman L, Schachat AP. Prevalence of lens opacities in the Barbados Eye Study. *Arch Ophthalmol.* 1997;115:105–111.

Williams A, Sloan FA, Lee PP. Longitudinal rates of cataract surgery. *Arch Ophthalmol.* 2006;124:1308–1314.

Other studies have linked the risk of developing cortical opacities and PSC with higher body mass index (BMI) at baseline and have shown increased risk with increasing BMI over time. The AREDS report no. 5 found that persons with moderate nuclear opacities were more likely to be female, nonwhite, and smokers, and to have large macular drusen. Moderate nuclear opacities were less common in people with higher educational status, in those with a history of diabetes (only patients with mild background diabetic retinopathy [BDR] were included in the study), and in those taking nonsteroidal anti-inflammatory drugs. Moderate cortical opacities were associated with dark iris color, large macular drusen, weight gain, higher sunlight exposure, and the use of thyroid hormone; they were less common in people with higher educational status.

Although reported risk factors for cataract development are not consistent, studies repeatedly show that cataracts are more common in African Americans and that nuclear cataracts are more common in women, smokers, and those with less education. Cigarette smokers of both sexes have repeatedly been shown to have an increased risk of developing nuclear lens opacities. Some smoking-related damage to the lens may be reversible, and smoking cessation reduces the risk of cataract by limiting total dose-related damage to the lens.

Age-Related Eye Disease Study Research Group. Risk factors associated with age-related nuclear and cortical cataract: a case-control study in the Age-Related Eye Disease Study. AREDS report no. 5. *Ophthalmology*. 2001;108:1400–1408.

Christen WG, Glynn RJ, Ajani UA, et al. Smoking cessation and risk of age-related cataract in men. *JAMA*. 2000;284:713–716.

Chylack LT Jr, Wolfe JK, Singer DM, et al. The Lens Opacities Classification System III. The Longitudinal Study of Cataract Study Group. *Arch Ophthalmol.* 1993;111:831–836.

Hiller R, Podgor MJ, Sperduto RD, et al. A longitudinal study of body mass index and lens opacities. The Framingham Studies. *Ophthalmology.* 1998;105:1244–1250.

Hiller R, Sperduto RD, Podgor MJ, et al. Cigarette smoking and the risk of development of lens opacities. The Framingham Studies. *Arch Ophthalmol.* 1997;115:1113–1118.

Klein BE, Klein R, Linton KL. Prevalence of age-related lens opacities in a population. The Beaver Dam Eye Study. *Ophthalmology*. 1992;99:546–552.

Leske MC, Chylack LT Jr, He Q, et al. Risk factors for nuclear opalescence in a longitudinal study. LSC Group. *Am J Epidemiol.* 1998;147:36–41.

Leske MC, Chylack LT Jr, Wu SY, et al. Incidence and progression of nuclear opacities in the Longitudinal Study of Cataract. *Ophthalmology*. 1996;103:705–712.

Sommer A, Tielsch JM, Katz J, et al. Racial differences in the cause-specific prevalence of blindness in east Baltimore. *N Engl J Med.* 1991;325:1412–1417.

CHAPTER 7

Evaluation and Management of Cataracts in Adults

When an ophthalmologist evaluates a patient for cataract surgery, it is essential that he or she determine whether the lens opacity is the principal cause of the visual decline and whether the cataract correlates with the degree of visual loss and the impact on the patient's activities of daily living (ADLs). The following issues may be considered in the evaluation and management of cataract:

- Will lens removal provide sufficient functional improvement to warrant surgery?
- Is the patient sufficiently healthy to tolerate surgery?
- Is the patient or another responsible person capable of participating in postoperative care?
- Is the lens opacity secondary to a systemic condition, or is it an impediment to the diagnosis or treatment of another ocular condition?

Because cataract surgery is, in the vast majority of cases, an elective procedure, the ophthalmologist should allow sufficient time to obtain the answers to these questions. The following sections provide an outline that can help accomplish this task. Ultimately, it is important that both patient and physician be satisfied that surgery is the appropriate choice for improving vision.

Clinical History: Signs and Symptoms

Decreased Visual Acuity

Many cataract patients are self-referred. In this situation, the clinical history is straightforward, and the patient tells the ophthalmologist which activities have been curtailed or abandoned. Some patients learn of their decline in visual acuity only after being examined. Still others deny they are having any problems until their limitations are demonstrated or privileges are withdrawn because they are no longer visually competent.

Different types of cataract may have different effects on visual acuity, depending on incident light, pupil size, and degree of myopia (Table 7-1). The presence of even small posterior subcapsular cataracts (PSCs) can greatly disturb reading acuity even

Table 7-1 Effect of Cataract on Visual Acuity

	Growth Rate	Glare	Effect on Distance	Effect on Near	Induced Myopia
Cortical	Moderate	Mild	Mild	Mild	None
Nuclear	Mild	Mild	Moderate	None	Moderate
Posterior subcapsular	Rapid	Marked	Mild	Marked	None

though distance vision is relatively unaffected. In contrast, the induced myopic shift from oil droplet cataracts may worsen distance clarity while preserving reading vision. The overall effect of the cataract on visual function is probably a more appropriate way to determine visual disability than is Snellen acuity alone.

After obtaining a thorough history from the patient, the clinician performs a complete visual examination, beginning with a careful refraction. Early development of nuclear sclerotic cataract may increase the dioptric power of the lens, commonly causing a mild to moderate degree of myopia. Asymmetric development of lens-induced myopia may produce disabling anisometropia. Specific testing of vision under conditions other than those of the refraction lane may simulate the situations in which the patient has difficulty performing important ADLs.

Glare

Cataract patients often report sensitivity to glare, which may vary in severity from a decrease in contrast sensitivity in brightly lit environments to disabling glare in the daytime or with oncoming car headlights. This increased sensitivity is particularly prominent with PSCs and, occasionally, anterior cortical lens changes. Glare testing attempts to measure the degree of visual impairment caused by the presence of a light source located in the patient's visual field. It is important to use a consistent, reliable method to determine glare sensitivity and to document the resultant loss of visual acuity. (Some third-party payers require that an insured person's visual acuity decline to a specified level or that visual loss due to glare be documented before they will approve cataract surgery reimbursement.)

Altered Contrast Sensitivity

Contrast sensitivity is the ability to detect subtle variations in shading. It is tested with the use of specially designed cards, on which are figures that vary in contrast, luminance, and spatial frequency. Because patients with ocular abnormalities have altered contrast sensitivity in reduced luminance, measurement of contrast sensitivity may provide a more comprehensive estimate of the visual resolution of the eye. A significant loss in contrast sensitivity may occur without a similar loss in Snellen acuity. However, abnormal contrast sensitivity is not a specific indicator of visual loss due to cataract. If a reproducible technique is used to measure contrast sensitivity, it offers another source of documentation of the visual impairment.

Rubin GS, Bandeen-Roche K, Huang GH, et al. The association of multiple visual impairments with self-reported visual disability: SEE project. *Invest Ophthalmol Vis Sci.* 2001;42:64–72.

Shankar H, Pesudovs K. Critical flicker fusion test of potential vision. *J Cataract Refract Surg.* 2007;33:232–239.

Vianya-Estopà M, Douthwaite WA, Noble BA, Elliott DB. Capabilities of potential vision test measurements: clinical evaluation in the presence of cataract or macular disease. *J Cataract Refract Surg.* 2006;32(7):1151–1160.

Myopic Shift

The development of cataract may increase the dioptric power of the lens, commonly causing a mild to moderate degree of myopia. Hyperopic presbyopic patients find their need for distance glasses diminishes as they experience this so-called *second sight.* This phenomenon is encountered with nuclear sclerotic cataracts and disappears when the optical quality of the crystalline lens further deteriorates. Asymmetric development of lens-induced myopia may produce intolerable anisometropia, prompting consideration of cataract extraction.

Monocular Diplopia or Polyopia

Occasionally, nuclear changes are localized to the inner layers of the lens nucleus, resulting in multiple refractile areas at the center of the lens. Such areas may best be seen as irregularities in the red reflex on retinoscopy or direct ophthalmoscopy. This type of cataract can result in monocular diplopia or polyopia, including ghost images and occasionally a true second image. Monocular diplopia can also occur with other ocular media opacities or other disorders of the eye (see also BCSC Section 5, *Neuro-Ophthalmology*). If acuity improves on a pinhole test, the clinician can rule out nonrefractive causes of visual loss.

Medical Management

Several nonsurgical approaches may be attempted to improve visual function in patients with cataracts. For example, careful refraction might improve spectacle correction for distance and near vision. Brighter illumination will improve the contrast of reading material, and higher spectacle adds may be helpful for reading. In patients with small axial cataracts, pupillary dilation, either pharmacologically or by laser pupilloplasty, may improve visual function by allowing more light to pass through peripheral portions of the lens.

Pharmacologic reversal of cataracts is a subject of ongoing research. Although progress is being made, no commercially available medication has been proven to delay or reverse cataract formation in humans. Aldose reductase inhibitors, which block the conversion of glucose to sorbitol, have been shown to prevent cataracts in animals with experimentally induced diabetes. Other possible agents to slow or reverse the growth of cataracts are under investigation and include sorbitol-lowering agents, aspirin, and glutathione-raising agents. Antioxidant vitamins E, C, beta carotene, and zinc do not slow cataract progression.

McNeil JJ, Robman L, Tikellis G, Sinclair MI, McCarty CA, Taylor HR. Vitamin E supplementation and cataract: randomized controlled trial. *Ophthalmology.* 2004;111:75–84.

Sackett CS, Schenning S. The age-related eye disease study: the results of the clinical trial. *Insight.* 2002;27:5–7.

Low Vision Aids for Cataract

Some patients with limited visual function from cataract may be helped by optical aids when surgical management is not feasible. Handheld monoculars of 2.5×, 2.8×, and 4× facilitate spotting objects at a distance, whereas high-add spectacles, magnifiers, closed-circuit televisions, and telescopic loupes may be used for reading and close work.

Cataracts reduce contrast and cause glare. The shorter wavelengths cause the most scatter; the color, intensity, and direction of lighting also affect glare. If a patient experiences problems in a particular lighting situation, the ophthalmologist may suggest reducing light transmission from 400–550 nm or increasing lumens directed at reading material and away from the patient's eyes.

For patients whose visual function could be aided or enhanced by visual rehabilitation, the American Academy of Ophthalmology (AAO) provides *SmartSight,* a Web site, which is available at http://one.aao.org/SmartSight.

Indications for Surgery

The most common indication for cataract surgery is the patient's desire for improved vision. The decision to operate is not based solely on a specific level of reduced acuity. Rather, the physician determines whether the patient's reduced visual function is expected to improve sufficiently to warrant cataract surgery. First, a detailed history must document the patient's subjective visual disability. Several questionnaires, such as the Visual Function Index (VF-14) or the Activities of Daily Vision Scale (ADVS), are available as adjunctive measures of impairment. Some governmental agencies and industries have minimum standards of visual function for tasks such as driving, flying, and operating complex equipment. A patient whose best-corrected visual acuity does not meet these visual requisites may need to consider cataract surgery. The eye surgeon must determine, through discussion with the patient and family, as well as through analysis of the results of subjective and objective testing, whether cataract surgery is advisable.

When a patient has bilateral visually significant cataracts, surgery is performed first in the eye with the more advanced cataract. In fragile patients with active or severe systemic illness, or in those with other ocular diseases contributing to reduced acuity, it may be appropriate to operate first on the eye with better visual potential, should only one surgical procedure be anticipated.

Patients undergoing second-eye cataract surgery show significant improvements not only in acuity and patient-reported visual ability but also in measures of bilateral visual function such as stereopsis and contrast sensitivity. The decision to proceed with cataract surgery on the second eye must be individualized to the patient's needs and visual potential just as it was for the first eye. Also, symptomatic anisometropia, which may occur as a result of the initial cataract surgery, may be unsatisfactorily addressed by nonsurgical treatment and disabling enough to the patient to justify surgery on the second eye. Before proceeding with the second surgery, the physician and patient should allow sufficient time to confirm the success and safety of the first operation.

Common indications for surgery in a patient with a monocular cataract include loss of stereopsis, diminished peripheral vision, disabling glare, or symptomatic anisometropia. The presence of cataract in one eye directly influences driving performance and accident avoidance.

Medical indications for cataract surgery include phacolytic glaucoma, phacomorphic glaucoma, phacoantigenic uveitis, and dislocation of the lens into the anterior chamber. An additional indication for surgery is the presence of a cataract sufficiently opaque to obscure the view of the fundus and impair the diagnosis or management of other ocular diseases such as diabetic retinopathy or glaucoma.

Castells X, Alonso J, Ribo C, et al. Comparison of the results of first and second cataract eye surgery. *Ophthalmology.* 1999;106:676–682.

Castells X, Comas M, Alonso J, et al. In a randomized controlled trial, cataract surgery in both eyes increased benefits compared to surgery in one eye only. *J Clin Epidemiol.* 2006;59(2):201–207.

Owsley C, McGwin G Jr, Sloane M, Wells J, Stalvey BT, Gauthreaux S. Impact of cataract surgery on motor vehicle crash involvement by older adults. *JAMA.* 2002;288:841–849.

Rosen PN, Kaplan RM, David K. Measuring outcomes of cataract surgery using the Quality of Well-Being Scale and VF-14 Visual Function Index. *J Cataract Refract Surg.* 2005; 31(2):369–378.

Talbot EM, Perkins A. The benefit of second eye cataract surgery. *Eye.* 1998;12:983–989.

Preoperative Evaluation

The following information should be obtained in order to determine whether cataract surgery is warranted. The parameters suggested should be tailored to the specific patient's situation.

General Health of the Patient

A complete medical history is the starting point for the preoperative evaluation. The ophthalmic surgeon should work closely with the patient's primary care physician to achieve optimal management of all medical problems, especially diabetes mellitus, ischemic heart disease, chronic obstructive pulmonary disease, bleeding disorders, or adrenal suppression caused by systemic corticosteroids. The ophthalmologist should be aware of drug sensitivities and use of medications that might alter the outcome of surgery, such as immunosuppressants and anticoagulants. The ophthalmologist should inquire specifically about the use of systemic sympathetic α_{1A}-antagonist medications (including prazosin, terazosin, doxazosin, and tamsulosin) used for the treatment of benign prostatic hypertrophy, as they are strongly associated with intraoperative floppy iris syndrome (IFIS) and with fluctuations in pupil size during cataract surgery. All α_{1A}-blockers can bind to postsynaptic nerve endings of the iris dilator muscle for a prolonged period, causing excessive iris mobility. This effect may occur after only one dose of the medication and may persist indefinitely even after discontinuation of the drug. The ophthalmic surgeon may avoid intraoperative complications by employing methods to maximize pupil size, including administration of intracameral phenylephrine, insertion of iris hooks or expanders, and use of ophthalmic viscosurgical devices.

Medication allergies should be documented and patients questioned regarding sensitivity to sedatives, narcotics, anesthetics, iodine, and latex. Factors limiting the patient's ability to cooperate in the operating room or to lie comfortably on the operating room table (eg, deafness, claustrophobia, restless leg syndrome, head tremor, or musculoskeletal disorders) will influence the choice of topical, local, or general anesthesia.

Chadha V, Borooah S, Tey A, Styles C, Singh J. Floppy iris behaviour during cataract surgery: associations and variations. *Br J Ophthalmol.* 2007;91:40–42. Epub 2006 Aug 30.

Chang DF, Campbell JR. Intraoperative floppy iris syndrome associated with tamsulosin. *J Cataract Refract Surg.* 2005;31(4):664–673.

Parssinen O, Leppanen E, Keski-Rahkonen P, Mauriala T, Dugue B, Lehtonen M. Influence of tamsulosin on the iris and its implications for cataract surgery. *Invest Ophthalmol Vis Sci.* 2006;47:3766–3771.

Pertinent Ocular History

The ocular history will help the ophthalmologist identify conditions that could affect the surgical approach and the visual prognosis. Trauma, inflammation, amblyopia, glaucoma, optic nerve abnormalities, or retinal disease might affect the visual outcome after cataract removal. Active uveitis should be controlled as well as possible before cataract surgery so that the risk of complications from postoperative inflammation, such as macular edema and iris adhesion to the lens implant, can be minimized. Patients with Fuchs uveitis are an exception to this concern, although the risk of severe postoperative glaucoma must be considered. A family history of retinal detachment is a risk factor for postoperative retinal detachment. Previous vitrectomy for the treatment of retinal disease or vitreous hemorrhage may cause intraoperative chamber fluctuations that increase the risk of posterior capsule disruption and loss of nuclear fragments posteriorly. The surgeon should make an extra effort to preserve superior conjunctiva in glaucoma patients who may require future filtration surgery.

Past records document the patient's visual acuity prior to the development of cataract. If the patient has had cataract surgery in the fellow eye, it is important to obtain information about the operative and postoperative course. If problems such as elevated intraocular pressure, vitreous loss, cystoid macular edema, endophthalmitis, or hemorrhage occurred in the first operation, the surgical approach and postoperative follow-up could be modified for the second eye in order to reduce the risk of similar complications.

If the patient has had refractive surgery, it is necessary to determine what procedure was performed, what the original refraction and original keratometry were, whether any intraoperative complications occurred, and whether the postoperative refraction is stable. This information is useful in both predicting the lens implant power and determining the surgical approach. (Refer to Chapter 8 for a complete discussion of calculating IOL power after corneal refractive surgery.)

Social History

The decision to undertake cataract surgery is based not only on the patient's visual acuity but also on the ramifications of reduced vision on the individual's quality of life. The surgeon should be aware of the patient's occupation, lifestyle, and any possible chemical dependencies, including nicotine and illicit (recreational) drugs, as all of these may affect postoperative recovery.

Measurements of Visual Function

Visual Acuity Testing

It is useful to measure Snellen acuity under lighted and darkened examination conditions. While visual acuity testing in the ophthalmologist's office is commonly performed in a darkened room, diminished Snellen acuity from a symptomatic cataract may sometimes be demonstrated only in a lighted room. Distance and near visual acuity must be tested and a careful refraction performed so that best-corrected visual acuity can be determined. In some patients, pinhole visual acuity is better than acuity obtained with refractive correction. Visual acuity may improve after pupillary dilation, especially in patients with PSCs.

Refraction

Careful refraction must be performed on both eyes. This assessment is useful in planning the IOL power necessary to obtain the desired postoperative refraction. If the fellow eye has a clear lens and a high refractive error that requires spectacle correction, obtaining a similar refractive result in the surgical eye avoids problems with postoperative anisometropia. Alternatively, a contact lens may be worn in the phakic eye. If the fellow eye has a cataract or if the patient expresses a desire to see at a distance (or at near) without spectacle correction, it may be preferable to plan the implant power to achieve postoperative emmetropia (or myopia). With the advent of multifocal lenses, additional discussions concerning greater spectacle independence and the risks of and alternatives to these lenses may be needed. In any event, the surgeon should carefully counsel patients proceeding with cataract surgery about the potential changes they will experience in their postoperative requirements for glasses.

Brightness Acuity

When a patient complains of glare, it is important to test distance and near visual acuity in a well-lighted room. Testing can be done with a nonprojected eye chart in ambient light conditions or with a projected eye chart and an off-axis bright light directed at the patient. Various instruments are available to standardize and facilitate this measurement. Patients with significant cataracts commonly show a decrease of 3 or more lines under these conditions, compared with the results when visual acuity is tested in the dark.

Contrast Sensitivity

Various methods have been developed to test contrast sensitivity in the ophthalmologist's office. Patients with cataracts may experience diminished contrast sensitivity even when Snellen acuity is preserved. (See also BCSC Section 3, *Clinical Optics*.)

Visual Field Testing

Confrontation visual fields should be tested in all cataract patients. In patients with optically dense cataracts that block the ophthalmoscopic view of the retinal periphery, light projection is used to test the peripheral visual field. Visual field testing may help the ophthalmologist identify visual loss resulting from disease processes besides cataract. Patients with a history of glaucoma, optic nerve disease, or retinal abnormality may benefit from static or kinetic visual field evaluation to document the degree of visual field loss. Preoperative visual field loss does not preclude improvement in visual function following cataract surgery. Progressive cataracts may induce diffuse visual field depression that disappears after surgery.

External Examination

The preoperative evaluation of a patient with cataract should include the body habitus and any abnormalities of the external eye and ocular adnexa. Such conditions as extensive supraclavicular fat, kyphosis, ankylosing spondylitis, generalized obesity, or head tremor may impact surgical approach.

The presence of enophthalmos or prominent brow may affect the surgical approach and the chosen route of anesthesia. The effects that entropion, ectropion, or eyelid-closure abnormalities may have on the tear film and ocular surface should be considered prior to cataract surgery and the condition treated, if necessary. Blepharitis, as manifested by collarettes, marginal eyelid thickening, and inspissation of meibomian gland secretions, should be treated before cataract surgery. Acne rosacea should be brought under control. The tear film should be examined for abnormalities in the aqueous or lipid layers; and abnormal tear dynamics, exposure keratitis, or decreased corneal sensation should be addressed. Active nasolacrimal disease should be treated, particularly if there is a history of periodic inflammation, infection, or obstruction.

Motility

The clinician should evaluate ocular alignment and test the range of movement of the extraocular muscles. Cover testing should be performed to document any muscle deviation. Abnormal motility may suggest preexisting strabismus with amblyopia as a cause of visual loss. The patient must be made aware that a significant tropia from disruption of fusion might result in diplopia following surgery. The presence of amblyopia may also limit the amount of improvement that can be expected from surgery.

Pupils

Evaluation of the pupillary response to light and accommodation is important. In addition to checking direct and consensual constriction of the pupil to light, the ophthalmologist should perform a swinging flashlight test to detect a relative afferent pupillary defect that would indicate extensive retinal disease or optic nerve dysfunction. Although a patient with a relative afferent pupillary defect in the cataractous eye may still obtain improved vision following cataract surgery, the visual outcome may be limited by optic nerve dysfunction. Proper patient expectations must therefore be set when this finding is present.

Small-optic IOLs may be inappropriate for a patient who has a large pupil in moderate or dim illumination, as the edge of the optic may fall short of the pupil border, allowing light to pass around the optic edge, with resultant glare or dysphotopsias. It is helpful to assess pupillary size after dilation because small pupils (eg, in patients with diabetes, posterior synechiae, pseudoexfoliation syndrome, or a history of systemic α_{1a}-antagonist or long-term topical miotic use) may increase the surgical risk. To maximize safety in this situation, the surgeon should prepare with specialized surgical techniques and instruments.

Slit-Lamp Examination

Conjunctiva

The conjunctiva is examined for scarring and the presence of a filtering bleb. Symblepharon or shortening of the fornices could be associated with underlying systemic or ocular surface diseases. Vascularization or scarring from previous chemical injury or ocular surgery may indicate compromised healing and limit surgical exposure.

Cornea

To evaluate the health of the cornea before cataract surgery, the clinician should assess corneal thickness and look for the presence of cornea guttata. When possible, specular reflection with the slit lamp may provide an estimate of the endothelial cell count and morphology. Marked abnormalities of the endothelial layer or a corneal thickness greater than 640 μm with accompanying stromal edema suggests that retaining corneal clarity after cataract surgery may be difficult. Although such conditions are not contraindications to surgery, these potential problems and their sequelae should be discussed with the patient. The ophthalmologist should perform surgery so as to minimize trauma to the endothelium. Irregularity of Descemet's membrane associated with cornea guttata may limit visual acuity following surgery. In patients with long-term contact lens wear, a history of corneal dystrophy, chlamydial infection, arcus, superficial punctate keratitis, pannus, or stromal opacities may limit the surgical view into the anterior segment during cataract extraction.

The proliferation of refractive surgical procedures has important implications for lens implant calculations and postoperative refraction. For example, obtaining the patient's original keratometry readings (those done before refractive surgery) can aid the cataract surgeon with more precise implant calculations. In addition, corneal topography is useful for evaluating the contour of the cornea for irregular astigmatism and for achieving more accurate keratometry readings. Special techniques for IOL power calculation and selection must be made for the patient who has undergone refractive surgery (see Chapter 8 for further discussion). Also, weakened or thinned areas in the cornea should be identified so that they can be avoided during surgery.

Anterior Chamber

A shallow anterior chamber may indicate anatomically narrow angles, nanophthalmos, an intumescent lens, or forward displacement of the lens–iris diaphragm by posterior pathology (eg, a ciliary body tumor). Knowing the depth of the anterior chamber and the axial thickness of the lens aids in surgical planning (anterior limbal, corneal, or scleral tunnel).

Preoperative gonioscopy should rule out angle abnormalities, including the presence of peripheral anterior synechiae, neovascularization, or a prominent major arterial circle. Use of a 3-mirror lens helps in evaluating the lens zonules for traumatic or genetic dehiscence. Gonioscopy is essential if anterior chamber IOL implantation is anticipated. The ophthalmologist should note the presence of peripheral anterior synechiae or abnormal iris vessels in the event that an angle-supported implant is required.

Iris

The presence of iridodonesis or exfoliation at the margin of the undilated pupil indicates weakened zonular attachments to the lens, or absence of them, and alters surgical approach. As discussed in the preceding sections, the clinician should measure pupil size and note the presence of synechiae after dilation. If the pupil dilates poorly, radial iridotomy, sector iridectomy, posterior synechiolysis, sphincterotomy, or iris retraction may be necessary in order to provide adequate exposure of the lens during surgery.

Crystalline Lens

The appearance of the lens should be carefully noted both before and after dilation of the pupil. The impact of "oil droplet" nuclear cataracts and small PSCs is best correlated with visual symptoms before dilation of the pupil. After the pupil is dilated, nuclear density can be evaluated, exfoliation syndrome can be detected, and opacities and distortion of the retinoscopic reflex can be visualized more easily.

The clinician should evaluate the clarity of the media in the visual axis in order to assess the lenticular contribution to the visual deficit. A thin slit beam of white light is focused on the posterior capsule. The light is then changed to cobalt blue; if the posterior capsule is no longer illuminated (as a result of blue-light scatter), the contribution of the lens opacity to visual acuity is most often 20/50 or worse. Dense brunescent nuclear sclerotic cataracts may permit remarkably good visual acuity, especially at near, whereas vacuolar cataracts detected through the red reflex can cause surprisingly severe visual loss. When dense cortical opacification is present, the intraoperative use of capsular dye to enhance visualization of the capsulorrhexis should be considered.

The position of the lens and the integrity of the zonular fibers must also be evaluated. Decentration of the lens, phacodonesis, or excessive distance between the lens and the pupillary margin indicates zonular disruption from causes such as subluxation of the lens as a result of previous trauma, metabolic disorders, or hypermature cataract. An indentation or flattening of the lens periphery may indicate focal loss of zonular support. If there is zonular laxity, the surgeon should be prepared to alter surgical technique, including the use of capsular tension rings or conversion to ECCE.

Ozturk F, Osher RH. Capsular staining: recent developments. *Curr Opinion Ophthalmol.* 2006;17:42–44.

Pandey SK, Werner L, Escobar-Gomez M, Roig-Melo EA, Apple DJ. Dye-enhanced cataract surgery. Part 1: anterior capsule staining for capsulorrhexis in advanced/white cataract. *J Cataract Refract Surg.* 2000;26:1052–1059.

Limitations of Slit-Lamp Examination

Some visually significant cataracts may appear nearly normal upon slit-lamp biomicroscopy. Examination of the lens with the retinoscope, however, may reveal lens-related visual changes. By examining the retinoscopic reflex, the clinician may detect posterior subcapsular opacities, refractile nuclear changes, or even diffuse cataracts. Similarly, examination using the direct ophthalmoscope through a +10 D lens at a distance of 2 feet will enhance the portions of the cataractous lens that are producing optical aberrations. This technique is particularly useful in identifying "oil droplet" cataracts.

Fundus Evaluation

Ophthalmoscopy

The ophthalmologist must perform a full fundus examination by direct and indirect ophthalmoscopy to evaluate the macula, optic nerve, retinal vessels, and retinal periphery. Particular attention should be paid to early macular degeneration, which may limit visual rehabilitation after an otherwise uneventful cataract extraction. The indirect ophthalmoscope is not useful for judging the visual significance of cataract. Although the direct ophthalmoscope is more useful in judging media clarity, the examiner must keep in mind that it, too, provides light that is more intense than that available to the patient under ambient lighting conditions.

Patients with diabetes should be examined carefully for the presence of macular edema, retinal ischemia, and background and proliferative retinopathy. Retinal ischemia may progress to posterior or anterior neovascularization, especially if the surgeon uses an intracapsular technique or ruptures the posterior capsule during extracapsular surgery. Careful examination of the retinal periphery may reveal the presence of vitreoretinal traction or preexisting retinal holes that may warrant preoperative treatment. Intracapsular surgery and primary discission of the posterior capsule are associated with a significantly higher incidence of retinal detachment and cystoid macular edema postoperatively.

Optic Nerve

The optic nerve should be examined for cupping, along with pallor and other abnormalities. Visual acuity, measurement of intraocular pressure, and the results of confrontation visual field testing and the pupillary examination will help determine whether other adjunctive testing is warranted.

Fundus Evaluation With Opaque Media

If cataract density prevents direct visualization of the posterior segment of the eye, instruments other than direct and indirect ophthalmoscopes may be used to evaluate the retina. B-scan ultrasonography of the posterior segment of the eye is useful whenever it is impossible to visualize the retina because of a dense cataract. Ultrasonography can elucidate whether a retinal detachment, vitreous opacity, posterior pole tumor, or staphyloma is present. (See also BCSC Section 3, *Clinical Optics*.) Light projection, 2-point discrimination, gross color vision, Maddox rod projection, or the presence of entoptic phenomena may also be useful in detecting retinal pathology. Electroretinography and visual evoked response are warranted in specific circumstances (see the section Special Tests).

Special Tests

Potential Acuity Estimation

Potential acuity estimation can be helpful in assessing the lenticular contribution to visual loss. Laser interferometry and the potential acuity meter are two of several methods by which postoperative acuity can be estimated.

In *laser interferometry,* twin sources of monochromatic helium–neon laser light create a diffraction fringe pattern on the retinal surface. Transmission of this pattern is mostly independent of lens opacities. It is possible to estimate retinal visual acuity by varying the spacing of the pattern; however, the area of the pattern subtending the retina is considerably larger than the fovea. For this reason, small foveal lesions that limit visual acuity may not be detected. The *potential acuity meter* projects a numerical or Snellen vision chart through a small entrance pupil. The image can be projected into the eye around lenticular opacities.

Laser interferometry and potential acuity meter determinations can be useful in estimating visual acuity potential after cataract extraction. Both are much more predictive in eyes with moderate lens opacities than in those with severe lens opacities. However, these tests can be misleading in the presence of several disorders, including age-related macular degeneration, amblyopia, macular edema, glaucoma, small macular scars, and serous retinal detachment. An accurate clinical examination of the eye is as good a predictor of the visual outcome as laser interferometry or potential acuity testing.

McGwin G Jr, Scilley K, Brown J, Owsley C. Impact of cataract surgery on self-reported visual difficulties: comparison with a no-surgery reference group. *J Cataract Refract Surg.* 2003;29(5):941–948.

Superstein R, Boyaner D, Overbury O. Functional complaints, visual acuity, spatial contrast sensitivity, and glare disability in preoperative and postoperative cataract patients. *J Cataract Refract Surg.* 1999;25(4):575–581.

Tests of Macular Function

Because cataracts can obstruct the ophthalmoscopic view of the fundus, direct examination may be difficult. The following tests measure retinal function rather than retinal appearance.

Maddox rod

In patients with dense cataracts that preclude adequate visualization of the fundus preoperatively, Maddox rod testing aids in evaluating macular function. Any large scotoma, represented as a loss of the red line of the Maddox glass as viewed by the patient, should raise the possibility of significant macular disease. (See also BCSC Section 3, *Clinical Optics*, on cylindrical lenses.)

Photostress recovery time

The photostress recovery time can be used to estimate macular function. After a penlight is shined directly into a normal eye (the "photostress"), a recovery period is necessary before the patient can identify the Snellen letters 1 line larger than that individual's baseline visual acuity (the photostress recovery time). Normal photostress recovery time averages 27 seconds, with a standard deviation of 11 seconds. Photostress recovery time is 50 seconds or less in 99% of normal eyes. Prolonged photostress recovery time is an indication of macular disease.

Glaser JS, Savino PJ, Sumers KD, McDonald SA, Knighton RW. The photostress recovery test in the clinical assessment of visual function. *Am J Ophthalmol.* 1977;83:255–260.

Blue-light entoptoscopy

During a blue-light entoptoscopy examination, the patient is asked to view an intense, homogeneous blue-light background. Under these conditions, the white blood cells coursing through the perifoveal capillaries produce shadows. If the patient sees the shadows, macular function is probably intact. However, this test has limited utility because many patients find the instructions difficult to comprehend.

Loebl M, Riva CE. Macular circulation and the flying corpuscles phenomenon. *Ophthalmology.* 1978;85:911–917.

Sinclair SH, Loebl M, Riva CE. Blue field entoptic phenomenon in cataract patients. *Arch Ophthalmol.* 1979;97:1092–1095.

Purkinje's entoptic phenomenon

Like blue-light entoptoscopy, Purkinje's entoptic phenomenon test is also subjective. A rapidly oscillating point source of light is shined through the patient's closed eyelids. The patient's ability to detect shadow images of the retinal vasculature provides a very rough indication that the retina is attached.

Electroretinography and visual evoked response

In rare cases where other testing is inconclusive, electroretinography (ERG) or visual evoked response (VER) testing can be done to evaluate retinal and/or optic nerve function. These tests are discussed fully in BCSC Section 12, *Retina and Vitreous.*

Preoperative Measurements

Several measurements, discussed in the following sections, should be taken preoperatively, especially if implantation of an IOL is planned.

Biometry

Accurate measurement of ocular axial length using A-scan ultrasonography or optical coherence biometry is required to calculate the appropriate IOL power. In addition, corneal power must be determined by manual keratometry or corneal topography. (IOL power determination is discussed in greater detail in Chapter 8.)

Corneal Topography

In contrast to manual keratometry, corneal topography provides a map of corneal contour. Using a method similar to that of the Placido disk, it provides additional information about the corneal surface as well as corneal power. Corneal topography is particularly helpful if the patient has irregular astigmatism or early keratoconus or has previously undergone keratorefractive surgery; if a toric IOL may be implanted; or if the surgeon plans to perform limbal relaxing incisions at the same time as cataract extraction. (Refer to Chapter 8 for a discussion on estimating central keratometry after refractive surgery.)

Corneal Pachymetry

Corneal pachymetry, a method to measure corneal thickness, is useful for assessing indirectly the function of the endothelium. Ultrasonic pachymeters are usually more reliable than optical pachymeters. In general, central corneal thickness greater than 640 μm in patients with endothelial dysfunction is associated with an increased risk of postoperative corneal decompensation.

Specular Microscopy

Specular microscopy is used to determine the number of cells per square millimeter of corneal endothelium. Because cataract surgery causes some loss of endothelial cells, the risk of postoperative corneal decompensation is increased if preoperative endothelial cell counts are low.

Abnormal endothelial cell morphology, including enlargement (polymegethism) and irregularity (pleomorphism), may limit the cornea's ability to withstand stress. (See BCSC Section 8, *External Disease and Cornea*.)

Patient Preparation and Informed Consent

In planning cataract surgery, the surgeon should evaluate the patient's ability to comply with prescribed postoperative care. The surgeon must inform the patient (and caregivers, if present) of the importance of using eyedrops, maintaining proper ocular hygiene, and keeping required appointments postoperatively. It is helpful to include a family member or friend in preoperative discussions to reinforce the patient's memory. The patient should understand activity restrictions during the immediate postoperative period, although the advent of small-incision surgery has significantly minimized postoperative limitations on activity. The surgeon should assess the patient's ability to function with only the fellow eye in the event that visual rehabilitation of the surgical eye is prolonged.

Before deciding to proceed with cataract surgery, the patient should have a clear understanding of the indications for and alternatives to surgery, as well as the likelihood of significant visual improvement. The patient should also have a clear understanding of the risks and benefits of cataract surgery. In addition, the surgeon and patient should discuss

- the role of preexisting ocular and medical disorders on visual outcome
- the desired postoperative refractive status and the limitations of pseudophakic correction
- the risk of serious, sight-threatening complications
- the risk of common intraoperative and postoperative complications
- the anticipated time course for activity limitations and reasonable expectations for the patient's return to regular daily activities
- the frequency and duration of postoperative eye medications
- the proposed date for providing the final optical correction

If patients and their caregivers are adequately prepared before surgery, they can anticipate a routine postoperative course and understand problems that may develop. Written or audiovisual materials may be useful adjunctive sources of information.

Cataract in the Adult Eye. Preferred Practice Pattern. San Francisco: American Academy of Ophthalmology; 2001.

CHAPTER 8

Surgery for Cataract

In this chapter, we will briefly review the past, examine the present, and look forward to the future of cataract surgery.

The Remote Past

Ancient and Medieval Techniques

The first documented treatment of cataract is couching (from the French verb *coucher,* "to put to bed"), which has a colorful history, starting from about the fifth century BC, and which physicians in parts of the developing world continue to use today (Fig 8-1). Couching was practiced in India, and its usage spread throughout the Roman Empire, medieval Europe, and sub-Saharan Africa. The procedure was an outgrowth of the limited understanding of ocular anatomy. The "crytalloides" (or lens) was thought to rest in the middle of the eye, in front of which was a clear space. An abnormal "humor" developed and flowed in front of the lens (the word *cataract* also means "waterfall"). The couching procedure sought to displace the abnormal material from its position in front of the "crystalloides."

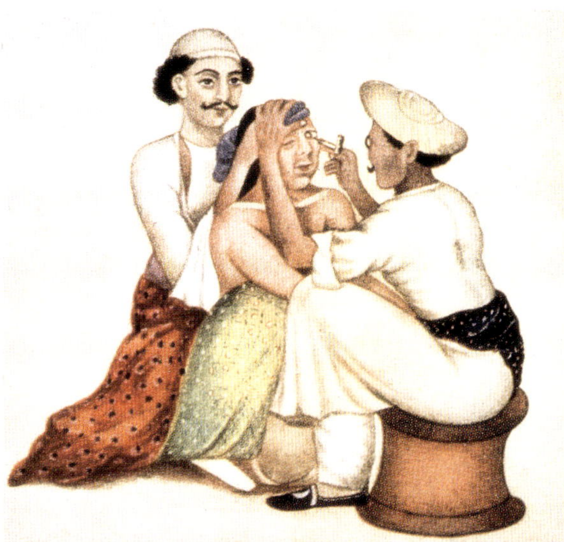

Figure 8-1 Couching. *(Reproduced from Duke-Elder S.* Diseases of the Lens and Vitreous; Glaucoma and Hypotony. *St Louis: Mosby; 1969.)*

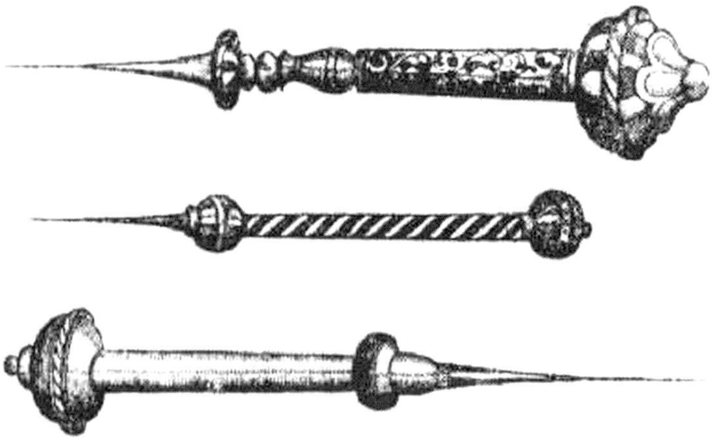

Figure 8-2 Couching needles. *(Courtesy of the Royal College of Ophthalmologists.)*

Couching was performed most commonly on patients with mature cataracts. The patient was seated and positioned so that sunlight would stream over the surgeon's shoulder, illuminating the patient's head. Techniques involved the use of 1 or 2 instruments. Basically, an incision was made somewhere posterior to the corneoscleral junction. A knife or needle (Fig 8-2) was used for the entry, and a needle or rod was used to push the cataractous lens inferiorly. An assistant to the physician restrained the patient. The speed of dislocation was related to both the skill of the surgeon and the status of the zonule. "Patching" with soft wool soaked variably in egg white, breast milk, or clarified butter was applied postoperatively.

How miraculous it must have seemed, particularly to the patient, who began the day as a blind person needing to be led to the procedure area, and who, by procedure's end, was able to see enough to walk in familiar surroundings. Not only was the patient rehabilitated, but the burden on the patient's family was reduced significantly. This immediate outcome was responsible for the procedure's popularity. The lack of sterilization and the inflammation that would occur from the retained lens with its disrupted capsule resulted in complications that developed after the surgeon had gone on to another town.

A variant technique, described by the Iraqi ocularist Ammar (AD 996–1020), involved suction aspiration of the cataract through a hollow needle. Syrians in the 12th and 13th centuries also tried this method but abandoned it because of lack of efficacy.

Corser N. Couching for cataract: its rise and fall. In: *Proceedings from the Ninth Annual History of Medicine Days.* Calgary: University of Calgary; 2000:35–41.

Sood NN, Ratnaraj A. Couching for cataract: hazards and management. *Am J Ophthalmol.* 1968;66(4):687–693.

Early Extracapsular Cataract Extraction

By 1600, anatomists had correctly identified the true position of the lens, and opacification of the lens had become the new definition of *cataract.* This simple statement belies the controversies these new understandings generated between anatomists and surgeons; however, the more "modern" view required a more "modern" therapeutic response.

Jacques Daviel (1696–1762) is justifiably credited with propelling cataract surgery toward the modern era. He restricted his practice to ophthalmology, and his decision to remove rather than displace the cataract was followed by the development of instruments to allow this revolutionary procedure. In Daviel's method of cataract extraction, an incision was made through the inferior cornea and enlarged with scissors. The cornea was elevated, the lens capsule incised, the nucleus expressed, and the cortex removed by curettage (Fig 8-3). Each operation took a few minutes and was performed without either anesthesia or aseptic technique. Presciently, Daviel's writings mention removal of the anterior lens capsule after creation of a circular opening.

Daviel's extracapsular cataract extraction (ECCE) was an innovation and an improvement over couching, but the technique, burdened by its moment in time, raised the following issues: wound healing; uveal, vitreous, or retinal prolapse; lens remnant–induced inflammation; and infection. Secondary procedures were common, particularly opening pupillary membranes that resulted from capsular opacification (discission). In fact, all the complications of cataract surgery that occur in small numbers in the modern era (as discussed in Chapter 9, Complications of Cataract Surgery) occurred at greater frequencies so that Daviel described a 50% success rate with his method.

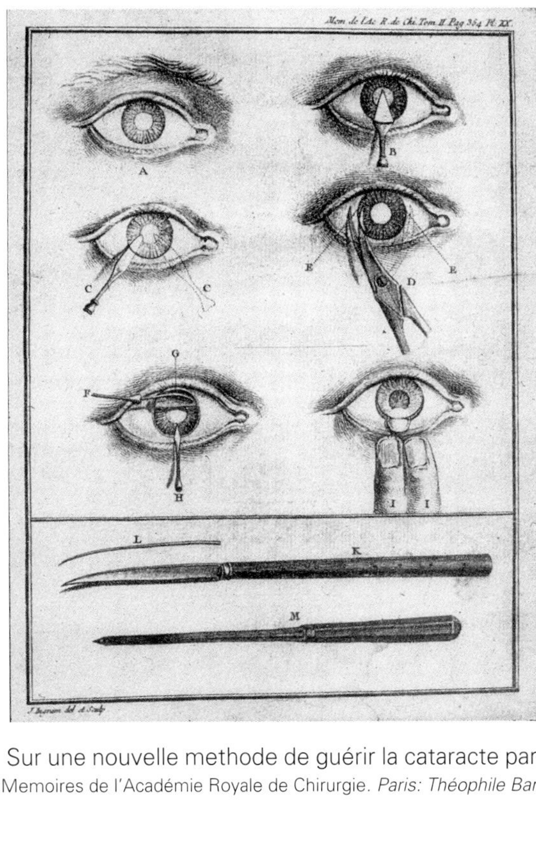

Figure 8-3 Daviel J. Sur une nouvelle methode de guérir la cataracte par l'extraction du cristalin. *(From Louis M, et al.* Memoires de l'Académie Royale de Chirurgie. *Paris: Théophile Barrois Lejeuene; 1787.)*

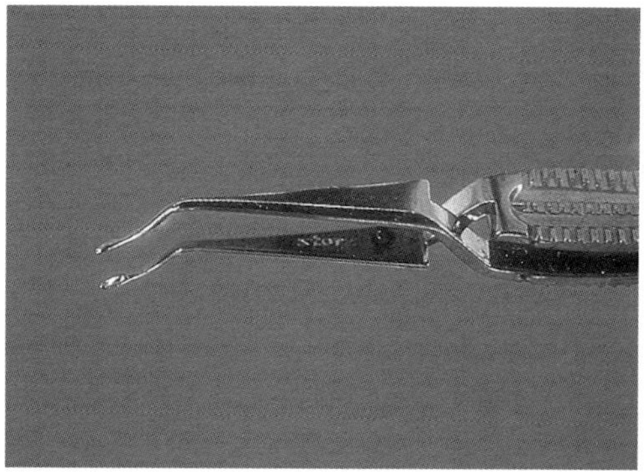

Figure 8-4 Kalt forceps.

Regardless, extracapsular surgery became the new "standard of care," and technological developments improved surgical outcomes. Albrecht von Graefe (1828–1870) improved upon extracapsular technique by developing a knife that created a better-apposed incision. This innovation decreased the rate of infection and uveal prolapse. Problems related to retention of lens material and posterior capsule persisted.

What if the lens could be removed in its entirety?

Rucker CW. Cataract: a historical perspective. *Invest Ophthalmol.* 1965;4:377–383.

Early Intracapsular Cataract Extraction

Samuel Sharp first performed a successful intracapsular cataract extraction (ICCE) in 1753, by removing a cataractous lens, capsule intact, through a limbal incision using pressure from his thumb. Intracapsular cataract extraction had arrived.

One of the chief problems to be solved in the development of ICCE was how to lyse or break the zonular fibers. Lieutenant Colonel Henry Smith, an Englishman stationed in India, used external manipulation with a muscle hook to break the inferior attachments mechanically and expel (express) the cataractous lens from the eye through a limbal incision. The lens would "tumble": the inferior pole of the lens would exit the eye before the superior pole. (Compare this intracapsular maneuver with the modern "phaco-flip" technique, described later in this chapter.) His technique, called the *Smith-Indian operation,* was used in 50,000 cases over a 25-year period at the end of the 19th and beginning of the 20th century.

Another method of lens removal was direct extraction. Toothless forceps, developed by ophthalmologists such as Verhoeff and Kalt, were used to grasp the lens capsule (Fig 8-4). The cataract was then gently pulled from the eye with a side-to-side motion that broke the zonular insertion. Suction cup–like devices called *erysiphakes* were devised by Stoewer and by Ignacio Barraquer (1884–1965) to remove the lens with traction or tumbling (Fig 8-5).

The Recent Past

Modern Advances in Intracapsular Surgery

In relatively short order, fine suture material, the binocular operating microscope, and modern sterilization techniques increased surgical success and reduced the number and

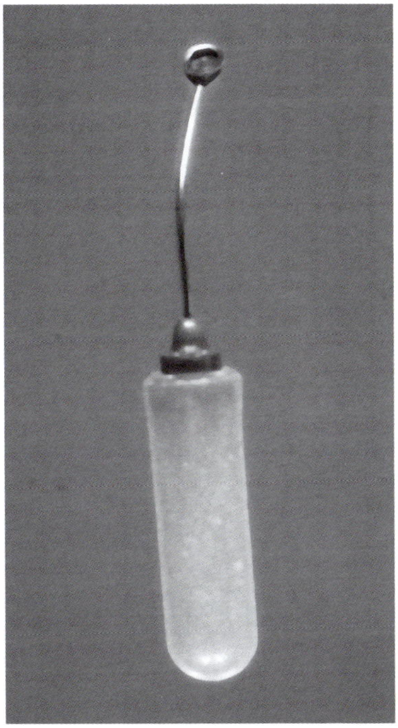

Figure 8-5 Barraquer erysiphake.

severity of complications. Chemical dissolution of the zonular fibers with the enzyme α-chymotrypsin was first reported by Joaquin Barraquer in 1957. The traditional capsule forceps and erysiphake had given way to the cryoprobe for lens extraction. The cryoprobe is a hollow metal-tipped probe that is cooled by compressed nitrous oxide and then applied to the lens surface. As the temperature of the metal drops below freezing, an iceball forms, and the lens adheres to the probe (Fig 8-6). Gentle to-and-fro maneuvers during delivery of the lens help strip anterior vitreous membrane attachments from the lens, break remaining zonular adhesions, and reduce vitreous loss.

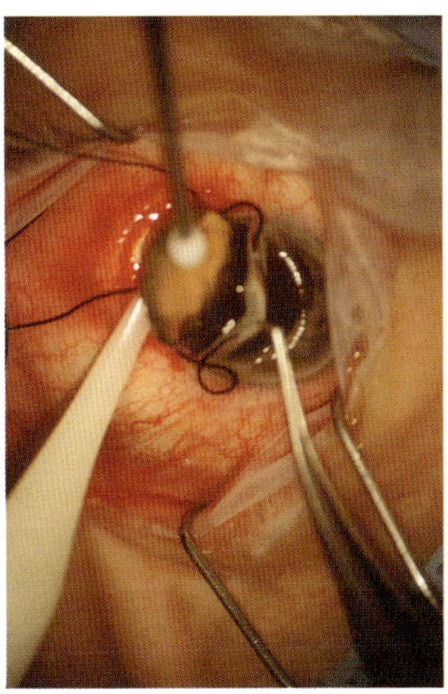

Figure 8-6 Cryoextraction of cataract (ICCE). Lens lifted out of the eye. *(Courtesy of Lisa F. Rosenberg, MD.)*

ICCE evolved into a very successful operation. Modern ICCE still plays a role in less-advantaged parts of the world because of the following:

- Less-sophisticated instrumentation is required (operating loupes instead of operating microscopes; nonautomated extraction devices such as cryoprobes, capsular forceps, or erysiphakes), allowing ICCE to be performed in a wide range of conditions.
- Visual rehabilitation, with the use of temporary aphakic spectacles, is usually possible soon after surgery.

Even in the best of surgical facilities, modern ICCE may be advantageous in patients with subluxed or dense brunescent lenses or in those with pseudoexfoliation.

Absolute contraindications include cataracts in children and young adults and cases of traumatic capsule rupture. Relative contraindications include high myopia, Marfan syndrome, morgagnian cataracts, and vitreous presenting in the anterior chamber. A general description of modern ICCE is in the Appendix at the end of this chapter.

Problems after ICCE are related to the following:

- *Size of the incision.* Consequences include delayed healing, greater induced astigmatism, delayed dispensing of refractive correction. Problems include wound leaks, suture irritation, suture abscess, filtering blebs, and iris or vitreous incarceration as a result of elevated internal pressure on the incision.
- *Bending of the cornea or inadvertent corneal touch with the cryoprobe or cataractous lens during extraction.* Endothelial cell loss and corneal edema can occur as a result.
- *Loss of a barrier between the anterior and posterior segments.* Forward movement of the vitreous plays a role in the development of postoperative cystoid macular edema (CME) and rhegmatogenous retinal detachment, both of which are more common after ICCE than after ECCE or phacoemulsification.
- *Limitations of IOL choice and position.* An anterior chamber lens can be used. There is no capsular bag or capsule remnant to secure a posterior chamber lens. A posterior chamber lens would have to be either sutured to the iris or secured transsclerally.

Because of these drawbacks, ECCE again became the preferred technique.

Blodi FC. Cataract surgery. In: Albert DM, Edwards DD, eds. *The History of Ophthalmology.* Cambridge, MA: Blackwell Scientific; 1996:165–177.

Gorin G. *History of Ophthalmology.* New York: Raven Press; 1982.

The Renaissance of Extracapsular Extraction

The shift from ICCE procedures to new methods of ECCE technique was driven by developments that decreased the rate of potentially blinding complications. One such development was leaving the posterior lens capsule intact, which enabled anterior and posterior compartments of the eye to maintain their separation, thus eliminating forward movement of the vitreous. The risk of potentially blinding complications such as aphakic retinal detachment, CME, and decompensation of the cornea was reduced.

To avoid the complications previously seen with ECCE, modern extracapsular surgery required complete removal of cortical lens material left after the nucleus was removed. Technology once again responded with the introduction of irrigation and aspiration of cortical material, first with manual systems and then with systems that provided variable suction and gravity flow of fluid to keep the anterior chamber formed. Increased knowledge of aqueous humor composition and corneal endothelial metabolism led to the development of balanced salt solution (BSS) and to this solution's importance as a tool for the extracapsular surgeon. Ophthalmic viscosurgical devices, a most important advance for the surgeon using phacoemulsification, aided the extracapsular surgeon as well.

The Modern ECCE Procedure

The "rediscovery" of ECCE by nucleus expression was a major leap forward in modern cataract surgery. Selection of this technique depends on the instrumentation available, the surgeon's level of experience, the size of the pupil, and the status of the zonule.

ECCE involves removal of the lens nucleus and cortex through an opening in the anterior capsule, with the capsular bag left in place. This technique has a number of advantages over ICCE. Because it is performed through a somewhat smaller incision, it results in

- less trauma to the corneal endothelium
- less induced astigmatism
- a more stable and secure incision

In addition, the posterior capsule remains intact, which

- reduces the risk of intraoperative vitreous loss
- allows better anatomical position for IOL fixation
- reduces the incidence of CME, retinal detachment, and corneal edema
- provides a barrier restricting the exchange of some molecules between aqueous and vitreous
- reduces bacterial access to the vitreous cavity
- eliminates the short-term and long-term complications associated with vitreous adherence to the iris, cornea, and incision

Primary (concomitant) or secondary (subsequent) IOL implantation, filtration surgery, corneal transplantation, and wound repair are all technically easier and safer when an intact posterior capsule is present.

Equipment

A wide range of instruments is available for each step of modern ECCE, from opening the capsule to dissecting and extracting the lens nucleus, removing the lens cortex, and polishing the lens capsule. The *cystitome* is an instrument used for anterior capsulotomy (the opening of the anterior capsule of the lens). Cystitomes can be fashioned from 23–27-gauge needles: the needle is bent at its hub and at the place where the beveled tip begins. Prefabricated cystitomes are also commercially available.

Blunt *cannulas* are used to irrigate and aspirate fluid, as well as to aspirate cortical lens material during surgery; they are available in various sizes and configurations. Cannulas

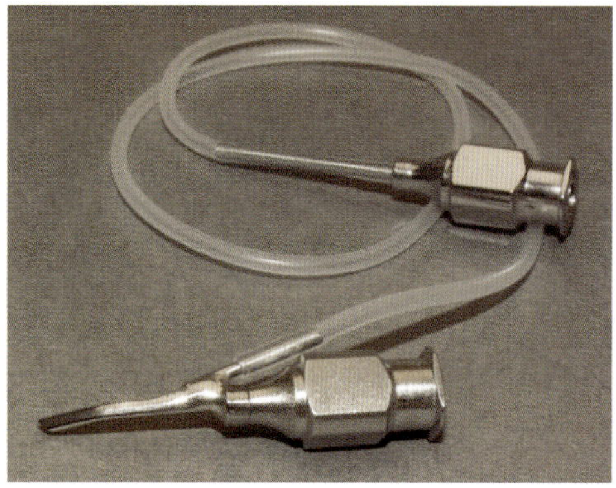

Figure 8-7 Simcoe irrigating/aspirating cannula. *(Photo by Carol Everhart Roper. Courtesy of Accutome, Inc.)*

have an opening at the side or end of the tip to direct fluid flow. The gauge of the opening is determined by the intended function of the instrument. Smaller ports develop high suction and adhesion and are better for grasping and withdrawing material, whereas larger ports allow irrigation and aspiration of thicker substances such as ophthalmic viscosurgical devices and lens cortex. A coaxial, double-lumen cannula is commonly used for extracapsular surgery: one lumen irrigates BSS into the chamber while the second lumen aspirates lens material from the chamber (Fig 8-7). Irrigation is gravity fed from a solution bottle; fluid flow is regulated with adjustment of the bottle height and the flow restrictor slide. The infusion may be constant, or the surgeon can employ a foot switch connected to a pinch valve. Aspiration may simply involve a syringe connected to the cannula, or it may be part of a pump system controlled by a foot pedal. Such automated systems are discussed further in the section on phacoemulsification later in this chapter.

A general description of the modern extracapsular cataract surgical procedure is in the Appendix at the end of this chapter.

Ophthalmic Viscosurgical Devices

Ophthalmic viscosurgical devices (OVDs) are also referred to as *viscoelastic agents*. Their introduction has had a profound influence on the evolution of extracapsular and phacoemulsification surgery, and their use has decreased the incidence of corneal edema as a complication of phaco surgery.

OVDs contain one or more of the following substances in varying concentrations: sodium hyaluronate, chondroitin sulfate, or hydroxypropyl methylcellulose.

Sodium hyaluronate is a biopolymer that occurs in many connective tissues throughout the body. It has a high molecular weight (2.5–4 million daltons) and low protein content and carries a single negative charge for the disaccharide unit. Hyaluronate has a half-life of approximately 1 day in aqueous and 3 days in vitreous.

Chondroitin sulfate is a viscoelastic biopolymer similar to hyaluronate but possessing a sulfated group with a double-negative charge. Chondroitin sulfate is commonly obtained from shark cartilage.

Hydroxypropyl methylcellulose (HPMC) does not occur naturally in animal tissues, but cellulose is widely distributed in plant fibers such as cotton and wood. The structure of the commercial product is a cellulose polymer modified by the addition of hydroxypropyl and methyl groups to increase the hydrophilic property of the material. Methylcellulose is a nonphysiologic compound that does not appear to be metabolized intraocularly. It is eventually eliminated in the aqueous but can easily be irrigated from the eye.

Physical Properties

The physical properties of OVDs are the result of chain length and molecular interactions both within chains and between chains and ocular tissue.

Viscosity describes a resistance to flow or shear force. The higher the molecular weight, the more the compound resists flow. A compound with high viscosity holds its shape better than does a compound with low viscosity. The viscosity of an OVD at rest is a function of concentration, molecular weight, and the size of the flexible molecules in the material.

Viscoelasticity means that the substance reacts as an elastic compound or gel when energy is transmitted at a high frequency. At low-frequency energy, the substance reacts primarily as a viscous compound. OVD can be slowly introduced into the eye with a 23-gauge cannula and yet can maintain the intraocular space even if the incision is open while manipulations occur in the anterior chamber. The degree of elasticity increases with increasing molecular weight and chain length.

Pseudoplasticity is the ability of an OVD to transform from a gel to a liquidlike substance when under pressure. In clinical terms, at 0 shear force, an OVD is a lubricant and coats tissues well, but under the influence of stress, it functions like a liquid.

Surface tension relates to the coating ability of an OVD. Lower surface tension provides better coating and a low contact angle.

Cohesive and *dispersive* describe the general behaviors of any OVD. Cohesive OVDs adhere to themselves and are generally high-molecular-weight agents with high surface tensions and high pseudoplasticity. Dispersive agents, conversely, are substances with little tendency for self-adherence, with generally low molecular weights and good coating abilities (low surface tension). Practically speaking, cohesive agents tend to be easily aspirated and are rapidly removed from the eye, whereas dispersive agents are removed less rapidly. Examples of cohesive agents include Healon, Healon GV (Advanced Medical Optics [AMO], Santa Ana, CA); Amvisc, Amvisc Plus, OcuCoat (Bausch & Lomb, Rochester, NY); and Provisc (Alcon, Ft Worth, TX). Examples of dispersive agents are Viscoat (Alcon) and Vitrax (AMO).

Healon 5 (AMO) consists of sodium hyaluronate 2.3% and has higher viscosity than Healon or Healon GV. Surgeons have found Healon 5 useful in challenging cases, including for deepening shallow chambers; for viscomydriasis of small pupils; and for stabilization of the anterior chamber in patients with the intraoperative floppy iris syndrome. With lower flow settings, Healon 5 resists aspiration and maintains anterior chamber depth. With higher flow settings, Healon 5 breaks up and resembles a dispersive OVD. The removal of Healon 5 requires more time and attention to avoid postoperative IOP elevations.

Characteristics of OVDs

The *space maintenance ability* of OVDs keeps the anterior chamber formed despite the presence of one or more incisions. With expansion of the chamber, manipulations can be made away from the corneal endothelium and posterior lens capsule. A cohesive OVD can be used to enlarge a marginally dilated pupil (viscomydriasis). It can also be used to keep the plane of the anterior capsule flat to assist a controlled continuous curvilinear capsulorrhexis (discussed later in this chapter). Lens implantation is less traumatic to the zonules and the posterior capsule when the capsular bag is inflated with an OVD. In the presence of an open posterior lens capsule, a dispersive OVD can be injected over the tear to keep the vitreous from moving anteriorly. Injection of an OVD through the pars plana can elevate lens fragments that have fallen into the anterior vitreous through a posterior capsule tear; these fragments can then be emulsified or removed manually.

Because of its dispersive nature, the OVD can be used for coating the endothelium in cases that require more time, phaco power, or both. Care must be taken to completely remove intraocular OVD to reduce the risk of an ocular hypertensive period related to angle outflow obstruction.

The *optical clarity* of an OVD has allowed surgeons to use a layer of OVD on the surface of the cornea. When slightly moistened with BSS, the agent coats the epithelium. This maneuver prevents drying and eliminates the need to irrigate the corneal surface. It also provides a slightly magnified view of anterior segment structures.

Buratto L, Giardini P, Bellucci R. *Viscoelastics in Ophthalmic Surgery*. Thorofare, NJ: Slack, Inc; 2005:5.

Lane SS, Lindstrom RL. Viscoelastic agents: formulation, clinical applications, and complications. In: Steinert RF, ed. *Cataract Surgery: Technique, Complications, and Management.* Philadelphia: Saunders; 1995:37–45.

Oshika T, Eguchi S, Oki K, et al. Clinical comparison of Healon5 and Healon in phacoemulsification and intraocular lens implantation: randomized multicenter study. *J Cataract Refract Surg*. 2004;30(2):357–362.

Anesthesia for Cataract Surgery

Historically, cataract surgery was performed without anesthesia. Karl Koller used topical cocaine anesthesia of the limbus in the late 1800s. Retrobulbar anesthesia was first described in 1884 by Herman Knapp, who injected 4% cocaine for ocular anesthesia prior to enucleation surgery. The modern technique of retrobulbar anesthesia, described in 1945 by Walter Atkinson, allowed the evolutionary advances of peribulbar and sub-Tenon anesthesia.

Retrobulbar anesthesia (Figs 8-8, 8-9), used with or without regional anesthesia of cranial nerve VII (facial nerve), provides excellent ocular akinesia and anesthesia. Complications of retrobulbar anesthesia are uncommon but include retrobulbar hemorrhage; globe penetration; optic nerve trauma; inadvertent intravenous injection associated with cardiac arrhythmias; and inadvertent intradural injection with associated seizures, respiratory arrest, and brain stem anesthesia (these complications are discussed more fully in BCSC Section 1, *Update on General Medicine*). A surgeon should know how to perform a *lateral cantholysis* to release a tense retrobulbar hemorrhage.

In *peribulbar anesthesia,* a shorter (1″) 25- or 27-gauge needle is used to introduce anesthetic solution external to the muscle cone, underneath Tenon's capsule, via single or

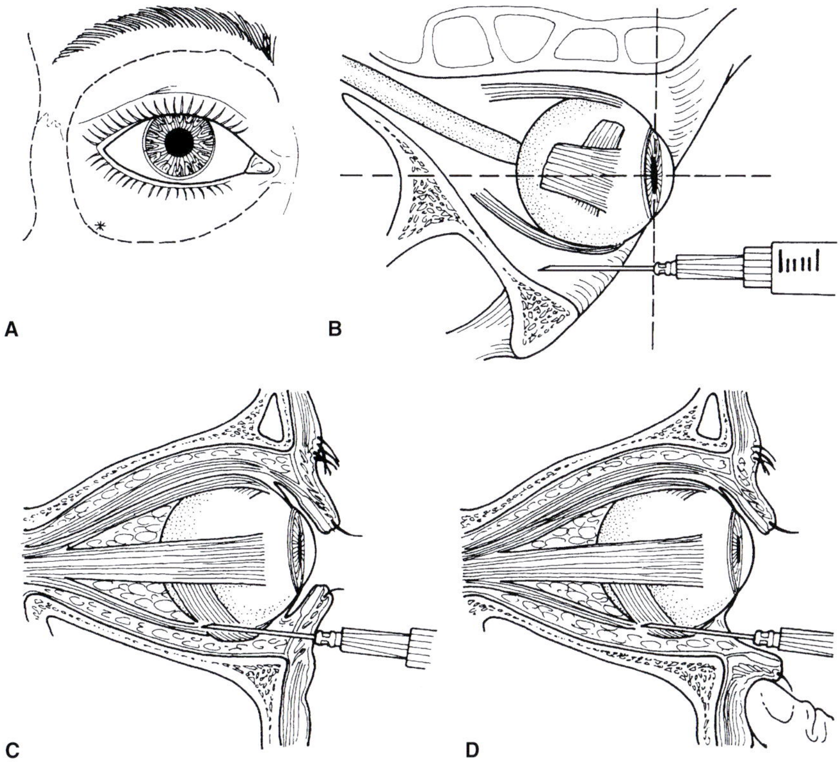

Figure 8-8 Peribulbar anesthesia. **A,** A 27-gauge 20- to 25-mm sharp disposable needle enters the orbit at the lower temporal orbital rim *(asterisk),* slightly up from the orbital floor and very close to the bone. **B,** The needle passes backward in a sagittal plane and parallel to the orbit floor **(C** and **D),** passing the globe equator to a depth controlled by observing the needle/hub junction reaching the plane of the iris **(B).** The technique is equally applicable to the transcutaneous **(C)** or transconjunctival **(D)** route. *(Reproduced with permission from Jaffe NS, Jaffe MS, Jaffe GF.* Cataract Surgery and Its Complications. *6th ed. St Louis: Mosby; 1997.)*

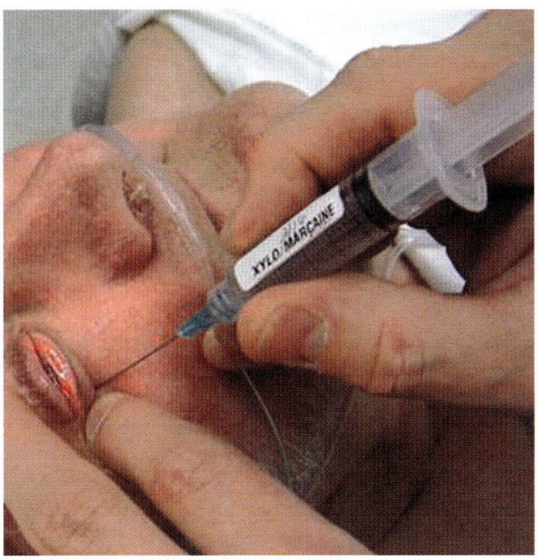

Figure 8-9 Retrobulbar injection. *(Courtesy of Ken Mitchell, MD.)*

multiple injection sites. Theoretically, peribulbar anesthesia eliminates the risk of complications such as optic nerve injury and central nervous system spread of anesthesia from intradural injection (Fig 8-10; also see Fig 8-8B). However, the risk of globe penetration is not eliminated, and the peribulbar method is slightly less effective than the retrobulbar for providing akinesia and anesthesia. In addition, the onset of effect is slower.

Topical anesthesia has evolved as a natural extension of phacoemulsification with foldable IOLs. Advantages of topical anesthesia include no risk of ocular perforation, extraocular muscle injury, or central nervous system depression. Vision returns almost immediately, and patients are able to leave the operating room without being patched because no eyelid block is used.

Topical anesthesia is administered as topical proparacaine or tetracaine drops, cellulose pledgets, or lidocaine jelly. Topical anesthetic agents are used with or without intravenous sedation. Topical anesthesia may be supplemented with the *intracameral* use of preservative-free lidocaine. Only nonpreserved lidocaine, generally 1%–2%, should be used for anterior chamber instillation, as some preservative agents can be toxic to intraocular structures. Transient amaurosis due to a direct retinal effect has been reported following the use of intracameral anesthetics, more commonly in patients with open posterior capsules or previous vitrectomy. Topical anesthesia should be reserved for the cooperative cataract patient who, with a dilated pupil, can tolerate the microscope light.

The type of anesthesia appropriate for the individual patient should be considered carefully. A general discussion of the advantages and risks of the different types of anesthesia should accompany the informed consent process. A discussion of what the patient will experience in the operating room will increase the likelihood of achieving a more relaxed patient on the day of surgery.

Subconjunctival lidocaine (Xylocaine) can be used to augment topical anesthesia in patients who experience sensation after administration of topical tetracaine or intracameral lidocaine. A 30-gauge needle is used to inject the lidocaine posterior to the phaco incision.

Sub-Tenon (Fig 8-11) infusion of lidocaine (Xylocaine) can be used to provide anesthesia and moderate akinesia during surgery. Lidocaine is administered through a cannula or catheter placed into a small posterior incision, under conjunctiva and Tenon's capsule.

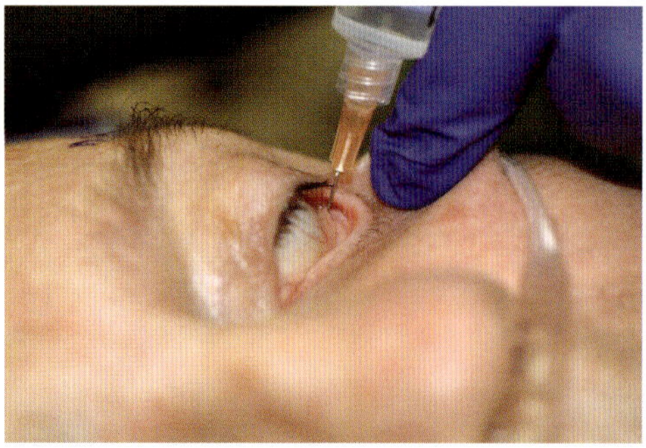

Figure 8-10 Peribulbar injection via conjunctiva. *(Courtesy of Ken Mitchell, MD, and Dan Skufca, MD.)*

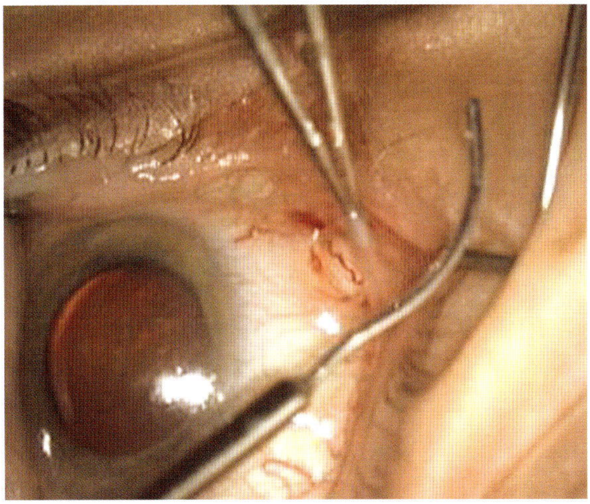

Figure 8-11 Sub-Tenon injection. *(Courtesy of University of Iowa, Dept. of Ophthalmology.)*

A *facial nerve block* (Fig 8-12), common in the era of large-incision ICCE/ECCE, is not generally needed with small-incision surgery. However, patients with essential or reactive blepharospasm may require a facial block to avoid complications during surgery.

General anesthesia, with clearance from the patient's primary care physician or an anesthesiologist, is appropriate to consider for pediatric patients and for patients who

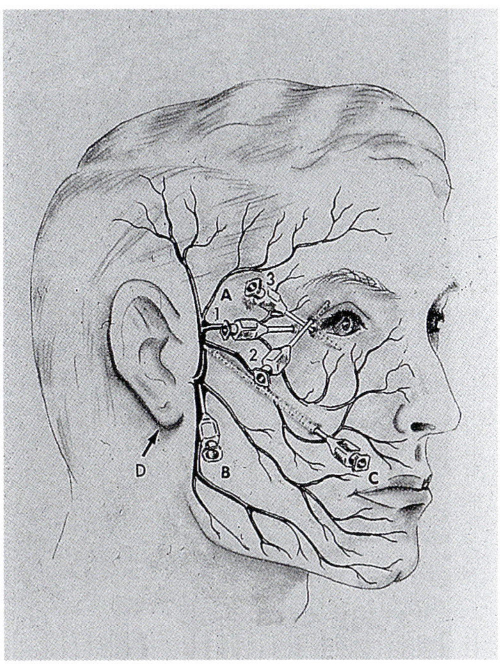

Figure 8-12 Akinesia of orbicularis oculi. *A,* Van Lint akinesia. *B,* O'Brien akinesia. *C,* Atkinson akinesia. *D,* Nadbath-Ellis akinesia. *(Reproduced with permission from Jaffe NS, Jaffe MS, Jaffe GF.* Cataract Surgery and Its Complications. *5th ed. St Louis: Mosby; 1990.)*

have any condition that would prevent their cooperation during surgery, including head tremor, deafness, neck or back problems, restless legs syndrome, or claustrophobia.

Boulton JE, Lopatatzidis A, Luck J, Baer RM. A randomized controlled trial of intracameral lidocaine during phacoemulsification under topical anesthesia. *Ophthalmology.* 2000;107:68–71.

Pang MP, Fujimoto DK, Wilkens LR. Pain, photophobia, and retinal and optic nerve function after phacoemulsification with intracameral lidocaine. *Ophthalmology.* 2001;108: 2018–2025.

Phacoemulsification

Originally, all extracapsular techniques involved nuclear expression, but in 1967 Charles Kelman, MD, developed phacoemulsification (phaco), which differed from conventional ECCE with nuclear expression by the size of the incision and the method of nucleus removal. Initially, Kelman met with considerable resistance from his colleagues.

Phacoemulsification uses an ultrasonically driven tip to fragment the nucleus of the cataract and to emulsify these fragments. The technique also uses a surgeon-controlled automated aspiration system to remove the cortical material through a small needle introduced through a very small incision. Phacoemulsification results in a lower incidence of wound-related complications, faster healing, and more rapid visual rehabilitation than procedures that require larger incisions. This technique also creates a relatively closed system during both phacoemulsification and aspiration, thereby controlling anterior chamber depth and providing safeguards against positive vitreous pressure and choroidal hemorrhage.

One problem for the early phaco surgeon was related to the proximity of the phaco needle to the corneal endothelium. The development of OVDs resolved this problem. Injection of these devices allowed space to be maintained between the phaco tip and the endothelium. The risk of corneal edema rapidly decreased with the usage of OVDs.

Another stumbling block was that after the nucleus was emulsified and the cortical material was aspirated, the incision had to be opened to accommodate the early polymethylmethacrylate anterior chamber and posterior chamber lenses, which were rigid and which required an opening slightly larger than the optic. In the 1980s, Thomas Mazzocco, MD, developed and implanted the first foldable IOL made of silicone; other designs followed, with IOLs in both silicone and acrylic. The development of foldable IOLs that could be inserted through 2.75–4.0-mm incisions enabled the phaco surgeon to keep the incision small. Many more surgeons transitioned to phacoemulsification and small-incision surgery, and phacoemulsification of cataract with insertion of a foldable IOL became the most common and the preferred type of cataract surgery in the developed world.

Ultrasonics Terminology

The following are terms commonly used in phaco surgery:

Cavitation The formation of gas bubbles arising from the solution in response to pressure changes at the phaco tip; these bubbles expand and contract. Implosion of the bubbles causes localized intense heat and pressure liberation at the tip, resulting in emulsification of lens material. Continuous cavitation, produced by continuous ultrasound, is less efficient than the transient cavitation of pulsed ultrasound delivery.

Chatter Chatter occurs when the ultrasonic stroke overcomes the vacuum, or "holding power." This causes the nuclear fragments to be repelled by the ultrasonic tip until the vacuum reaches high enough levels to neutralize the ultrasonic tip's repulsive energy and once again attracts the material. This back and forth movement of lens material from the tip inhibits "followability" (defined under Vacuum Terminology). A reduction in phaco power can diminish chatter by decreasing the stroke length of the tip excursion, thereby reducing forces pushing the fragment away from the tip.

Duty cycle During pulsed phacoemulsification, the period when phaco power is being delivered. If the time of "power on" equals the time of "power off," the duty cycle is 50%.

Frequency In phacoemulsification, how fast the phaco needle moves back and forth. The frequency of ultrasonic handpieces is between 27,000 hertz (Hz) and 60,000 Hz.

Inflow The introduction of BSS into the eye through the tubing and handpiece by depressing the foot pedal to position 1 (see the section Phaco Instrumentation).

Load In ultrasonics, the mass of nuclear material in contact with the phaco tip. Responding to the load requires that the system and the ultrasonic tip maintain constant stroke length or power. Because load is constantly changing, the system must be able to adapt to changing conditions. If the system cannot, then the cutting efficiency will be compromised.

Piezoelectric crystal A type of transducer used in ultrasonic handpieces that transforms electrical energy into mechanical energy. Linear motion is generated when a tuned, highly refined crystal is deformed by the electrical energy supplied by the console.

Power The ability of the phaco needle to vibrate and cavitate the adjacent lens material. Power is noted as a linear percentage of the maximum stroke length of which the needle is capable. Phaco power is produced when the foot pedal is depressed to position 3.

Stroke The linear distance that the tip traverses to produce an impact on lens material. This impact is measured by the velocity of tip movement at an ultrasonic frequency between 27,000 Hz and 60,000 Hz, and by the stroke length, which varies among the various devices from 2 to 4 mils (0.002″–0.004″).

Tuning The method used to match the optimum driving frequency of the ultrasonic board within the console with the operating frequency of the phaco handpiece in a specific medium (eg, BSS).

Ultrasonic Frequencies above the range of human audibility, or greater than 20,000 Hz. In phacoemulsification, the term *ultrasonic* is used because the phaco needle moves back and forth in excess of 20,000 Hz.

Vacuum Terminology

A review of the following terms may help the reader to understand concepts related to the removal of nuclear and cortical material.

Aspiration The withdrawal of fluid and lens material from the eye; produced by depressing the foot pedal to position 2 and continuing in position 3.

Aspiration flow rate The flow of fluid through the tubing, measured in milliliters per minute (mL/min). In a peristaltic system, the flow is determined by the speed of the pump. Other factors influencing flow include compliance, venting, and tubing size.

Followability The ability of a fluidic system to attract and hold nuclear or cortical material on the distal end of an ultrasonic or irrigation/aspiration handpiece until vacuum forces achieve evacuation.

Occlusion An obstruction of the aspiration port or aspiration tubing. When lens material occludes the tip, vacuum builds until the material is evacuated.

Rise time The rate at which vacuum builds once the aspiration port has been occluded. Rise time is directly related to the aspiration flow rate, which is related to the pump speed. The faster the aspiration flow rate (or pump speed), the faster the rise time.

Surge A phenomenon that occurs when vacuum has built up because of an occlusion and the occlusion is suddenly broken, leading to the fluid in the higher-pressure (positive) anterior chamber tending to rush into the lower-pressure (negative) phaco tip. If the negative surge exceeds the inflow capability of the irrigation line, anterior chamber depth fluctuations may occur and iris or posterior capsule may be drawn into the tip. Changes made in phaco equipment in order to limit surge include the following: higher fluid inflow, lower vacuum, low-compliance tubing of thinner diameter, a smaller tip, coiled aspiration tubing, and occlusion mode software. In addition, improvements in software allow automatic modification of aspiration and flow.

Vacuum Aspiration level, or vacuum, is a parameter measured in millimeters of mercury (mm Hg) or inches of water and defined as the magnitude of negative pressure created in the tubing. Vacuum determines how well particulate material that has occluded the phaco tip will be held to it.

Venting Also known as "exposing to the air," the process whereby negative pressure or vacuum is equalized to atmospheric levels to minimize surge.

Phaco Instrumentation

All current phaco machines have in common foot pedal controls with at least 3 positions. Position 1 allows entry of fluid into the handpiece through the irrigation port. Position 2 engages the aspiration mode at a constant or variable rate, depending on the settings selected by each surgeon. Position 3 adds the phaco power at a variable or fixed level.

The instruments used in phacoemulsification involve both ultrasonics and vacuum and fluid dynamics. The phaco handpiece has been likened to a jackhammer/vacuum/garden hose instrument that allows breaking the nucleus of the crystalline lens into fragments and aspirating them from the eye. Irrigation both cools the handpiece and keeps the anterior chamber formed.

The mechanical energy is produced by a to-and-fro oscillation of the tip at a frequency that is preset for each machine. The amplitude of the movement, or stroke length, is variable; it is measured in mils (1 mil = 1/1000 of an inch). It is the stroke length of the phaco tip that is changed when the power is changed. As the tip moves forward, compression of gas atoms in solution occurs; as the tip moves backward, expansion of gas atoms occurs and bubbles of gas form. The bubbles are subject to the same compression and expansion. When the bubbles implode, they release heat and shock waves (cavitation) that contribute at the tip to activity that disassembles the nucleus. Cavitation can be enhanced by changes in the needle shape. For example, the distal bend in the angled Kelman tip adds a nonaxial vibration to the primary oscillation. The nonaxial vibration augments the axial vibration and produces at the cutting tip an elliptical motion that increases the mechanical breakdown of nuclear material (Fig 8-13).

Phaco tips vary according to the angle of the tip and the size of the lumen. Phaco tips are available in 0°, 15°, 30°, 45°, 60°, and combined 30°/60° (turbo) beveled tips (Fig 8-14). In general, the surgeon chooses the bevel angle of the phaco tip based on personal preference. The angle also influences the direction of spread of the cavitation force. Tips with steeper bevels are better for cutting nuclear material (eg, using continuous phacoemulsification during sculpting). A tip with a greater bevel has an oval-shaped port with a larger surface area. Because pressure is defined as force per unit area, the tips with the greater surface area can generate greater adherence of nuclear material (Fig 8-15).

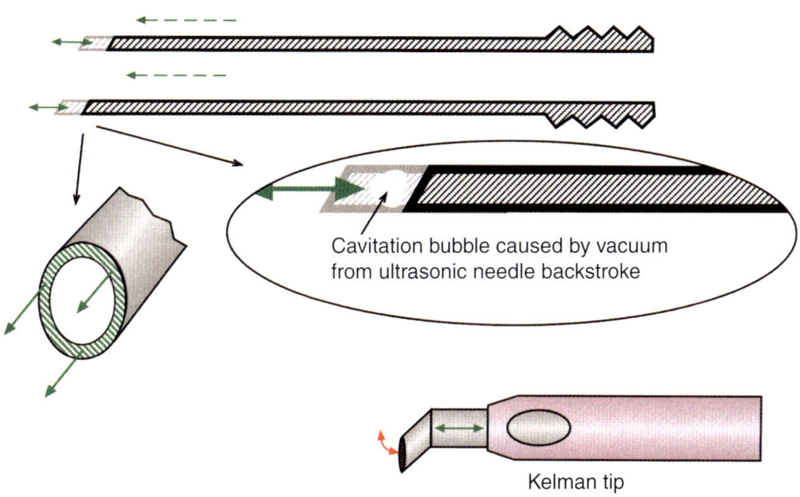

Figure 8-13 Cavitation is affected by the angle of the phaco tip as well as by different needle shapes. *(Reprinted with permission from Seibel BS.* Phacodynamics: Mastering the Tools and Techniques of Phacoemulsification Surgery. *3rd ed. Thorofare, NJ: Slack; 1999.)*

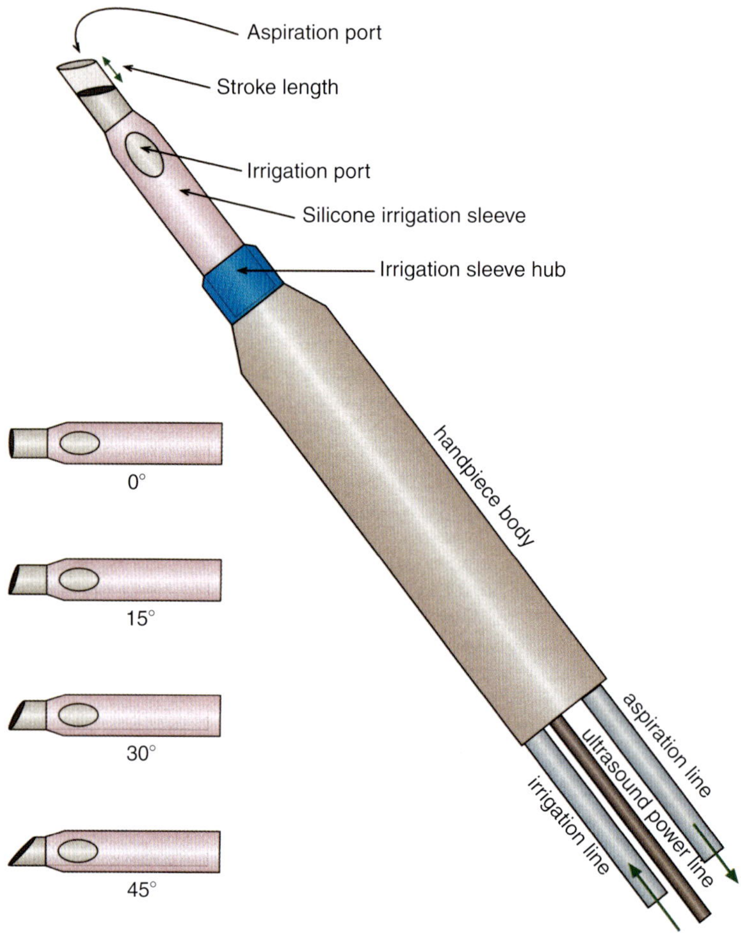

Figure 8-14 Parts of a phaco handpiece; smaller drawings depict the different tip bevels available. *(Reprinted with permission from Seibel BS.* Phacodynamics: Mastering the Tools and Techniques of Phacoemulsification Surgery. *3rd ed. Thorofare, NJ: Slack; 1999.)*

Phaco Power Delivery

Continuous phacoemulsification describes the constant delivery of phaco power when the machine is in foot position 3. *Panel control* ultrasound allows the power to be set from 0%–100%; the set level of power is delivered when the foot pedal is depressed throughout the position 3 excursion. With *surgeon-controlled* ultrasound, the surgeon controls the amount of phaco power delivered by varying the excursion of the foot pedal while in position 3. Continuous phaco power delivery may be used for sculpting deep grooves in the lens nucleus (eg, for "divide and conquer" or phaco "stop and chop" techniques).

The delivery of phaco power is a double-edged sword. Certainly, cavitation, shock waves, shear forces, and heat buildup at the tip may all facilitate nucleus disassembly. However, the classic longitudinal stroke of the tip tends to push nuclear fragments away even as the aspi-

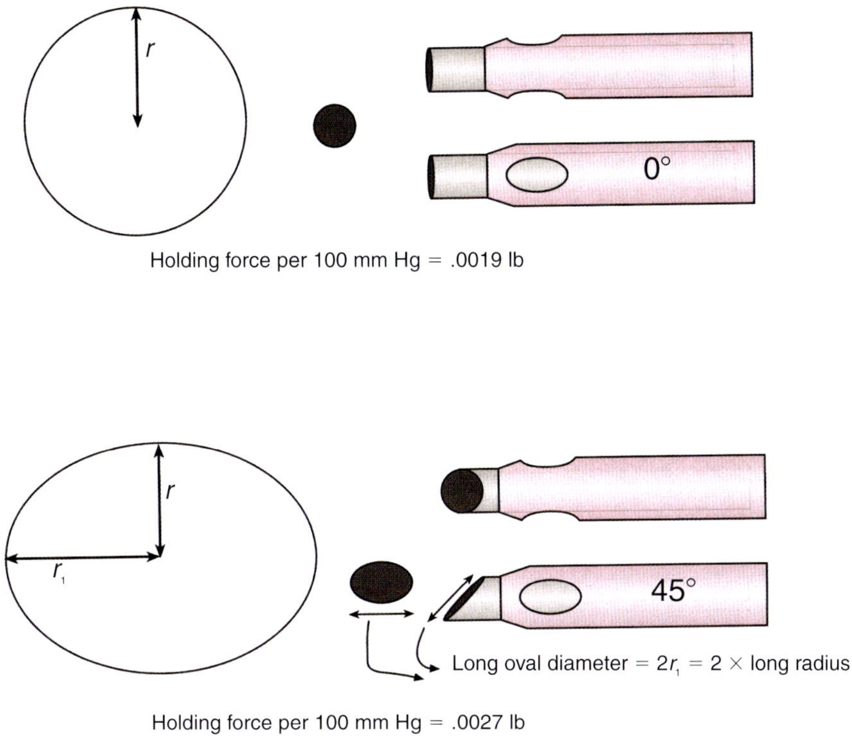

Figure 8-15 Drawing depicts the relationship between the phaco tip bevel and holding force. *(Reprinted with permission from Seibel BS.* Phacodynamics: Mastering the Tools and Techniques of Phacoemulsification Surgery. *3rd ed. Thorofare, NJ: Slack; 1999.)*

ration attracts them (chatter). In addition, continuous cavitation is less energy efficient than transient cavitation. Lastly, heat buildup from phaco power delivery may cause wound burns.

In an attempt to deliver phaco power more efficiently, modes such as pulse and burst were developed.

- Pulsed phacoemulsification involves setting the number of pulses per second while in position 3. The term *pulse* describes an interval of phaco power turned on alternating with the same interval during which phaco power is off. The amount of power delivered depends on the foot pedal excursion in position 3. The delivery of phaco power for only a portion of the cycle reduces repulsion of material by the vibrating tip and improves followability.
- Burst mode phacoemulsification involves delivery of preset power (0–100) in single bursts that are separated by decreasing intervals as the foot pedal is depressed through position 3. At the end of the position 3 excursion, the power is no longer delivered in bursts but is continuous. Burst mode allows the phaco needle tip to bury into the lens, an essential step for chopping techniques.

Additional advances in the control of phaco power delivery are discussed in the section Advances in Energy Delivery.

Irrigation

The fluid dynamics of phacoemulsification require constant irrigation through the irrigation sleeve around the ultrasound tip, with some egress of fluid through the incisions. BSS was designed to resemble aqueous humor. Its biocompatibility, along with its sterility, was a major impetus for the development of automated irrigation and aspiration.

Constant irrigation maintains anterior chamber depth and cools the phaco probe, preventing heat buildup and subsequent damage to adjacent tissue. Use of chilled irrigation fluid has been advocated by some, who claim that the cold fluid cools the probe more effectively, constricts blood vessels, maintains corneal clarity better, and may even stabilize the blood–aqueous barrier. Some surgeons put epinephrine in the BSS irrigating bottle to maintain pupillary dilatation. Others put antibiotics in the bottle as prophylaxis against endophthalmitis (see the section Antimicrobial Prophylaxis).

Liou SW, Yang CY. The effect of intracameral adrenaline infusion on pupil size, pulse rate, and blood pressure during phacoemulsification. *J Ocul Pharmacol Ther*. 1998;14(4):357–361.

Aspiration

The aspiration system of phacoemulsification machines varies according to pump design. The 3 types of pumps are peristaltic, diaphragm, and Venturi.

The peristaltic pump consists of a set of rollers that move along flexible tubing, forcing fluid through the tubing and creating a relative vacuum at the aspiration port of the phaco tip (Fig 8-16). Vacuum response time with this type of pump is relatively rapid; linear control is achieved as the speed of the rollers is increased.

The diaphragm pump consists of a flexible diaphragm overlying a fluid chamber with 1-way valves at the inlet and outlet. The diaphragm moves out, creating a relative vacuum in the chamber that shuts the exit valve, causing the fluid to flow into the chamber. The diaphragm then moves in, which increases the pressure in the chamber and closes the intake valve while opening the exit valve (Fig 8-17). This type of pump system produces a slower rise in vacuum. With continued occlusion of the aspiration port, however, the vacuum will continue to increase in an exponential manner.

The Venturi pump (Fig 8-18) creates a vacuum based on the Venturi principle: a flow of gas or fluid across a port creates a vacuum proportional to the rate of flow of the gas. This system produces a rapid, linear rise in vacuum and allows for instantaneous venting to the atmosphere that immediately stops the flow through the port.

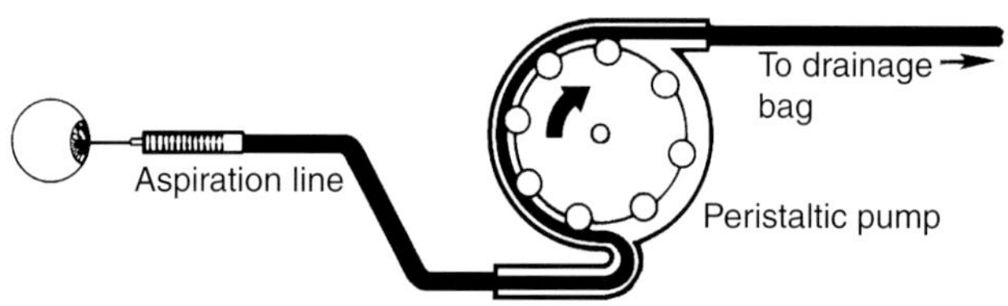

Figure 8-16 The peristaltic pump. *(Redrawn with permission from* Practical Phacoemulsification: Proceedings of the Third Annual Workshop. *Montreal, Quebec: Medicopea International, Inc; 1991:43–48.)*

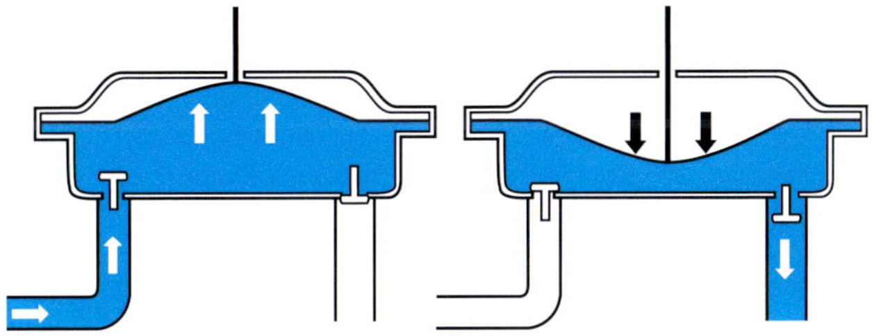

Figure 8-17 The diaphragm pump. *(Redrawn with permission from* Practical Phacoemulsification: Proceedings of the Third Annual Workshop. *Montreal, Quebec: Medicopea International, Inc; 1991:43–48.)*

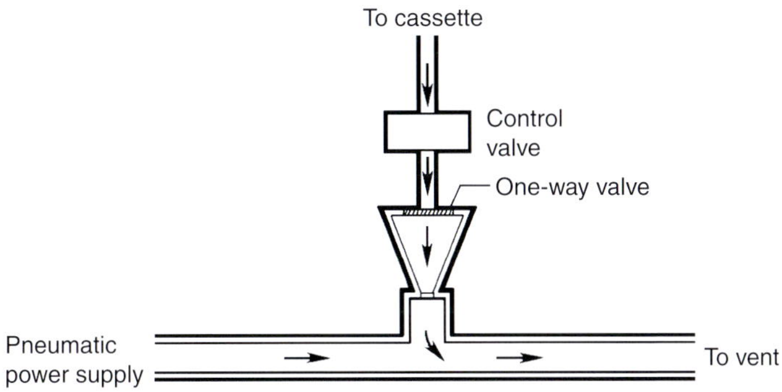

Figure 8-18 The Venturi pump. *(Redrawn with permission from* Practical Phacoemulsification: Proceedings of the Third Annual Workshop. *Montreal, Quebec: Medicopea International, Inc; 1991:43–48.)*

In general, all of these pumps are effective. The vacuum rise time (the amount of time required to reach a given level of vacuum) varies among the different pump designs (Fig 8-19). In planning a specific technique, the surgeon should consider the rise time of the instrument to be used. Further, the vacuum rise time is inversely proportional to the aspiration flow rate. The faster the flow rate, the shorter the rise time will be. Conversely, as the aspiration flow rate is decreased by half, from 40 to 20 mL/minute, the vacuum rise time is doubled, from 1 to 2 seconds (Fig 8-20).

Making the Transition

Most cataract surgeons skilled in ECCE have already chosen to develop phacoemulsification skills and to offer small-incision surgery to the vast majority of their patients. Residents in training often start with ECCE to develop their microsurgical skills and to hone their use of fine suture material. They soon advance to learning phacoemulsification, which is taught as the preferred method of cataract surgery in residency programs in the United States.

In making the transition from ECCE to phacoemulsification, the surgeon should alter technique slowly and cautiously and should perform phaco only after completing a training course that includes instruction on proper patient selection, specific surgical techniques, and instrument parameters. A surgeon wishing to make a smooth transition

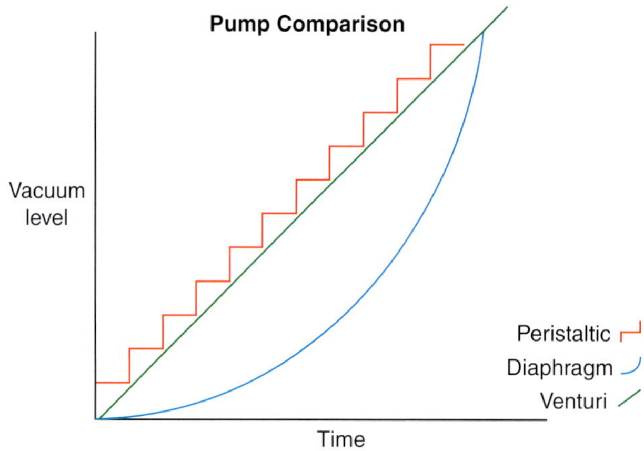

Figure 8-19 Comparison of vacuum rise times in the peristaltic, diaphragm, and Venturi pumps. *(Redrawn with permission from* Practical Phacoemulsification: Proceedings of the Third Annual Workshop. *Montreal, Quebec: Medicopea International, Inc; 1991:43–48.)*

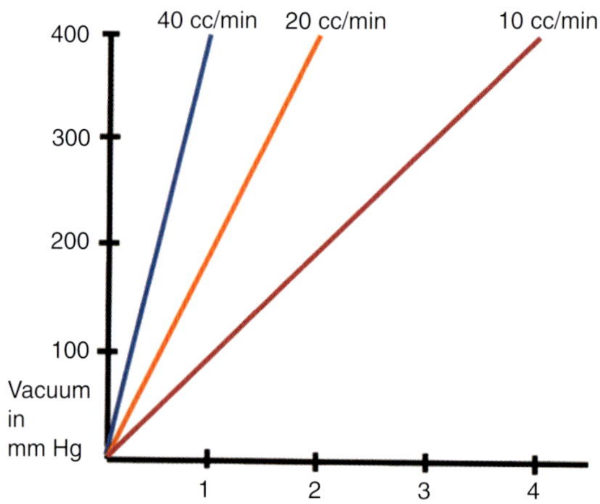

Figure 8-20 Graph depicts the relationship between aspiration flow rate and vacuum rise time. *(Reprinted with permission from Seibel BS.* Phacodynamics: Mastering the Tools and Techniques of Phacoemulsification Surgery. *3rd ed. Thorofare, NJ: Slack; 1999.)*

to phacoemulsification should meet with experienced phaco surgeons and ask a skilled surgeon to observe his or her first few cases.

Ideally, the first patient should be a cooperative individual who can lie still for a longer than average time (eg, no hip or back problems or restless legs), because the first phaco cases will probably take longer than the ECCEs with which the transitioning surgeon is familiar. Patients with large pupils should be selected, and the nuclei should be of moderate density (2–3+). The corneas should be free of dense arcus and should be without significant cornea guttata. Eyes of normal axial lengths are preferable to short eyes, with their crowded anterior chambers, or to long eyes, which have low scleral rigidity. The beginning phaco surgeon should avoid performing surgery on the patient who has only 1 functional eye. Eyes with exfoliation syndrome should be avoided because the zonular fibers in these cases are weak and the pupils may not dilate well. Patients with subluxated or dislocated lenses are cases for only the most proficient of experienced phaco surgeons.

In a similar fashion, progression can be made from a capsulotomy to a capsulorrhexis as the surgeon's level of comfort with the technique increases. Options for phaco incisions include limbal, posterior scleral tunnel, and clear corneal locations. Once confidence is gained, transition to a temporal approach can be considered. During the learning process, it is not advisable to change all of these parameters at once. If problems are encountered during surgery, the surgeon should be prepared to convert to standard ECCE.

The transitioning surgeon should pay careful attention to the patient's orbital anatomy. Shallow orbits and prominent eyes allow better surgical exposure. Using an approach from the superior limbus in patients with deep orbits or tight palpebral fissures, the surgeon must rotate the eye downward. The phaco handpiece must be held in a more vertical orientation. Visualization and manipulation of the handpiece become more awkward. Ultimately, transitioning surgeons may want to operate on patients with deep orbits or tight fissures only after they have mastered the temporal clear corneal incision.

A Basic Phaco Procedure Outline

As with conventional ECCE, pupillary dilation with mydriatic/cycloplegic drops is essential. For an experienced phaco surgeon, pupil-stretching techniques or special iris retractors can be used to open miotic pupils unresponsive to pharmacologic dilation (see Special Circumstances, Use of Pupillary Expansion).

Exposure of the Globe

During surgery, the eyelids are usually held apart with a lid speculum. When selecting the speculum, the surgeon should make sure that it will accommodate the phaco handpiece and other instruments. For a surgeon seated for a superior approach phacoemulsification, a bridle suture may be placed to help position the globe. The bridle suture is especially helpful to the beginning phaco surgeon for stabilizing the globe and exposing the bulbar conjunctiva to create a conjunctival flap.

Paracentesis

A 15° sharp blade is used to create a small paracentesis, placed approximately 2 or 3 clock-hours away from the site where an incision will be made for the phaco handpiece. A straight entry plane is made parallel to the iris and to the left for a right-handed surgeon, to the right for a left-handed surgeon. An OVD is then instilled to protect intraocular structures and allow more control during creation of the phaco incision.

Scleral Tunnel Incisions

The superiorly placed scleral tunnel incision with an internal corneal lip is frequently used by beginning phaco surgeons. Small, posteriorly placed superior stepped scleral tunnel incisions reduce the incidence of both early and late surgically induced astigmatism.

Although a limbal-based conjunctival flap can be used, a fornix-based conjunctival flap is preferable because it affords an unobstructed view of the sclera and limbus without manipulation. After creating the conjunctival flap, the surgeon clears the overlying Tenon's capsule from the sclera and applies light bipolar cautery to achieve hemostasis. Excessive cautery is to be avoided because it may cause scleral shrinkage and postoperative astigmatism.

The initial scleral step incision should be made perpendicular to the scleral surface at a depth of approximately 0.3 mm and placed 1.0–3.0 mm posterior to the surgical limbus. The initial incision length should be 2.75–7.00 mm, depending on the style of IOL to be implanted. Foldable IOLs can be inserted through incisions of 2.75–3.20 mm, whereas all polymethylmethacrylate (PMMA) IOLs require openings slightly larger than the diameter of the optic. The scleral incision is usually linear (tangential to the limbus), but it may be curvilinear (following the limbus or following the curve opposite the limbus) or chevron-shaped. The surgeon then uses a blade to enter the scleral groove at a chosen depth and dissects anteriorly, parallel to the corneoscleral surface and into clear cornea, developing a tunnel incision (Fig 8-21). The

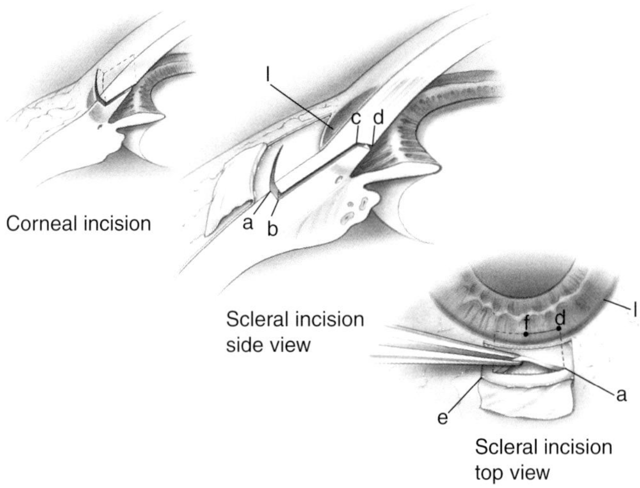

Figure 8-21 Two types of phacoemulsification incisions. Detail for scleral incision, side view: *a to b:* Initial groove is 1/3–1/2 of scleral depth; if groove is too deep, bleeding may increase and entry into anterior chamber is likely to be too posterior, causing iris prolapse. *a to l:* Incision is traditionally 2–3 mm posterior to limbus. *b to c:* Tunnel is traditionally dissected past vascular arcade; if too long, ultrasound tip mobility is restricted and corneal striae decrease visibility. *c to d:* Short third plane is made by changing angle of blade prior to entering anterior chamber. In scleral incision, top view: *e to a:* Length of incision is determined by size of IOL. *f to d:* Initial opening into anterior chamber is usually 3.0–3.25 mm; after phacoemulsification, it is fully opened for IOL insertion. If opening is too small, irrigation flow is decreased, chamber tends to shallow, and heat buildup may cause burn. If opening is too large, excessive fluid egress causes chamber shallowing and iris may prolapse. *(Reproduced with permission from Johnson SH.* Phacoemulsification. Focal Points: Clinical Modules for Ophthalmologists. *San Francisco: American Academy of Ophthalmology; 1994, module 6. Illustration by Christine Gralapp.)*

tunnel incision is carried forward, just anterior to the vascular arcade. If the scleral groove is entered too deeply, the scleral flap will be very thick, and the blade may penetrate the anterior chamber earlier than anticipated, closer to the vascular iris root. If the scleral groove is entered superficially, the scleral flap will be very thin and prone to tears or buttonholes. Either metal or diamond knives may be used for fashioning the scleral tunnel, but beginning surgeons may benefit from the added resistance and the tactile feedback provided by a metal blade.

To enter the anterior chamber from beneath the scleral flap, the surgeon uses a keratome sized to match the phaco tip width. The keratome is inserted in the tunnel until it reaches the clear cornea beyond the vascular arcade. The heel of the keratome is elevated, and the tip of the keratome is pointed posteriorly, aiming toward the center of the lens and creating a dimple in the peripheral cornea. The keratome is then slowly advanced in this posterior direction, creating an internal corneal lip as it enters the anterior chamber. The stepped incision creates a valve that allows the incision to be self-sealing once the anterior chamber is re-formed. If the scleral tunnel incision is too long, the surgeon may have problems manipulating the phaco tip within the anterior chamber. In addition, corneal striae and distortion may reduce visibility as the surgeon manipulates the phaco tip.

The subsequent closure of a step, or tunnel, incision at the end of the case depends not on radial compression of the anterior and posterior lips of the incision but rather on reapproximation of the surfaces of the tunnel flap. Various suture closures of scleral incisions are illustrated in Figure 8-22.

With the continuing evolution of techniques for self-sealing incisions and the use of foldable IOLs, many surgeons have elected not to suture the incision at all in small-incision cases. Long-term evaluation of the results and stability of this type of incision closure have shown that small scleral tunnel and clear corneal incisions, both with and without suture closure, heal quickly, are relatively stable, and induce minimal astigmatism. Even though no-stitch cataract surgery has many advantages, the surgeon should always be ready to place a suture if the incision closure appears to be inadequate.

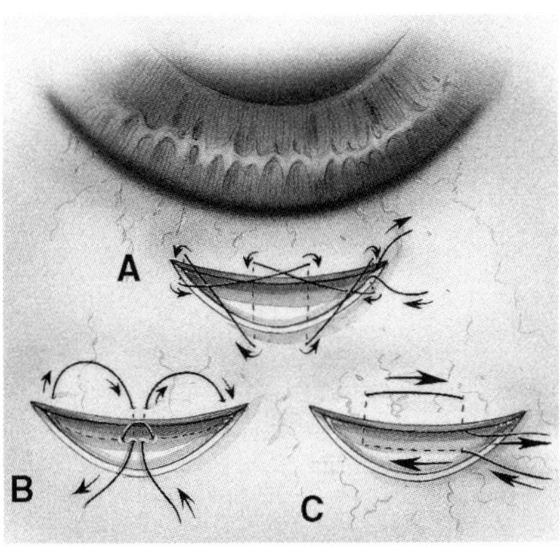

Figure 8-22 Wound closure techniques. **A,** Classic radial running x-closure must be keratometrically monitored (preferably quantitatively rather than qualitatively) during tying to avoid undesired postoperative astigmatism. Alternatively, horizontal suturing techniques using multiple bites **(B)** or a single bite **(C)** have been devised to try to decrease the induced astigmatism. *(Reproduced with permission from Johnson SH.* Phacoemulsification. Focal Points: Clinical Modules for Ophthalmologists. *San Francisco: American Academy of Ophthalmology; 1994, module 6. Illustration by Christine Gralapp.)*

Clear Corneal Incision

Phaco surgeons most often use a clear corneal incision (Fig 8-23). These small incisions are typically 2.7–3.2 mm wide, just large enough to accommodate the foldable IOL after phacoemulsification. They usually have little or no effect on preexisting astigmatism. Globe stabilization is important in clear corneal incisions, especially if the procedure is performed with topical anesthesia. Fixation rings, 0.12-mm toothed forceps, or instruments supplying counterpressure can be used to stabilize the globe as the incisions are made. The incisions can be made superiorly, temporally, or at the steepest axis of the cornea, depending on the surgeon's preference.

One approach for the clear corneal incision is a multiplanar incision using a vertical corneal groove. In the technique introduced by Langerman, a diamond or metal knife is used to create a 0.3-mm-deep groove perpendicular to the corneal surface. Another blade is inserted in the groove, and its tip is then directed tangential to the corneal surface, thereby creating a 1.5-mm tunnel through the clear cornea into the anterior chamber. This multiplanar incision architecture is usually watertight. A variation on the multiplanar incision involves making a deeper vertical groove and creating a hinge.

Another approach is the beveled, multiplanar self-sealing incision, as advocated by Shimuzu and Fine. A beveled 3-mm diamond blade is flattened against the eye, and the tip is used to enter the cornea just anterior to the vascular arcade. The blade is advanced tangentially to the corneal surface until the shoulders of the blade are fully buried in the stroma. The point of the blade is then redirected posteriorly so that the point and the rest of the blade enter the anterior chamber parallel to the iris. This technique ideally creates a 3 × 2-mm corneal incision that is watertight. Disposable steel blades can also be used

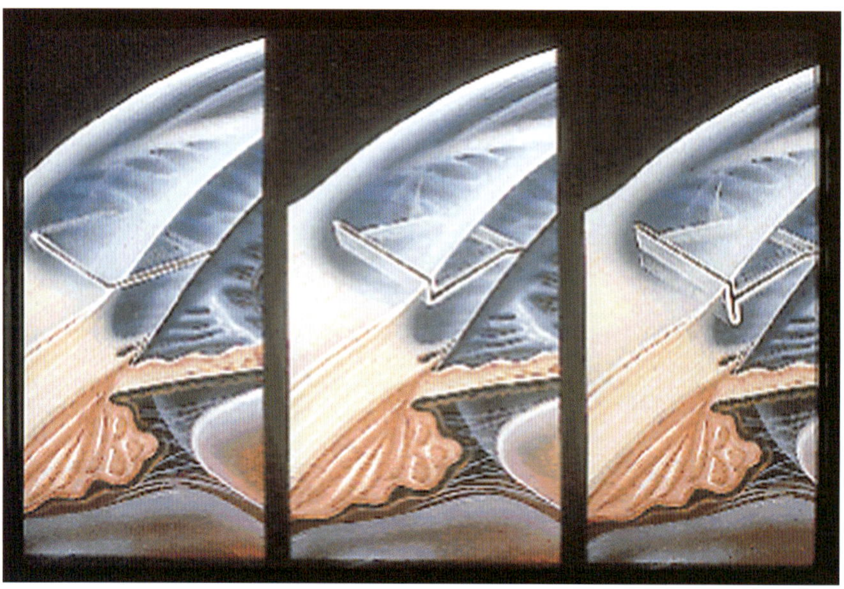

Figure 8-23 Architecture of clear corneal incisions. Single plane *(left)*, shallow groove *(center)* and deep groove *(right)*. *(Reprinted with permission from Fine IH.* Clear Corneal Lens Surgery. *Thorofare, NJ: Slack; 1999.)*

to create these incisions. Newer beveled, trapezoidal diamond blades (Fig 8-24) have been developed for self-sealing clear corneal incisions. Such blades can be advanced in one motion and in one plane, from clear cornea into the anterior chamber. The blade is oriented parallel to the iris (0°), and the tip is placed at the start of the clear cornea, just anterior to the vascular arcade. The blade is tilted up and the heel down so that the blade is angled 10° from the iris plane and then advanced into the anterior chamber in one smooth, continuous motion. Regardless of which type of clear corneal incision is used, the goal is to keep the incision just large enough to accommodate the folded IOL with its inserter, generally 2.7–3.2 mm.

A third approach is the "near clear" approach, in which the incision begins within the vascular arcade. Proponents of this approach cite better closure and reduced incidence of induced astigmatism. However, slight bleeding may occur during surgery, and a subconjunctival hemorrhage may be present postoperatively.

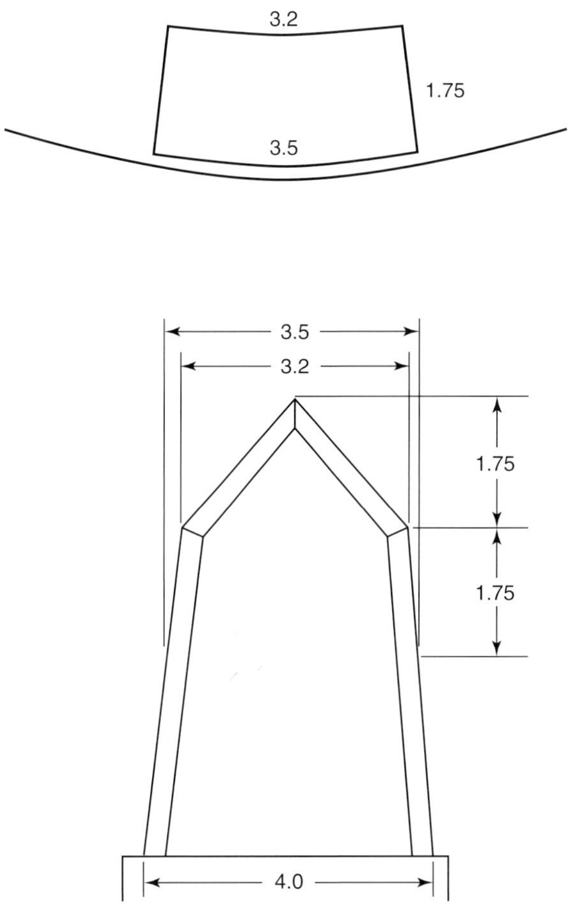

Figure 8-24 *Below,* Dimensions and shape of a beveled trapezoidal diamond blade used in clear corneal incisions and *(above)* contour of the incision made with this knife. *(Reprinted with permission from Fine IH, Fichman RA, Grabow HB.* Clear-Corneal Cataract Surgery and Topical Anesthesia. *Thorofare, NJ: Slack; 1993.)*

The temporal approach clear (or "near clear") technique has the following advantages:

- avoids dissection of Tenon's capsule and of conjunctiva, which decreases the risk of bleeding (eg, in patients on anticoagulants)
- creates a self-sealing incision that does not usually require sutures and allows for rapid visual rehabilitation
- offers better accessibility because brow obstruction is eliminated with a temporal approach
- offers an excellent red reflex
- spares the superior conjunctiva for subsequent surgery (eg, glaucoma filtering procedures or aqueous shunt surgery)
- avoids the need for a traction suture
- permits use of topical anesthesia, which brings its own set of advantages

However, the surgeon should also be aware of the disadvantages of temporal approach surgery, which include the following:

- need for the surgeon to adapt to a different surgical position
- lack of forehead support for the surgeon's hands (although a wrist rest can be used)
- development of corneal striae intraoperatively if incision extends too far anteriorly, with reduced visualization
- need to enlarge the incision for use of nonfoldable IOLs (eg, anterior chamber IOL [ACIOL])
- difficulty in converting to a manual expression ECCE technique
- proximity of instruments to the corneal endothelium during surgery
- possible corneal thermal burns
- higher incidence of endophthalmitis in some studies (thought to be related to inadequate incision closure)

Ernest PH, Neuhann T. Posterior limbal incision. *J Cataract Refract Surg.* 1996;22(1):78–84.

Fine IH. Corneal tunnel incision with a temporal approach. In: Fine IH, Fichman RA, Grabow HB, eds. *Clear-Corneal Cataract Surgery and Topical Anesthesia.* Thorofare, NJ: Slack; 1993:50–51.

Langerman DW. Architectural design of a self-sealing corneal tunnel, single-hinge incision. *J Cataract Refract Surg.* 1994;20(1):84–88.

Masket S. Cataract incision and closure. *Focal Points: Clinical Modules for Ophthalmologists.* San Francisco: American Academy of Ophthalmology; 1995, module 3.

Masket S. Horizontal anchor suture closure method for small incision cataract surgery. *J Cataract Refract Surg.* 1991;17(suppl):689–695.

Nagaki Y, Hayasaka S, Kadoi C, et al. Bacterial endophthalmitis after small-incision cataract surgery: effect of incision placement and intraocular lens type. *J Cataract Refract Surg.* 2003;29(1):20–26.

Shepherd JR. Induced astigmatism in small incision cataract surgery. *J Cataract Refract Surg.* 1989;15(1):85–88.

Continuous Curvilinear Capsulorrhexis

After the incision has been made, the next step is to open the capsule. Although a can-opener capsulotomy can be used with phacoemulsification, continuous-tear curvilinear capsulorrhexis (CCC) is the capsular opening that allows a wider range of safer phaco techniques (Fig 8-25). CCC resists radial tears that could extend around and open the posterior capsule, setting the stage for the development of complications. In addition, CCC stabilizes the nucleus, allowing maneuvers to disassemble the nucleus within the capsular bag. Disassembling the nucleus in the capsular bag decreases endothelial trauma. CCC also helps stabilize and center the lens implant. Further, CCC transfers the haptic forces circumferentially and prevents lens implant decentration if YAG posterior capsulotomy is performed. A CCC sized just smaller than the IOL optic may allow a tighter contact between the posterior surface of the posterior chamber IOL and the posterior capsule, possibly reducing posterior capsule opacification. Lastly, certain lens implants designed to provide multifocality require a CCC of a certain size.

The surgeon begins a CCC with a central linear cut in the anterior capsule, using a cystitome needle or capsulorrhexis forceps with special tips for grasping and tearing the anterior capsule. At the end of the linear cut, the needle is either pushed or pulled in the direction of the desired tear, allowing the anterior capsule to fold over upon itself. The surgeon then engages the free edge of the anterior capsule with either forceps or the

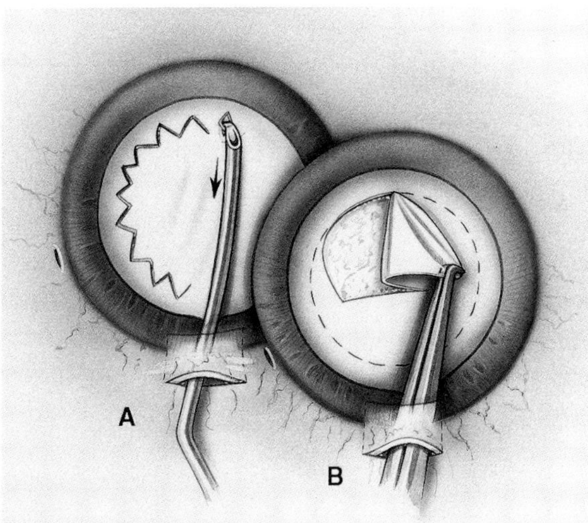

Figure 8-25 Anterior capsulotomy techniques. **A,** In the "can-opener" incision, punctures are made peripherally and pulled centrally so that the torn edges connect. Each puncture site has the potential for a radial tear if stressed. **B,** In the capsulorrhexis, tearing is begun within the area to be excised and finished from the outside in. When stress lines in the free flap appear between forceps and the tear site, best control is maintained by regrasping the flap near the tear site. Positive vitreous pressure makes the tear travel peripherally; filling the anterior chamber with an OVD will counteract the posterior vitreous pressure and make it easier to complete the capsulorrhexis tear. *(Reproduced with permission from Johnson SH.* Phacoemulsification. Focal Points: Clinical Modules for Ophthalmologists. *San Francisco: American Academy of Ophthalmology; 1994, module 6. Illustration by Christine Gralapp.)*

capsulotomy needle, and the flap is carried around in a circular manner as the surgeon directs the tension toward the center of the lens.

The tear should not be allowed to turn inward, as this results in a central opening that is too small; nor should the tear turn outward, as this leads to an opening that is too large or to extension of the tear to the posterior capsule. An opening that is too small complicates most nucleus disassembly techniques and may contract postoperatively (capsular phimosis). The overlapping anterior capsule is prone to opacify, especially in diabetic patients. A capsulorrhexis that is too large complicates endocapsular phacoemulsification techniques and may allow the IOL optic or haptic to dislocate anteriorly. For these reasons, many surgeons advocate a size that allows the capsular rim to cover the optic edge to reduce posterior capsule opacification.

For maximum control of the size, frequent regrasping of the flap near the tear is helpful. The forceps or cystitome can be used to change the direction of the tear and prevent a CCC that is too small or too large. OVD can be added to keep the lens surface flat to avoid extension peripherally. Any factor that causes shallowing of the chamber will also make the lens move forward, directing the tear "downhill" toward the periphery. The surgeon should check for pressure on the globe caused by the capsulotomy instrument, the surgeon's fingers, or the eyelid speculum. Inserting a second instrument (such as an iris spatula) through the paracentesis to press posteriorly on the lens may also help control the direction of the tear.

If the capsulorrhexis seems too small after phacoemulsification is completed, a decision must be made whether to enlarge it before or after IOL implantation. If a foldable lens is used, the capsular bag can be expanded with a cohesive OVD; the lens may then be inserted. The cystitome or microscissors can be used to cut the anterior capsule edge of the CCC and extend the new tear around so that it enlarges the original CCC.

In cases with loose zonules, creation of a CCC may be hampered by the lens nucleus and bag rotating along with the tear, dehiscing more zonules and setting the stage for complications. Use of capsular hooks may stabilize the bag to allow completion of the tear.

If a CCC cannot be completed, conversion to a can-opener anterior capsulotomy is an acceptable strategy. However, this type of anterior capsulotomy makes hydrodissection, hydrodelineation, and endocapsular phacoemulsification more challenging.

Mackool RJ. Capsule stabilization for phacoemulsification (letter). *J Cataract Refract Surg.* 2000;26(5):629.

Hydrodissection

Following capsulorrhexis, gentle injection of irrigating fluid, or hydrodissection, is performed to separate the peripheral cortex from the underlying posterior lens capsule. In addition to loosening the lens nucleus/cortex complex, this procedure facilitates nuclear rotation during phacoemulsification and hydrates the peripheral cortex, making it easier to aspirate after nucleus removal.

The surgeon places a bent, blunt-tipped 25- to 30-gauge cannula or flattened hydrodissection cannula attached to a 3–5-mL syringe under the anterior capsule flap. While carefully lifting the capsular flap, the surgeon injects BSS in a radial direction. Gentle posterior pressure centrally on the nucleus will express posterior fluid and prevent fluid pressure from rupturing the posterior capsule. Gentle irrigation should continue until the surgeon sees a wave of fluid moving under the nucleus and across the red reflex. In mature cataracts or in cases without a red reflex, careful hydrodissection should continue until nuclear rotation can be performed. Irrigation in the subincisional area may require a right-angled or J-shaped hydrodissection cannula.

If the nucleus is displaced into the anterior chamber, it can be reposited into the posterior chamber with OVD and application of slight pressure posteriorly on the nucleus. Alternatively, a supracapsular phacoemulsification technique may be selected in this situation. Hydrodissection is riskier after a can-opener capsulotomy has been performed, with zonules that are weakened, or in a patient who has posterior polar cataracts.

Hydrodelineation

Some surgeons also inject BSS into the substance of the nucleus to hydrodelineate, or separate, the various layers of the nucleus after hydrodissection. This technique separates the harder central endonucleus from the softer outer epinucleus, which can remain behind to act as a cushion to protect the underlying posterior capsule from inadvertent trauma during nucleus removal. In less brunescent cataracts, a fluid wave can be seen to separate the endonucleus from the epinucleus and produce the "golden ring" sign. Hydrodelineation is not effective in white or densely brunescent nuclei.

Nuclear Rotation

If hydrodissection has succeeded in breaking attachments between posterior cortex and posterior capsule, the surgeon should be able to rotate the endonucleus and epinucleus within the capsular bag. Phacoemulsification techniques are easier to perform when there is a freely rotating lens within the bag.

Difficulty in rotating the nucleus may occur with soft nuclei or may suggest either inadequate hydrodissection (which can be repeated) or loose zonules, which can cause the bag to rotate instead of the nucleus. Use of bimanual techniques through 2 paracenteses may allow rotation.

Instrument Settings for Phacoemulsification

Most methods of nucleus removal consist of several distinct steps, including sculpting, cracking or chopping, grasping, and emulsifying. With contemporary phaco machines, all the phaco parameters—power levels and intervals of delivery, aspiration flow rate, and vacuum—can be adjusted for each step of the procedure, giving the surgeon maximum control of the process. The vacuum is set to a level appropriate for the hardness of the nucleus. For example, harder cataracts require higher vacuum. If vacuum is set too low, lens chatter can occur, with large and small nuclear fragments bouncing around the anterior chamber. Higher vacuum improves the purchase of the phaco tip on the nuclear material and allows techniques with lower ultrasound power and shorter ultrasound time. Of course, higher vacuum might attract and tear iris and anterior or posterior capsule. It is suggested that the beginning phaco surgeon begin with power, pulse, burst, and vacuum levels recommended in courses, by surgical mentors, or by phaco instrument representatives.

Sculpting, the process of debulking the central nucleus, involves a shaving maneuver in which the tip of the phaco port is never fully occluded. Without occlusion, only incidental vacuum is generated. Only a portion of the phaco needle is in contact with the nucleus with each forward pass; thus, lens material can be removed in a controlled fashion. Aspiration is responsible for bringing the nuclear particles into the aspiration port and out of the eye. Sculpting is usually performed with modest vacuum, low aspiration flow, and low phaco power.

Vertical chopping techniques (discussed later) require a strong purchase of the nucleus with the phaco needle. High vacuum is required. Phaco power is best delivered in burst mode to prevent repulsion of the nucleus. Once the nucleus is impaled, position 2 is used with maintenance of high vacuum to allow chopping.

After the nucleus has been sculpted and cracked or chopped, the nuclear fragments are grasped and emulsified by occlusion of the phaco tip. Vacuum is essential at this point in the procedure to grasp the nuclear fragments and pull them to a "safe zone," between the posterior capsule and endothelium, before emulsification. Full occlusion of the phaco tip allows the vacuum to build up to its maximum preset level. Full vacuum draws nuclear material into the tip and allows it to be molded as it enters. The ultrasound power then emulsifies the material into smaller pieces. Vacuum functions to drive the emulsified nuclear material farther into the tip, and it also helps feed additional nuclear material into the tip. If the repulsive action of the ultrasound tip oscillating against the nuclear material is counterbalanced by the vacuum and the flow pulling the material inward, chatter is reduced.

A low flow rate is considered desirable because it provides greater stability to the anterior chamber. After each nuclear fragment is completely emulsified and aspirated and occlusion is broken, low flow is immediately resumed. With low flow, emulsification and aspiration occur at a slower, more controlled rate; with high flow, events occur more quickly, and iris and other intraocular tissue can be aspirated inadvertently.

Strategies for Irrigation and Aspiration

In phacoemulsification and in ECCE with manual expression, the same instruments and techniques are used for irrigation and aspiration of cortical material.

A plate of soft epinucleus or "transitional cortex" may rest on the posterior capsule. The phaco needle can be used to accomplish irrigation and aspiration without ultrasound; reduced vacuum and flow settings can be used to aspirate this material from the capsular fornix or posterior capsule. The irrigation/aspiration (I/A) system straight tip can be used with the port down and low vacuum to strip this material carefully from the posterior capsule.

The surgeon can remove peripheral cortical material of the lens by first rotating the port toward the equator of the lens capsule. The cortical material should be engaged under low suction and dragged to the center of the inflated capsular bag. The port is then rotated so that it is fully visible to the surgeon and can be stripped under greater suction.

Sometimes the surgeon finds it difficult to reach the subincisional cortex. In these cases, a 45°, right-angled (90°), or U-shaped (180°) aspiration cannula may be useful to engage and strip this cortical material. Another technique involves filling the anterior chamber with OVD and aspirating subincisional cortex with an aspiration cannula attached to a handheld syringe. The aspiration and irrigation functions may also be separated, and the aspiration port may be introduced through the paracentesis while irrigation through the phaco incision maintains the chamber.

Cortex resistant to aspiration can be separated from the capsular bag with OVD ("viscodissected") to allow a better purchase with the I/A handpiece. Another strategy leaves removal of subincisional cortex until after implantation of the IOL. The IOL can be rotated within the bag so the haptics will further loosen the cortex. The benefits of attempting to remove small amounts of residual cortex must be weighed against the risk of damaging the posterior capsule. Very small amounts of retained fine cortical strands may easily be resorbed postoperatively.

After removing the cataract and inserting the IOL, the surgeon should remove the OVD from the anterior segment. Some surgeons remove the OVD from behind the optic. Others push the optic down to release the OVD from the bag and allow its aspiration from the anterior chamber.

To produce a slightly firm eye, sterile BSS is used, via the paracentesis, to re-form the anterior chamber. The incision is examined for leakage. If the incision leaks, both sides of the corneal tunnel incision can be hydrated with sterile BSS injected through a syringe with a blunt 25- to 26-gauge irrigating tip. Hydration of the corneal incision causes temporary stromal swelling and increases the wound apposition between the roof and the floor of the tunnel, thereby eliminating any leakage. Some surgeons hydrate the stroma in all cases. If the incision leaks after stromal hydration, it requires a suture. Larger incisions that are used to allow insertion of a PMMA lens generally require suture closure.

Location of Emulsification

The nucleus may be emulsified at various locations within the eye, including the anterior chamber, iris plane, and posterior chamber. The location chosen for emulsification will determine which techniques are employed for nucleus management.

Anterior chamber

When the technique of phacoemulsification was first developed by Kelman, it involved prolapsing the nucleus into the anterior chamber. Visualization was excellent, and any decrease in pupil size after nuclear prolapse was less problematic. The risk of posterior capsule damage or rupture was minimized because of the greater distance between the lens and capsule. However, the risk of corneal endothelial trauma and resultant corneal edema was increased because of the proximity of the phaco needle to the endothelium. No OVDs were available at that time. Corneal edema was the major reason phacoemulsification did not attract early converts until the development of more "cornea friendly" techniques.

Iris plane

A later development was to perform phacoemulsification at the iris plane. In this location, the superior pole of the nucleus is prolapsed anteriorly (Fig 8-26A), and emulsification occurs halfway between the corneal endothelium and the posterior capsule, thereby reducing the risk of damage to either structure. Once prolapsed, the nucleus can be manipulated (Fig 8-26B) with less stress on the posterior capsule and zonular fibers. In patients with small pupils, this technique permits placement of the nucleus within the pupil, thus maintaining visualization and allowing for safe emulsification.

The iris plane location is often desirable for the beginning phaco surgeon and in cases with small pupils or compromised capsular or zonular integrity. The disadvantages of this technique include the difficulty in prolapsing the nucleus and potential damage to the corneal endothelium if the superior pole of the nucleus is emulsified too close to the cornea.

Posterior chamber

The posterior chamber is now the most common region for dismantling the nucleus (Fig 8-27). Nucleus removal from this location requires capsulorrhexis, hydrodissection,

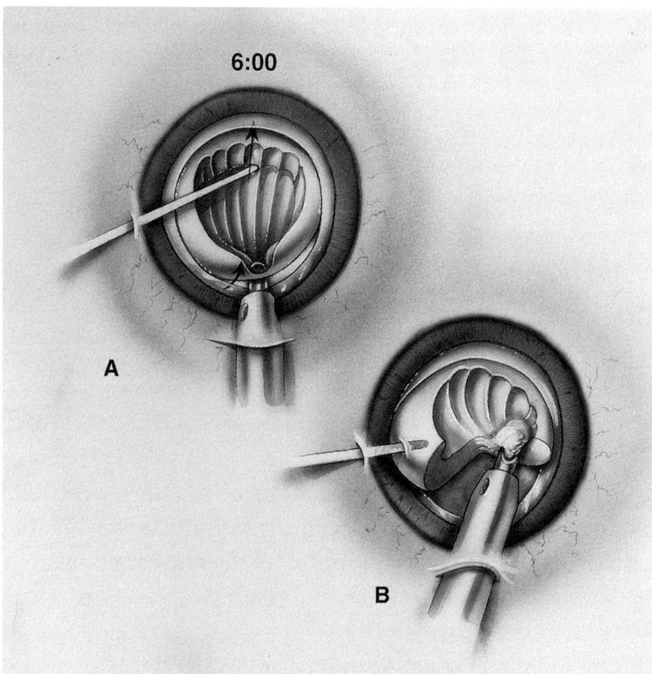

Figure 8-26 Emulsification of the nucleus as a whole at the iris plane, following central sculpting. **A,** Lens is subluxed by pushing the spatula against the ledge to move the lens toward 6 o'clock, leaving the anterior-posterior plane of the spatula unchanged. The anterior chamber is shallowed by stopping irrigation, allowing the superior lens equator to present anteriorly as the lens rotates around the stable spatula. The ultrasound tip is partially withdrawn to catch the posterior surface of the superior lens equator and help lift the lens. **B,** Nucleus is stabilized by sticking it with the spatula, and the ultrasound tip debulks the lens by quadrants. Both instruments are used to rotate the lens counterclockwise as the process continues. *(Reproduced with permission from Johnson SH.* Phacoemulsification. Focal Points: Clinical Modules for Ophthalmologists. *San Francisco: American Academy of Ophthalmology; 1994, module 6. Illustration by Christine Gralapp.)*

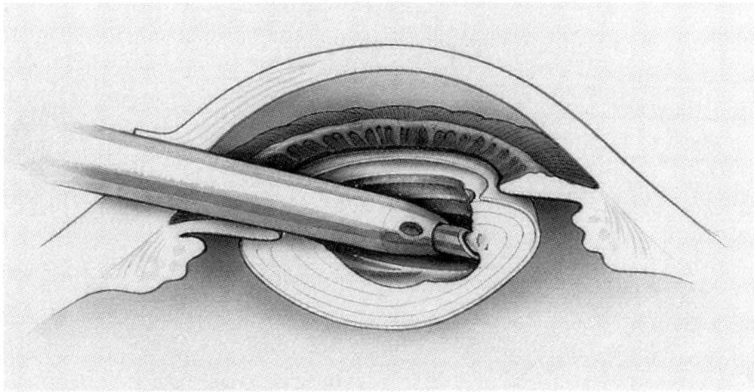

Figure 8-27 Central sculpting of the nucleus when managed as a whole. If the iris plane approach is used, the nucleus is sculpted to 1/2–2/3 its depth, leaving an inferior ledge; if the posterior chamber approach is used, the nucleus is sculpted deep centrally and thinned inferiorly to weaken the remaining lens material. *(Reproduced with permission from Johnson SH.* Phacoemulsification. Focal Points: Clinical Modules for Ophthalmologists. *San Francisco: American Academy of Ophthalmology; 1994, module 6. Illustration by Christine Gralapp.)*

and nucleus rotation. The advantages of posterior chamber phacoemulsification are the reduced risk of corneal endothelial trauma and the ability to minimize the size of the capsulorrhexis opening, which is useful with suboptimal dilation. The disadvantages include the need to emulsify close to the posterior capsule, the greater stress placed on the posterior capsule and zonular fibers when the nucleus is being manipulated, the technical difficulty in small-pupil cases, and the need to employ more sophisticated methods of nuclear splitting.

Supracapsular

Kelman initially used this technique, but he did so without protection of the endothelium through use of OVDs. The essence of this technique involves prolapsing the nucleus through the capsulorrhexis during hydrodissection and then either repositing the nucleus in the posterior chamber on top of the capsular bag (as suggested by William Maloney, MD) or leaving a pole anterior to the iris (recommended by David Brown, MD). This approach theoretically reduces the stress on the zonules during nucleus manipulation. It can be used in small-pupil cases. Both positions require medium to large capsulorrhexes.

The risks of this technique include a greater chance of aspirating and damaging the iris in the phaco tip (because the anterior capsule rim no longer separates the nucleus from the iris) and the inability to maintain control of the nuclear pieces as they are created, because they are no longer contained in the capsular bag.

One-Handed Technique of Nucleus Disassembly

This technique involves an adequate capsulorrhexis and one surgical incision. As no OVD is present before keratome entry, a diamond blade may be useful for its exquisite sharpness and ease in entering the anterior chamber. Hydrodissection, hydrodelineation, and nuclear rotation within the capsular bag are performed. The phaco needle is used to shave layer by layer through the nucleus from edge to edge, rotating the nucleus to access thicker regions (Fig 8-28). When the nucleus has been removed, the phaco needle can be used to remove the epinuclear envelope, with low phaco power and medium vacuum settings. Any residual cortex is removed with I/A.

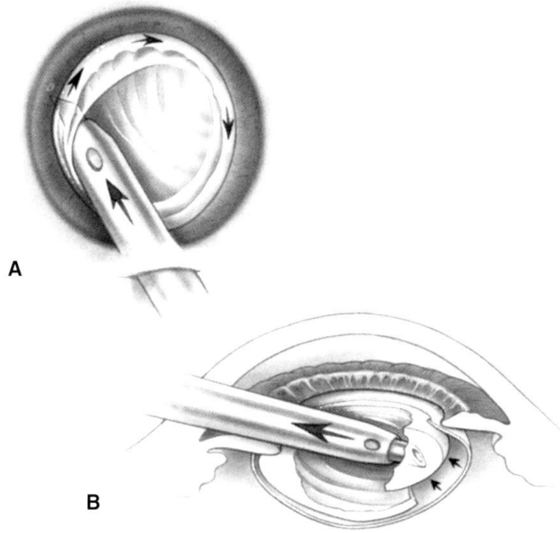

Figure 8-28 One-handed nuclear rotation **(A)** and nuclear rim removal **(B).** *(Reproduced with permission from Johnson SH.* Phacoemulsification. Focal Points: Clinical Modules for Ophthalmologists. *San Francisco: American Academy of Ophthalmology; 1994, module 6. Illustration by Christine Gralapp.)*

Two-Handed Techniques of Nucleus Disassembly

A popular approach of nucleus disassembly usually requires 2 instruments to subdivide the nucleus prior to its emulsification. This process allows for removal of the hard endonucleus first, within the capsular bag, using the epinucleus and cortex as a cushion to protect the underlying posterior capsule. The endonucleus is divided into several small pieces. This division process allows for a more controlled removal using less phaco power and time. This technique requires a CCC to provide an intact and very resilient capsular opening.

Phaco fracture technique

The most widely used 2-handed technique was developed by Howard Gimbel, MD (nucleofractis), and John Shephard, MD ("divide and conquer"), for removal of all but very soft cataracts. After adequate hydrodissection and hydrodelineation have been performed, a deep central linear groove or trough is sculpted in the nucleus, with continuous ultrasound used for sculpting. Any groove must be deep enough to allow subsequent cracking. Clues that the groove depth is adequate include smoothing of the striations in the groove, brightening of the red reflex in the groove, and sculpting to a depth of 2–3 phaco tip diameters.

At this point, nuclear cracking can be done to separate the nucleus into 2 pieces, or the deeply grooved nucleus can be rotated to create troughs to divide each half into quadrants. The phaco tip and second instrument are inserted into each groove and spread apart, with a cross action or parallel action, thereby achieving the complete separation of the pieces (Fig 8-29).

The second instrument can then be used to present either the peripheral rim or the apex of the quadrant to the phaco needle (Fig 8-30). This piece is engaged by the phaco tip,

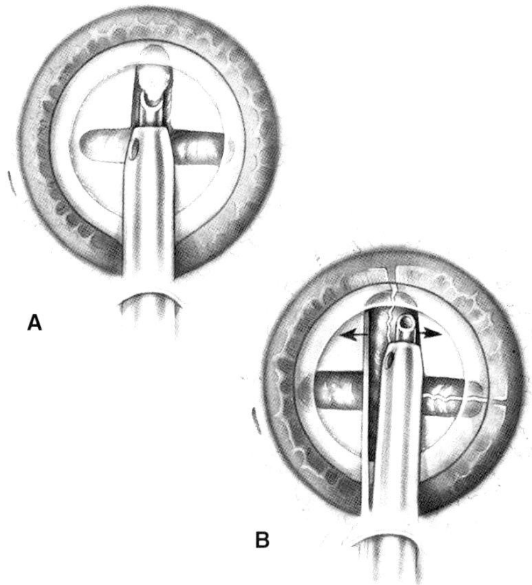

Figure 8-29 **A,** Sculpting grooves. **B,** Cracking with phaco needle and second instrument. *(Reproduced with permission from Johnson SH.* Phacoemulsification. Focal Points: Clinical Modules for Ophthalmologists. *San Francisco: American Academy of Ophthalmology; 1994, module 6. Illustration by Christine Gralapp.)*

and after adequate vacuum is attained, the nuclear quadrant is pulled toward the center of the capsular bag and emulsified. Each quadrant is sequentially removed in the same manner.

Gimbel HV. Divide and conquer nucleofractis phacoemulsification: development and variations. *J Cataract Refract Surg.* 1991;17(3):281–291.

Koch PS. *Converting to Phacoemulsification: Making the Transition to In-the-Bag Phaco.* 3rd ed. Thorofare, NJ: Slack, Inc; 1992.

Koch PS, Davison JA, eds. *Textbook of Advanced Phacoemulsification Techniques.* Thorofare, NJ: Slack, Inc; 1991.

Shepherd JR. In situ fracture. *J Cataract Refract Surg.* 1990;16(4):436–440.

Steinert RF, ed. *Cataract Surgery: Technique, Complications, and Management.* 2nd ed. St Louis: Mosby; 2004.

Chopping techniques

The *horizontal* phaco chop technique originally described by Nagahara does not entail creation of a central groove but instead advocates use of the natural fault lines in the lens nucleus for creation of a fracture plane. After burying the phaco tip in the center of the nucleus by using high vacuum, the surgeon inserts a phaco chop instrument under the anterior capsule flap, deeply engages the endonucleus in the periphery, and draws it toward the phaco tip, thereby cracking the nucleus into 2 pieces. The phaco tip is then buried in one of the nuclear halves, and the phaco chop instrument is used in the same fashion to create multiple small wedges of nucleus for emulsification.

Koch and Katzen modified this procedure by making a central groove and starting with division of the nucleus into 2 pieces through sculpting and cracking, with subsequent

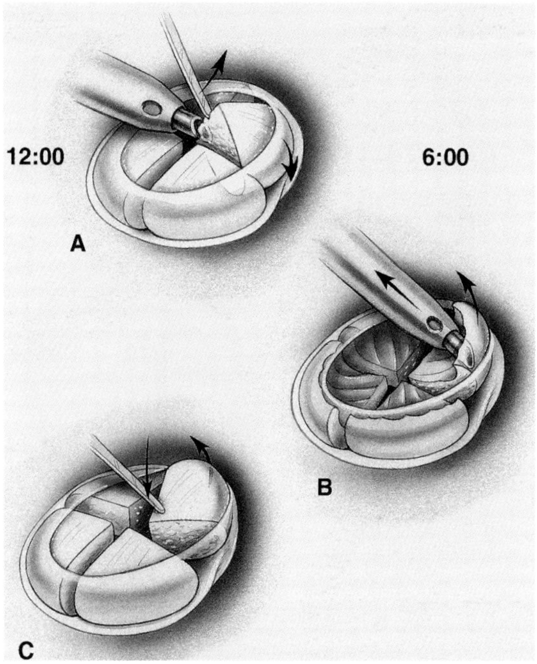

Figure 8-30 Quadrant removal techniques. **A,** Spatula lifts the apex of the quadrant, the ultrasound tip is embedded into the posterior edge, and aspiration centralizes the quadrant for emulsification. **B,** Quadrants are debulked centrally after splitting; the ultrasound tip is embedded into the cortical rim and aspiration is maintained to tumble the rim and remainder of the quadrant centrally. **C,** Spatula pushes the apex of the quadrant posteriorly so the rim moves to front and center. *(Reproduced with permission from Johnson SH.* Phacoemulsification. Focal Points: Clinical Modules for Ophthalmologists. *San Francisco: American Academy of Ophthalmology; 1994, module 6. Illustration by Christine Gralapp.)*

chopping of heminuclei ("stop and chop" phaco; Fig 8-31). The groove affords the surgeon more room to manipulate the nuclear pieces in the capsular bag. High levels of vacuum are necessary to maintain a firm grasp on the nucleus as it is being fragmented; in addition, the high vacuum allows more controlled removal of the pieces and reduces the use of ultrasound energy. Any remaining epinucleus and cortex are removed in standard fashion.

Classic horizontal chop entailed the challenge of placing the chopper under the capsular rim and around the equatorial nucleus without direct visualization, and "stop and chop" phaco required creation of a groove. *Vertical chopping* techniques that eliminate both of these challenges have been developed. After the center of the nucleus is impaled with the phaco tip using high vacuum and burst mode, a chopper with a sharp tip is buried within the nucleus, just adjacent to the phaco tip. The phaco tip lifts while the chopper depresses and the instruments are separated to effect the chop, which occurs along natural fault lines in the nucleus.

In practice, either the vertical or the horizontal chopping technique can be used with almost any other strategy for nucleus disassembly. Chopping is not appropriate for soft nuclei, for example, pure PSCs; vacuum aspiration with minimal or no phaco power may be more appropriate in these cases.

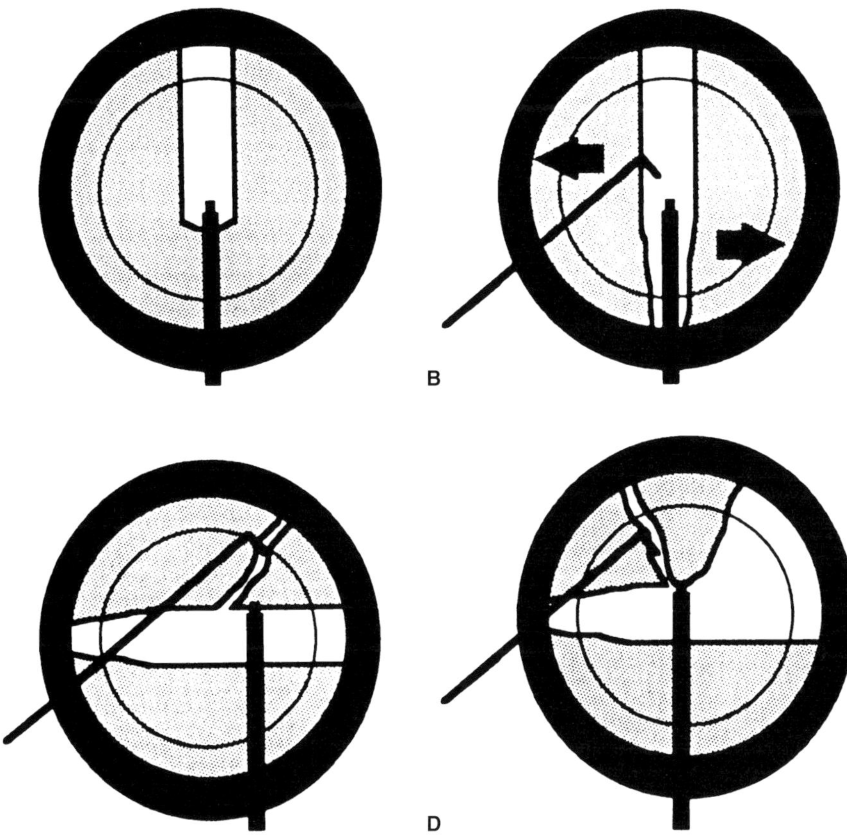

Figure 8-31 Stop and chop. **A,** Soft cataracts are prepared by sculpting a trench in the middle of the cataract, providing space for later manipulation. **B,** After sculpting is complete, the nucleus is fractured into halves with the phaco tip and the chopper. **C,** The phaco tip is driven into the nuclear half about a third of the way across from right to left. The chopper is buried in the periphery of the nucleus and pulled toward the phaco tip. When the instruments are close to each other, they are separated, and a small segment of the nucleus is chopped off. It is already impaled on the phaco tip and can be emulsified without further manipulation. **D,** The phaco tip is driven into the remaining nucleus and the same steps are repeated: bury the chopper, pull it toward the phaco tip, chop, separate, remove. This sequence is repeated until the entire nucleus is emulsified. *(Reproduced with permission from Koch PS, Katzen LE. Stop and chop phacoemulsification.* J Cataract Refract Surg. *1994;20:566–570. ©American Society of Cataract and Refractive Surgery.)*

Chang DF. *Phaco Chop: Mastering Techniques, Optimizing Technology, and Avoiding Complications.* Thorofare, NJ: Slack, Inc; 2004.

Koch PS. *Mastering Phacoemulsification: A Simplified Manual of Strategies for the Spring, Crack, and Stop and Chop Technique.* 4th ed. Thorofare, NJ: Slack Inc; 1994.

Endolenticular technique

Endolenticular phacoemulsification was developed as a "forward-looking" technique. A very small capsulorrhexis is made at the periphery of the anterior capsule. A small phaco needle is used to emulsify the lens entirely within the capsular bag. The retention of the anterior capsule during emulsification may reduce endothelial cell loss. The small capsulorrhexis can be enlarged to allow lens implantation into the capsular bag.

The prospect is to have a biocompatible, transparent material that can be injected into the bag after nuclear evacuation and that will allow compression and expansion, with ciliary body contraction transmitted via the intact zonules. Then, permanent tissue glue or a "plug" would close the capsulorrhexis. This sequence will allow a true rehabilitation of the senescent crystalline lens. Unfortunately, to date, that material and glue have yet to be developed and tested for use in humans.

Koopmans SA, Terwee T, Glasser A. Accommodative lens refilling in Rhesus monkeys. *Invest Ophthalmol Vis Sci.* 2006;47(7):2976–2984.

Nishi O, Nishi K. Accommodation amplitude after lens refilling with injectable silicone by sealing the capsule with a plug in primates. *Arch Ophthalmol.* 1998;116(10):1358–1361.

Advances in Energy Delivery

Technological advances have reduced the total amount of phaco energy delivered to achieve emulsification. This reduces the chances of incision burn.

Alcon Infiniti

Alcon (Ft Worth, TX) developed a series of alternatives to the longitudinal forward to-and-fro movements of traditional phacoemulsification. NeoSoniX technology produced a 2° clockwise-counterclockwise rotation of the tip at 100 Hz. The most current upgrade is OZil torsional technology, which incorporates a new handpiece capable of creating rotatory ultrasound movements of the phaco needle at 32 kilohertz (KHz) and longitudinal movements at 44 KHz. When combined with an angled phaco needle, these torsional movements create a side-to-side motion at the tip, enhancing the needle's cutting effectiveness with significantly reduced thermal energy generation. The to-and-fro movement at the tip allows emulsification on both excursions, with reduced repulsion of fragments, in contrast to longitudinal phacoemulsification. More efficient use of power results in less delivered energy and less heat, 2 of the goals of the new systems.

AMO Sovereign With WhiteStar

Digital "ultrapulsing" of ultrasound energy is a feature of the AMO Sovereign phacoemulsification system with WhiteStar technology (AMO, Santa Ana, CA). With digital ultrapulsing, the surgeon can select a duty cycle that allows sensitive control over the delivery of phaco power. By reducing the interval of phaco power delivery ("micropulsing"), the machine reduces total expended energy and heat production.

This marked reduction in heat has led to the use of *bimanual microphacoemulsification,* in which paracenteses are made, one for a small phaco needle without a surrounding irrigation sleeve and another to allow the introduction of instruments that provide irrigation, tear the capsule, complete the capsulorrhexis, hydrodissect, hydrodelineate, and chop. Bimanual microphacoemulsification is an advanced technique whose advantages will not be fully realized until IOLs that can be delivered through a 1.4-mm incision are widely available.

Alió JL, Rodriguez-Prats JL, Vianello A, Galal A. Visual outcome of microincision cataract surgery with implantation of an AcriSmart lens. *J Cataract Refract Surg.* 2005;31(8):1549–1556.

Bausch & Lomb Millennium

Millennium Microsurgical System (Bausch & Lomb, Rochester, NY) has a unique foot pedal that features dual-linear independent control of both aspiration and phaco power. High vacuum without commensurate phaco power permits chopping, with reduced total phaco power delivered. Custom Control Software (CCS) allows a choice of 5 ultrasound modes (continuous, pulse, single-burst, fixed-burst, and multiple-burst). In pulse mode, up to 120 pulses per second (PPS) are possible. The multiple-burst setting is capable of microburst (minimum 4 milliseconds [msec]), with a duty cycle limit that can be set to prevent continuous ultrasound even at full depression of the foot pedal. These features have allowed this platform to be used for bimanual microphacoemulsification.

STAAR Surgical Sonic WAVE

The Sonic WAVE phacoemulsification system (ultrasound alternative) (STAAR Surgical Company, Monrovia, CA) produces either sonic energy or ultrasound energy in a single unit. The Sonic WAVE blends low-frequency pulses (40–400 Hz) with new ultra vacuum technology. The CruiseControl chamber sequesters nuclear material from the aspiration line and reduces postocclusion surges. Again, higher vacuum permits nuclear dismantling with less power delivered during mechanical techniques such as chopping.

Fine IH, Packer M, Hoffman RS. Power modulations in new phacoemulsification technology: improved outcomes. *J Cataract Refract Surg.* 2004;30(5):1014–1019.

Alternate Technologies for Nucleus Removal

Sutureless Nonphaco Cataract Surgery

During the transition from ECCE to phacoemulsification, some surgeons developed techniques to extract the nucleus, either intact or in manually segmented pieces, preserving the smaller scleral tunnel incision. The procedure has continued to find advocates in developing countries.

Fry LL. The phacosandwich technique. In: Rozakis GW, Anis AY, et al, eds. *Cataract Surgery: Alternative Small Incision Techniques.* Thorofare, NJ: Slack Inc; 1990:71–110.

Gutiérrez-Carmona FJ. *Phaco Without the Phaco: ECCE and Manual Small-Incision Techniques for Cataract Surgery.* Kent: Anshan; 2005.

Kansas P. Phacofracture. In: Rozakis GW, Anis AY, et al, eds. *Cataract Surgery: Alternative Small Incision Techniques.* Thorofare, NJ: Slack Inc; 1990:45–70.

Keener GT. The nucleus division technique for small incision cataract extraction. In: Rozakis GW, Anis AY, et al, eds. *Cataract Surgery: Alternative Small Incision Techniques.* Thorofare, NJ: Slack Inc; 1990:163–195.

Laser Photolysis

Currently, the only FDA-approved laser system for cataract extraction is the Dodick Photolysis, Q-switched Nd:YAG system (A.R.C. Laser Corp, Salt Lake City, UT). It generates laser shock waves at 200–400 nanoseconds that strike a titanium target at the end of the aspirating handpiece. The system includes Venturi fluidics and a touch-screen control panel; it also includes an ultrasound handpiece port for emulsifying cataracts that are too dense for laser phacoemulsification.

Water Jet Phacolysis

The AquaLase Liquefaction Device is a water jet–based instrument that is available from Alcon (Ft Worth, TX) in the company's Infiniti System. With this system, 4-µL pulses of warmed BSS are delivered through a polymer tip to delaminate lens material without longitudinal rotary mechanical movement of the instrument. The polymer tip is soft and less likely to rupture posterior capsule than are metal phaco tips.

These technologies have been used for the removal of nuclei of modest grades of density. Their adoption may be limited as a result of the advances in the delivery of controlled phaco power discussed earlier.

Antimicrobial Prophylaxis

As endophthalmitis remains one of the worst complications of cataract surgery (see Chapter 9, Complications of Cataract Surgery), one goal of the preoperative preparation and intraoperative management of the patient is to reduce the introduction of pathogenic organisms into the anterior chamber.

Before Surgery

Preoperatively, the surgeon should identify and reduce infectious risk factors as much as possible—for example, through preoperative treatment of coexisting eyelid disorders such as conjunctivitis, blepharitis, hordeolum, or chalazion. An ocular prosthesis in the fellow eye may harbor bacteria, warranting evaluation of the socket and cleaning of the prosthesis prior to surgery. Systemic infections should be identified and treated before elective surgery. Immunocompromised patients may warrant administration of systemic antibiotics (such as oral fluoroquinolones) before and immediately after surgery.

Patients with cardiac valvular disease or orthopedic joint replacements may ask about the need to take systemic antibiotics before cataract surgery. Cataract surgery is not considered to be an invasive procedure that induces transient bacteremia, and antibiotic prophylaxis is not required.

Although no studies convincingly demonstrate the efficacy of topical antibiotics in reducing the risk of endophthalmitis in routine cataract surgery, some evidence supports an association between the use of preoperative topical antibiotics and a reduction in ocular surface bacterial counts, as well as a lower incidence of positive aqueous cultures after surgery. Many cataract surgeons give their patients topical antibiotics as prophylaxis before surgery; the dosage varies from administration for 2–3 days preoperatively to frequent dosing just prior to surgery.

Dajani AS, Taubert KA, Wilson W, et al. Prevention of bacterial endocarditis: recommendations by the American Heart Association. *JAMA*. 1997;277:1794–1801.

In Surgery

In the operating room, sterilization of the fornix has become an important goal. A 5% solution (not scrub or soap) of povidone-iodine placed in the conjunctival fornix prior to surgery has been associated with a reduction in bacterial colony counts cultured from the ocular surface at the time of surgery and a decreased risk of culture-proven endophthalmitis. In addition, preparation of the skin around the eye with a 5%–10% povidone-iodine solution reduced bacterial counts on the eyelid margins. If a patient is allergic to iodine, dilute alcohol, an alternate antiseptic such as Techni-Care (Care-Tech Laboratories, Inc, St Louis, MO), or saline may be used for skin preparation only. Extreme care should be paid to prevent corneal exposure to potentially toxic agents (eg, chlorhexidine). As lid margins may harbor pathogens, care should be taken to drape the lashes out of the operative field (Fig 8-32).

It is important not only to limit the number of times that instruments are introduced into the eye but also to check for signs of lint, cilia, and other debris on the tips of all instruments inserted. It is wise to reduce intraoperative manipulation as well. Meticulous wound closure is imperative. Despite all of these efforts, the conjunctiva may harbor

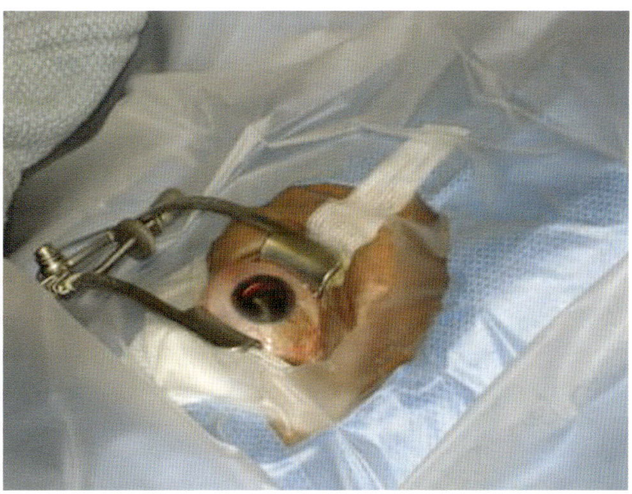

Figure 8-32 Sterile draping with lid margin coverage. *(Courtesy of Ken Mitchell, MD.)*

residual bacteria. Studies have documented that 7%–35% of cataract surgeries result in bacterial inoculation of the anterior chamber. That endophthalmitis is infrequent is a testament to the ability of the anterior chamber to clear itself of a potentially pathologic inoculum.

The surgeon should also recognize that the risk of endophthalmitis increases with a torn posterior lens capsule, vitreous loss, and prolonged surgery. Some surgeons place antibiotics in the irrigating solution or inject them into the anterior chamber at the end of surgery. A significant reduction in endopthalmitis with the use of intracameral cefuroxime has been reported. The injection of antibiotics under the conjunctiva or Tenon's capsule is an option as well. However, aminoglycosides should be avoided because of the risk of macular infarction after subconjunctival use.

Conflict surrounds the possibility of an increased risk of endophthalmitis after nonsutured clear corneal temporal approach cataract surgery. It has been shown that hypotony may cause the nonsutured incision to allow inflow of tear contents into the eye. For this reason, hydrating the stroma and leaving a slightly firm eye at the end of the case may reduce the risk of wound separation. Any question about wound leakage should prompt the use of suture closure.

After Surgery

Use of antibiotic eyedrops is often continued or instituted after routine cataract surgery. Although reduced bacterial counts have been documented with the administration of topical antibiotics, no clear-cut evidence has been presented to confirm a reduced incidence of endophthalmitis with their use.

Cooper BA, Holekamp NM, Bohigian G, Thompson PA. Case-control study of endophthalmitis after cataract surgery comparing scleral tunnel and clear corneal wounds. *Am J Ophthalmol.* 2003;136(2):300–305.

Miller JJ, Scott IU, Flynn HW Jr, Smiddy WE, Newton J, Miller D. Acute-onset endopthalmitis after cataract surgery (2000–2004): incidence, clinical settings, and visual acuity outcomes after treatment. *Am J Ophthalmol.* 2005;139(6):983–987.

Seal DV, Barry P, Gettinby G, et al. ESCRS study of prophylaxis of postoperative endophthalmitis after cataract surgery: case for a European multicenter study. *J Cataract Refract Surg.* 2006;32(3):396–406.

Modification of Preexisting Astigmatism

Cataract surgery has been called the most commonly performed refractive procedure in ophthalmology. Certainly, elimination of spherical refractive error through meticulous lens implant calculations is possible. Any preoperative astigmatism may be considered for reduction at the time of cataract surgery.

Because a cataract can induce refractive astigmatism, it is important for the surgeon to compare the preoperative refractive cylinder with K readings. If the refractive cylinder matches the power and axis by keratometry, cataract-induced astigmatism is negligible, and the refractive cylinder can be considered for reduction through surgery. Any discrepancy may be analyzed through computerized corneal imaging. If questions remain, it is wiser to defer astigmatism reduction until stable refractions are obtained in the postoperative period.

Surgical planning for refractive cataract surgery includes consideration of incision size and location, postoperative astigmatism reduction with photorefractive corneal surgery, intraoperative and postoperative limbal relaxing incisions, and use of toric IOLs. (Also see Section 13, *Refractive Surgery*).

Incision Size and Location

One prerequisite is to create a small incision that does not induce any corneal astigmatism. If a larger incision is required, placing it across the steeper axis of curvature may reduce preoperative astigmatism.

Astigmatic Keratotomy

Astigmatic keratotomy (AK) is a technique surviving from the incisional corneal refractive era (refractive keratotomy). Within the cornea, paired incisions were placed at varying distances from the apex of the steepest corneal meridian in order to decrease the curvature of that meridian and to increase the curvature of the meridian 90° away ("coupling"). Glare from spread of the incisional scar toward the pupil is a potential problem for the cataract surgical patient, for whom postoperative quality of vision is paramount. Any infection near the center of the cornea has serious consequences. For these reasons, AK has largely been supplanted by limbal relaxing incisions.

Limbal Relaxing Incisions

Limbal relaxing incisions (LRIs) have been advocated as an effective method for reducing 0.5–4.0 diopters (D) of astigmatism. Because of their placement at the limbus, LRIs have the potential advantage of preserving the optical qualities of the cornea, inducing less postoperative glare, minimizing discomfort, reducing overcorrections, and allowing quicker recovery of vision.

Surgeons planning to use a surgical technique that is unfamiliar to them should consider taking courses and performing practice surgeries. To improve outcomes, the surgeon should select a nomogram and track postoperative refractive results.

Before any injection anesthetic is given to the patient, the 6 and 12 o'clock meridians are marked in 1 of 2 ways, with the patient sitting upright: with a 25-gauge needle in the corneal epithelium; or with a spot, made by a purple skin marker, at the limbus. The steep axis is then identified with use of these landmarks or other natural landmarks if they exist. An incision is made at the limbus radially across the steep axis. One or more incisions are made depending on the nomogram of the surgeon's choosing. Some surgeons place the cataract incision within the LRI; others prefer to use a separate location. LRIs may also be done postoperatively in an office setting.

Budak K, Freidman NJ, Koch DD. Limbal relaxing incisions with cataract surgery. *J Cataract Refract Surg*. 1998;24(4):503–508.

Gills JP. *A Complete Guide to Astigmatism Management*. Thorofare, NJ: Slack, Inc; 2003.

Nichamin LD. Opposite clear corneal incisions. *J Cataract Refract Surg*. 2001;27(1):7–8.

Toric IOLs

Toric IOLs are designed to correct astigmatism. The *STAAR Toric* IOL (STAAR Surgical Company, Monrovia, CA), approved by the Food and Drug Administration (FDA) in 1998, was the first toric IOL available in the United States. Made of silicone, the STAAR Toric IOL is a plate-style lens, with an axis mark and large positioning holes on each plate that allow posterior and anterior capsule to fuse within the hole, reducing rotation of the lens. The IOL comes in 2 lengths: 10.8 mm and 11.2 mm. The labeled cylinder powers of 2.0 D and 3.5 D at the IOL plane achieve reduction of 1.4 D and 2.3 D at the corneal plane after implantation.

The FDA approved the *AcrySof Toric* IOL by Alcon in September 2005. This is a 1-piece acrylic lens with the toric power placed on the posterior surface of the IOL and with axis markings located at the base of each haptic to help the surgeon with alignment of the lens after implantation in the bag. The lens is available in 3 cylindrical powers that effect a correction of between 1.03 D and 2.06 D at the corneal plane.

The advantage of toric IOLs is the avoidance of extraincisional complications. In addition, better standardization of correction occurs with the IOLs than with incisional correction. The disadvantages of the toric IOL relate to possible lens rotation away from the desired axis. Rotation may be more likely when the IOL is implanted in a larger capsular bag. Each degree of rotation reduces the effect of astigmatism correction by approximately 3% and may induce higher-order aberrations. If needed, a second procedure to rotate the lens to the correct axis should be done early in the postoperative period before complete capsular fixation of the lens occurs.

Sun XY, Vicary D, Montgomery P, Griffiths M. Toric intraocular lenses for correcting astigmatism in 130 eyes. *Ophthalmology*. 2000;107(9):1776–1782.

Special Circumstances

Cataract Surgery in the Patient Taking Anticoagulants

Certain cataract surgery patients are at high risk of thromboembolic events and are under treatment with antiplatelet agents and/or anticoagulants. Studies have shown that intraocular hemorrhagic events are rare in patients maintained on anticoagulants and that medical complications are rare in patients who stop their treatment before surgery. The decision either to continue or to stop these agents should be made on an individual basis with advice from the patient's internist or general physician. All cataract surgeons should be competent to diagnose and manage conjunctival hematoma, retrobulbar hemorrhage with a tight orbit, and intraoperative choroidal hemorrhage (see Chapter 9, Complications of Cataract Surgery, and Chapter 10, Cataract Surgery in Special Situations).

Katz J, Feldman MA, Bass EB, et al. Risks and benefits of anticoagulant and antiplatelet medication use before cataract surgery. *Ophthalmology*. 2003;110(9):1784–1788.

Kearon C, Hirsh J. Management of anticoagulation before and after elective surgery. *N Engl J Med*. 1997;336(21):1506–1511.

Cataract Surgery in the Patient Taking Tamsulosin

Patients, particularly older men, should be asked about use of medication to help urine flow. Tamsulosin (Flomax) and other α_{1a}-adrenergic antagonists have been associated with the intraoperative floppy iris syndrome (IFIS). This syndrome is manifested by a pupil that may not dilate fully and may constrict during cataract surgery. The iris may billow and prolapse through the incision. The risk of capsule rupture and vitreous loss is increased. Strategies for management include the use of Healon 5, preoperative pupillary dilatation with atropine, intracameral epinephrine, iris hooks, and low aspiration flow rates. See Chapter 9, Complications of Cataract Surgery, for further discussion.

Chang DF, Campbell JR. Intraoperative floppy iris syndrome associated with tamsulosin. *J Cataract Refract Surg*. 2005;31(4):664–673.

Use of Capsule Staining

A continuous curvilinear capsulorrhexis is the gold standard for modern phacoemulsification. By backlighting the anterior capsule tear with the red reflex, the clinician can more easily create the CCC. The red reflex can be obtained via retroillumination with the operating microscope. However, when the red reflex is poor or absent (as in white cataracts, dense brunescent cataracts, anterior cortical or subcapsular cataracts, vitreous hemorrhage, and asteroid hyalosis), visualizing the anterior capsule tear can be a challenge. In these cases, staining the anterior capsule allows better visualization. When the capsule is stained, a stark contrast exists between it and the nonstained anterior subcapsular surface. For a discussion of dyes and other details, see Chapter 10, Cataract Surgery in Special Situations.

Use of Pupillary Expansion

A small, nondilatable pupil makes modern phacoemulsification and IOL implantation difficult. In the past, iris surgery was performed before lens extraction. Surgery may have included multiple sphincterotomies, radial iridotomy, or sector iridectomy. These techniques created permanent distortion of the pupil and reduced reactivity to light and accommodation. To reduce postoperative dysfunction, the technique of stretching the pupil using micro hooks placed 180° apart was developed; each hook can be placed under the iris margin and retracted to the limbal incision, thereby stretching the sphincter and resulting in an enlarged pupil. The procedure is used at the 12 and 6 o'clock positions and then the 3 and 9 o'clock positions. Alternatively, polypropylene iris hooks (Grieshaber, Schaffhausen, Switzerland) can be placed through paracenteses and used to expand the pupil; they are kept in place until after phacoemulsification and lens implantation are completed.

Another technique involves using one of many pupil expanders (eg, Graether Pupil Expander [Eagle Vision, Memphis, TN]; Morcher Pupil Dilator [Morcher, Stuttgart, Germany]; Beehler Iris Expander [Moria Instruments, Doylestown, PA]; Perfect Pupil [BD Ophthalmic Systems, Franklin Lakes, NJ]). Microscopic sphincter tears may be seen postoperatively with use of these techniques.

The term *viscomydriasis* describes the use of a cohesive OVD such as Healon 5 (AMO, Santa Clara, CA) to increase pupil size immediately before capsulorrhexis or during a later stage of phacoemulsification. A poorly dilating pupil should be identified before surgery so that strategies and equipment are available to the surgeon for that patient.

Capsulorrhexis Issues

Another problem that may be encountered during capsulorrhexis creation may relate to a crowded anterior segment, as seen in hyperopia, intumescent lenses, nanophthalmos, and pseudoexfoliation. A shallow chamber results in a more anterior summit of the lens, which requires the surgeon to make the cystitome or forceps cut "downhill," possibly making control difficult. A shallow chamber may be treated with the use of a cohesive OVD (eg, Healon 5), pupil expansion, or, for resistant cases, a pars plana removal of vitreous (see discussion under "Posterior Capsule Rupture").

An additional problem encountered during creation or propagation of the tear is loss of the chamber. There are several possible causes of this loss, including an incision that is too large, leakage of OVD, pressure from the lid speculum, blepharospasm, choroidal effusion or hemorrhage, and aqueous misdirection. If the wound is too large, it can be partially closed with a suture that will still allow introduction of the phaco tip and sleeve. OVD can be reinjected to deepen the chamber. A tight speculum can be adjusted. Blepharospasm can be controlled with a facial nerve block. A firm eye with a shallow chamber may be caused by aqueous misdirection or choroidal hemorrhage.

Intraoperative indirect ophthalmoscopy helps differentiate among these complications. Aqueous misdirection will result in shallowing of the chamber without an abnormality in the posterior segment and may be managed by a pars plana removal of vitreous. Indirect ophthalmoscopy may help in confirming an effusion or hemorrhage. The case should be stopped if a choroidal hemorrhage is diagnosed.

Loose Zonules

Lens instability can vary from complete dislocation to subtle zonular weakness discovered only during surgery. Patients with a history of trauma or previous intraocular surgery, pseudoexfoliation syndrome, high myopia, Marfan syndrome, idiopathic ectopia lentis, or Weill-Marchesani syndrome should prompt the surgeon to prepare preoperatively for intraoperative management. Patients may demonstrate iridodonesis or phacodonesis, best seen through an undilated pupil. Ideally, these cases are best managed by surgeons who are experienced in the advanced techniques mentioned in this section.

If possible, the CCC should be started away from the identified weakness. This may reduce the tendency to extend the dislocation during the start of the capsulotomy. Intraoperative clues to an unexpected zonular weakness include a seemingly stiff anterior capsule on cystitome tearing, a bag that appears to move as the anterior capsule tear is advanced, a nucleus that snaps back after being spun, a sudden deepening of the anterior chamber, or an abnormal displacement of the nucleus on grooving or on securing a purchase for chopping.

Modified iris hooks (Mackool Capsule Support System [FCI Ophthalmics, Marshfield Hills, MA]) are available that support the capsular bag by stabilizing the rim after the capsulorrhexis. Also available to stabilize and support the capsular bag are capsular tension rings (CTRs) (Fig 8-33), made by various manufacturers. They can be inserted before or after phacoemulsification, with either strategy having advantages and disadvantages. Insertion, either with forceps or a "shooter," requires skill since injury to the iris, capsulorrhexis rim, or posterior capsule can occur. CTRs are contraindicated in cases with radial tears or with posterior capsule rupture. In cases where zonular weakness is likely to continue after surgery (eg, pseudoexfoliation), a CTR is available with an eyelet to be sutured ab interno to the sclera, preventing late displacement.

Capsular placement of a posterior chamber lens can be performed after complete removal of the cataract and stabilization and centration of the capsular bag with a CTR. Alternatively, sulcus fixation or suture fixation to the iris or sclera can be used, as can an ACIOL.

Goldman JM, Karp CL. Adjunct devices for managing challenging cases in cataract surgery: pupil expansion and stabilization of the capsular bag. *Curr Opin Ophthalmol.* 2007; 18(1):44–51.

Hasanee K, Ahmed I. Capsular tension rings: update on endocapsular support devices. *Ophthalmol Clin North Am.* 2006;19(4):507–519.

Mature Cataracts

Mature cataracts are lenses so opaque that visualization of the posterior lens capsule is prevented. Types of mature cataracts include dense nuclear sclerotic cataracts (brunescent) and softer white cataracts. Both types deserve capsule staining. The surgeon should always retain the option to perform an ECCE or ICCE in cases with extremely dense nuclei. It may be prudent to prepare a small scleral shelf that will allow enlargement and use of a large-incision technique if phacoemulsification is unsuccessful.

Dense lenses should alert the surgeon to possible zonular weakness. Chopping techniques have the advantages of reducing cumulative phaco power and of avoiding pushing a dense lens into the capsular fornix, with resultant compromised zonular support.

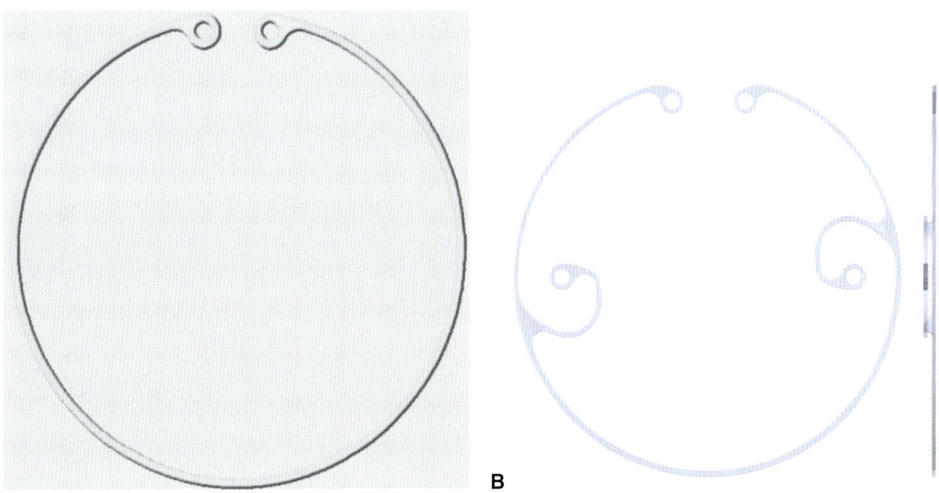

A B

Figure 8-33 **A,** Capsular tension ring (CTR). **B,** Eyelet for suture fixation. *(Courtesy of FCI Ophthalmics.)*

High-vacuum, low-power burst-mode settings may allow the phaco tip to penetrate enough to permit the use of horizontal or vertical chopping techniques. Advances in phaco technology (discussed previously) have resulted in shorter duty cycles and less heat production, reducing the risk of wound burn in these cases.

Soft opaque lenses may contain "lens milk," or liquefied cortex, that makes capsulorrhexis difficult. In these cases, after making the initial capsular tear, the surgeon may find it helpful to introduce the I/A handpiece for aspiration of the liquefied cortex before resuming completion of the tear. Dense lenses may have relative zonular weakness, and the surgeon should have mastered the techniques necessary to deal with capsular instability. Additional information can be found in Chapter 10.

Posterior Capsule Rupture

Every phaco or ECCE surgeon has encountered a ruptured posterior lens capsule. The management of a posterior capsule rupture should be a part of every surgeon's armamentarium. The rupture may occur early in the case from too vigorous a hydrodissection or late with insertion or rotation of the IOL. Suspicion of a posterior capsule tear should be aroused by a sudden, subtle deepening of the anterior or posterior chamber, a loss of aspiration ability when lens material is separated from the tip by vitreous, excessive movement of the nucleus, or a focal sharp red reflex zone within a section of sculpted nucleus.

Once a ruptured posterior lens capsule is discovered, it is important to avoid anterior chamber collapse with resultant forward movement of the vitreous. The surgeon should immediately return to foot position 1. Before removing the phaco needle, the surgeon should instill a dispersive OVD through the side port.

After the phaco needle is removed, an analysis of the amount and position of retained lens material should be made. Special care should be paid to preventing loss of nuclear material through the posterior capsule tear into the posterior segment. A decision should be made about whether to continue use of a small-incision technique or whether to enlarge the incision for an ECCE-like removal of lens material.

If significant nuclear material is present anterior to the tear, one small-incision technique that may be used involves elevation of the fragments with further OVD injection and insertion of a trimmed lens glide through the phaco incision and through the pupil to slide under the retained lens material. The phaco needle can then be re-inserted. With the bottle height lowered and low flow settings selected, emulsification of fragments over the glide can be performed. Cortex may be removed with I/A in the same fashion.

When nuclear material has fallen through the tear into the anterior vitreous, some beginning surgeons will perform the anterior vitrectomy, remove the cortex, and place a sulcus IOL but leave nucleus removal to a vitreoretinal colleague. More-experienced surgeons may use injection of an OVD such as Viscoat (Alcon) through a pars plana incision in order to center and elevate the fallen nuclear material. After making a conjunctival incision and measuring 3.5 mm posterior to the limbus, the surgeon uses a microvitreoretinal (MVR) blade (Alcon) to enter the vitreous cavity. The OVD cannula can be used to manipulate nuclear material into the posterior or anterior chamber. The surgeon can then perform phacoemulsification over a glide or remove material through a larger incision, using a loop.

After the retained lens nuclear material is removed, cleanup of vitreous and cortical material is accomplished via a 2-port anterior vitrectomy. Either an anterior or a posterior approach can be used. The irrigation flows through the paracentesis via a handheld or self-retained cannula. The vitrectomy guillotine cutter, now without the need for an irrigation sleeve, can be placed through the phaco incision, through a smaller additional paracentesis, or through the pars plana. The vitreous cutters available on most phaco machines will permit removal of vitreous and cortical material but not nuclear material. The irrigation bottle should be lowered, and aspiration and vacuum levels should be moderate; speeds from 200–800 cuts per minute may be selected. Use of high magnification will allow better visualization of the vitreous. Triamcinolone acetonide, preferably nonpreserved, can also be used to visualize the vitreous and allow better removal. Suture closure of the sclera over the pars plana incision is needed. A suture may also be required for the conjunctiva.

If an ECCE technique is to be used for removal of the lens material, the phaco incision can be carefully enlarged or a new incision constructed superiorly. A loop (and, if indicated, a glide) can be used to remove retained nuclear material. The incision can then be closed to the size of the original phaco incision. Vitreous and cortical cleanup is performed as outlined earlier.

If the visualization of the anterior chamber and the posterior chamber is good, lens implantation may proceed.

- If the posterior capsule tear is small and no zonular disinsertion is seen, a posterior chamber IOL (PCIOL) can be positioned with the haptics in the bag. If a large central posterior capsule tear is present, the optic can be gently pushed through the defect, with the haptics remaining in the bag.
- If the zonules are regionally and minimally compromised, the haptics of the PCIOL in the bag should be placed along the axis of the disinsertion in order to expand the bag in the region of the tear. A sufficiently large 3-piece IOL should be available for use, especially in patients with larger eyes. If enough zonules are significantly compromised, a CTR can be inserted before the PCIOL is implanted.
- A ciliary sulcus position can be chosen in the presence of a large posterior capsule defect and adequate anterior capsule support.
- The haptics of a longer 3-piece PCIOL can be sutured either to the iris or through and to the sclera, under a small scleral flap.
- An ACIOL (see the section Intraocular Lens Implantation) can be used if the capsule has been globally compromised.

Successful application of the skills discussed in this section to solving the problems at hand requires experience, preparedness, and stability.

Condon GP. Iris-sutured PCIOLs. *Cataract & Refractive Surgery Today*. May 2004:68–71.

Hu BV, Shin DH, Gibbs KA, Hong YJ. Implantation of posterior chamber lens in the absence of capsular and zonular support. *Arch Ophthalmol*. 1988;106:416–420.

Kwong Y, Yuen H, Lam R. Comparison of outcomes of primary scleral-fixation versus primary anterior chamber intraocular lens implantation in complicated cataract surgeries. *Ophthalmology*. 2007;114(1):80–85.

Osher RH, Snyder ME, Cionni RJ. Modification of the Siepser slip-knot technique. *J Cataract Refract Surg.* 2005;31(6):1098–1100.

Siepser S. The closed-chamber slipping suture technique for iris repair. *EyeWorld.* July 1997:3.

Stark WJ, Goodman G, Goodman D, Gottsch J. Posterior chamber intraocular lens implantation in the absence of posterior capsular support. *Ophthalmic Surg.* 1988;19:240–243.

Pars Plana Lensectomy

The posterior approach to lens extraction is performed through the pars plana, generally in combination with vitrectomy. See also BCSC Section 12, *Retina and Vitreous.*

Indications

The presence of a significant cataract with the urgent need for pars plana vitrectomy and/or retinal surgery is the general indication for this approach. Following trauma with lens rupture and vitreous disruption, this single approach is the best way to clean all of the vitreous and lens material from the eye. A pars plana approach may also facilitate removal of retained foreign bodies and management of perforating injuries. Crystalline lens removal may be essential in procedures for anterior proliferation of the hyaloid and in cases requiring anterior dissection of the vitreous for detachments with proliferative vitreoretinopathy. A posterior approach may be desirable in cases of symptomatic lens subluxation.

Contraindications

The most common contraindication for this approach is a nucleus too hard to be removed by this technique. A dense brunescent lens may be unsuitable for fragmentation through the pars plana; it may be preferable for the cataract surgeon to use an anterior approach and remove the lens first. Either combined surgery or sequential surgery may be performed.

Intraocular Lens Implantation

Historical Perspectives

Before 1949, cataract surgery resulted in aphakia, and patients were destined (unless highly myopic) to wear high hyperopic spectacles that were of considerable weight and that caused image magnification and distortion to the sides. Scleral contact lenses and eventual corneal contact lenses were used when available and possible.

The development of modern IOL implantation began in 1949. Harold Ridley, an English ophthalmologist, observed that PMMA fragments from airplane cockpit windshields were well tolerated in the anterior segment of the eyes of injured World War II pilots. He placed a disk-shaped PMMA lens into the posterior chamber of a 45-year-old woman after he performed an ECCE (Fig 8-34).

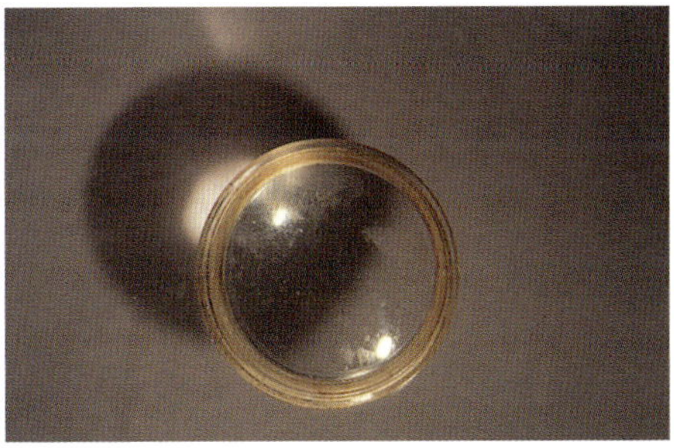

Figure 8-34 Original Ridley lens, first implanted by Harold Ridley in November 1949. *(Courtesy of Robert C. Drews, MD.)*

Ridley's lens corrected aphakic vision, but a high incidence of postoperative complications such as glaucoma, uveitis, and dislocation caused him to abandon his lens design. Though frustrated in his attempts, Ridley showed foresight in 3 important areas. First, he constructed his original lens of PMMA in a biconvex design. Second, he used extracapsular surgery for implantation of the lens. Third, he placed the lens in the posterior chamber. Ridley set the stage for a period of advances in cataract surgery that continues to this day, and he was knighted for his contributions.

Ophthalmologists in the 1950s were troubled by the serious complications associated with early IOL styles and by the fact that nearly all of the investigative work was done in humans, occasionally with very little scientific basis. Uncertainty concerning the long-term success and stability of these lenses limited their use. Yet the desire to manage aphakia without the problems and inconvenience of aphakic spectacles or contact lenses continued to inspire investigation into IOL implantation.

Extracapsular cataract surgery in the 1950s was crude by modern standards and was generally associated with retained lens cortex, which caused fibrosis and adhesions between iris and capsule. ICCE eliminated residual cortical material and became the preferred procedure. Because ICCE was more commonly performed in the early days of lens implantation, IOLs of that period featured optics with loops, struts, or holes for sutures required for fixation to the iris for support (Fig 8-35).

The anterior chamber angle was an alternate site for support of an IOL. The first ACIOLs (Fig 8-36) were rigid, and some patients complained of tenderness postoperatively. Fitting the length of the lens to the width of the chamber was difficult. The IOL length was selected by estimating anterior chamber width based on the horizontal corneal diameter. Because such estimation is crude even with modern instruments, complications arose. Oversized lenses and closed-loop IOLs caused pupillary distortion and contributed to uveitis-glaucoma-hyphema syndrome. ACIOLs that were too short would spin, decenter, and contact the corneal endothelium.

Complications associated with rigid ACIOLs spurred the development of the flexible-loop ACIOL. Additional advances included open support arms with 4-point fixation (Fig 8-37); these modifications have allowed ACIOLs to remain a treatment choice for cases with compromised capsular bags or for secondary IOL insertion.

As a result of the conversion to modern ECCE, IOL designs changed to allow placement in the posterior chamber and support from the lens capsule. ACIOLs were largely

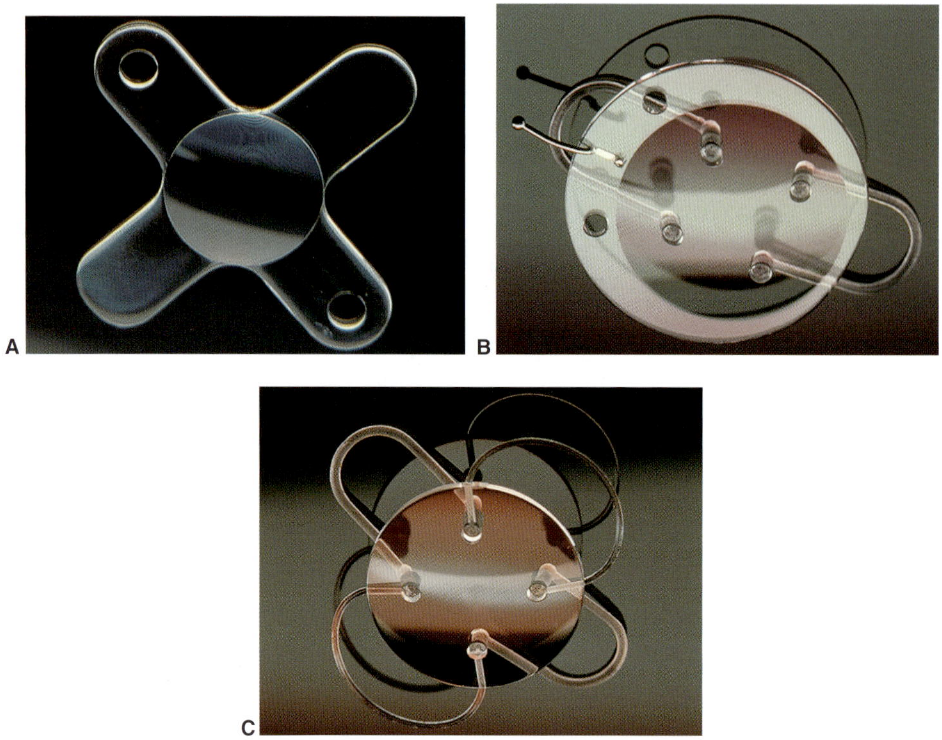

Figure 8-35 IOL styles for intracapsular surgery. **A,** Epstein lens made by Copeland; iris-supported with 2 opposing haptics placed anterior and posterior to the iris. **B,** Medallion lens with platinum clip designed by Worst; lens was implanted with polypropylene haptics posterior to the iris at 6 and 12 o'clock; peripheral iridectomy was made, and the platinum clip was bent back against the superior haptic to secure the lens against dislocation. **C,** Original iris-fixated lens designed by Fyodorov, as made in the United States; 2 looped haptics were placed posterior to the iris, and the optic and 2 opposing loops were placed anterior to the iris. *(Courtesy of Robert C. Drews, MD.)*

relegated to a backup role when capsule support was absent or when other problems precluded implantation of a PCIOL.

Apple DJ, Mamalis N, Olson RJ, et al. *Intraocular Lenses: Evolution, Designs, Complications, and Pathology*. Baltimore: Williams & Wilkins; 1989.

Posterior Chamber IOLs

The desire to place the IOL in the lens capsule was the impetus to expand research into posterior chamber lens implantation. Shearing took a flexible version of a 3-piece IOL that had closed loops and modified it by opening the loops and inserting the haptics into the capsular bag for posterior chamber placement. Subsequent modifications of this lens by Pierce, Sinskey, and Shearing allowed ECCE with posterior chamber lens implantation to become the standard for modern cataract surgery. The discovery that viscous sodium hyaluronate could protect the endothelium from critical damage during IOL implantation was a turning point in the acceptance of IOLs.

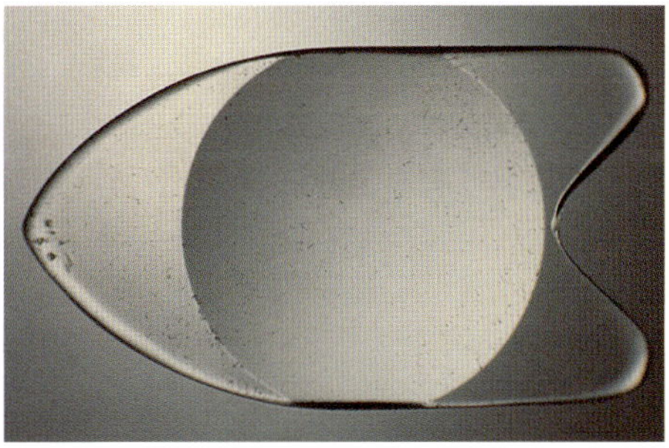

A

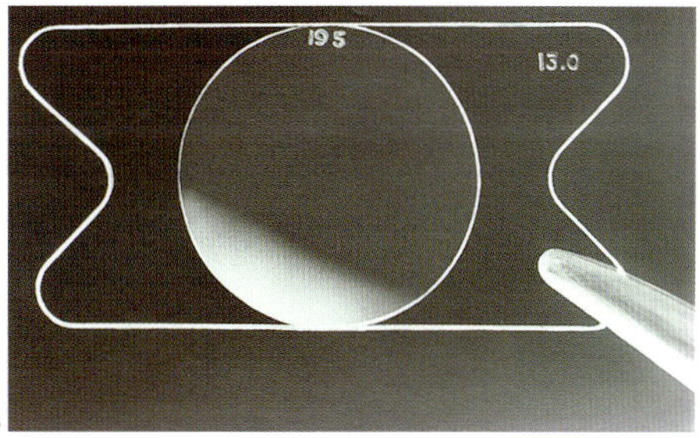

B

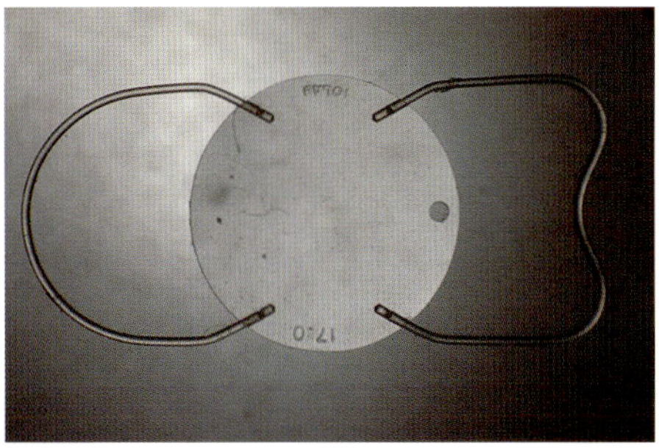

C

Figure 8-36 Early anterior chamber lens designs. **A,** Angle-supported lens designed by Strampelli; used from 1950 to 1955. **B,** Mark VIII lens designed by Choyce; rigid lens was implanted in anterior chamber angle either as a secondary lens implant or primarily after intracapsular cataract surgery. **C,** Azar 91Z lens; designed to be placed with rounded haptic in inferior chamber angle and notched haptic in superior chamber angle, with lens vaulted anteriorly. *(Courtesy of Robert C. Drews, MD.)*

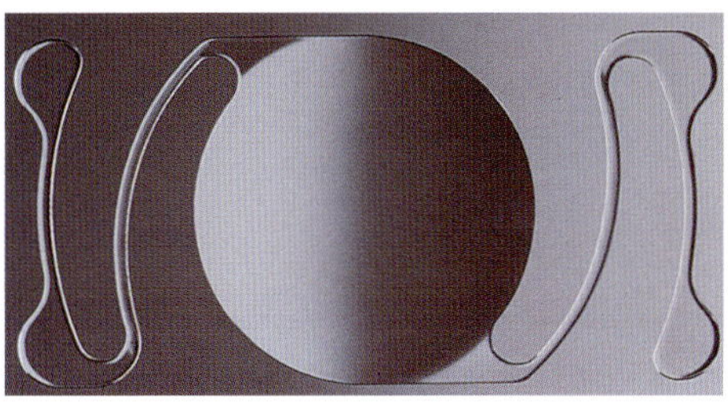

Figure 8-37 Kelman ACIOL with flexible 4-point fixation. *(Courtesy of Robert C. Drews, MD.)*

IOL optic geometry has evolved from the earlier plano-convex models to the newer biconvex design. Numerous changes in the shape of the posterior IOL surface and edge design were advanced to reduce late opacification of the posterior lens capsule and to facilitate laser capsulotomy. Other lens modifications include the incorporation of UV-absorbing chromophores into the material of the IOL to protect the retina from UV radiation. Special purpose lenses, such as those designed specifically for suture fixation in the ciliary sulcus, were also developed. These lenses have eyelets molded into the inside curve of the haptics to facilitate suture attachment. Other types of special-use IOLs include lenses designed with opaque flanges to decrease glare in clinical conditions such as aniridia and iris coloboma.

Mazzocco is generally given credit for developing a foldable IOL. His plate-style lens design (Fig 8-38) is still used for the correction of astigmatism at the time of cataract surgery and influenced the design of phakic refractive IOLs (see BCSC Section 13, *Refractive Surgery*). Foldable versions of the Shearing-style lens (Fig 8-39) soon followed. The obvious advantage of the foldable lens design is that it allows implantation of the IOL through a small incision. The availability of a small-incision lens was the factor that influenced

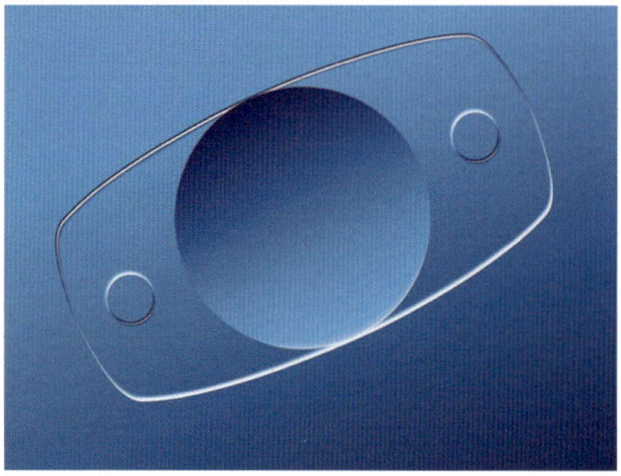

Figure 8-38 Mazzocco plate lens. *(Courtesy of STAAR Surgical.)*

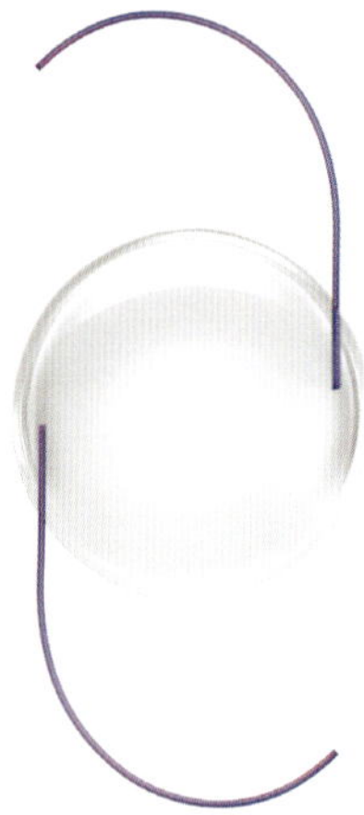

Figure 8-39 Modern 3-piece PCIOL. *(Courtesy of Bausch & Lomb Surgical.)*

the majority of ECCE surgeons to convert to using phacoemulsification. Although various materials have been evaluated, most foldable lenses are currently manufactured from either silicone or acrylic materials.

Although either silicone or acrylic materials are suitable for most patients, problems have been reported with silicone IOLs in patients undergoing vitrectomy with silicone oil injection. When cataract surgery is to be performed in a patient who is likely to require vitreoretinal surgery in the future (eg, a patient with high myopia, retinal detachment in fellow eye, or proliferative retinopathy), an IOL material other than silicone is preferred.

Hollick EJ, Spalton DJ, Ursell PG, et al. The effect of polymethylmethacrylate, silicone, and polyacrylic intraocular lenses on posterior capsular opacification 3 years after cataract surgery. *Ophthalmology.* 1999;106(1):49–54.

Multifocal Lenses

One of the drawbacks of IOLs as a replacement for the human crystalline lens has been the fixed focus of the IOL. Surgeons have had to ask their patients whether, after cataract surgery, they would prefer to see up close or in the distance without glasses. To address this issue, multifocal IOLs that provide refractive correction for both near and distance vision are available.

The original multifocal IOL concept was based on the principle that the pupil tends to constrict for near tasks, so the central portion of the lens was designed for near and the outer portion for distance. The obvious disadvantage is that distance correction is not available when bright lights constrict the pupil. Present designs address this problem by having central and outer zones for distance correction and intermediate zones for near. Other designs are supposed to move anteriorly with accommodative effort to allow near focusing. A combination of geometric optics and diffraction optics can also achieve a multifocal effect. The long-term effects of multifocal lenses are under investigation. The FDA has approved the following multifocal lenses for use in the United States:

- *AcrySof ReSTOR* (Fig 8-40) (Alcon, Ft Worth, TX) uses a central series of blended diffractive zones (apodized diffractive surface) designed to focus light from distant, intermediate, and near objects. Surgeons have reported that patients have acceptable distance and near vision with this lens, although intermediate vision may be less acute.
- *ReZoom* (Fig 8-41) is a multifocal aspheric refractive IOL that distributes light over 5 optical zones to provide near, intermediate, and distance vision. Its manufacturer, Advanced Medical Optics, brought the first multifocal IOL (Array) to the US market in the mid-1990s. The ReZoom lens, a second-generation multifocal, was approved by the FDA in March 2005. Surgeons have reported that patients have acceptable distance and intermediate-range vision with this lens.
- *Crystalens* (Fig 8-42) (Eyeonics, Inc, Aliso Viejo, CA) gained FDA approval in late 2003. The lens optic is attached to supportive flanges. Each flange has a "hinge" designed to allow the optic to move anteriorly with accommodative effort and to move posteriorly with accommodation relaxed. Patients have reported variability in achieving emmetropia and satisfactory accommodative range.

The advantages of these lenses include an increased range of vision with reduced dependence on glasses. The drawbacks of multifocal IOLs include reductions in contrast sensitivity and best-corrected visual acuity and the presence of glare and halos (see also BCSC Section 3, *Clinical Optics*). More "chair time" needs to be spent counseling these patients. Multifocal IOLs require very accurate biometry and IOL power calculations, and they may work best when implanted bilaterally in patients with minimal astigmatism. Patients with hyperopia may be less bothered by some visual aberrations than are patients with myopia. It is strongly recommended that a special consent process be used with this technology. The surgeon should have a strategy in place for managing postoperative residual refractive errors, including possible IOL exchange, performed preferably before capsular fibrosis increases the difficulty of explantation.

Javitt JC, Steinert RF. Cataract extraction with multifocal intraocular lens implantation: a multinational clinical trial evaluating clinical, functional, and quality-of-life outcomes. *Ophthalmology*. 2000;107(11):2040–2048.

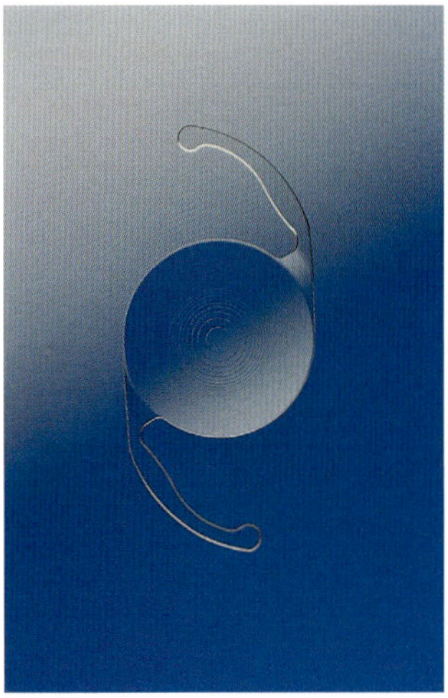

Figure 8-40 AcrySof ReSTOR lens. *(Courtesy of Alcon Laboratories, Inc.)*

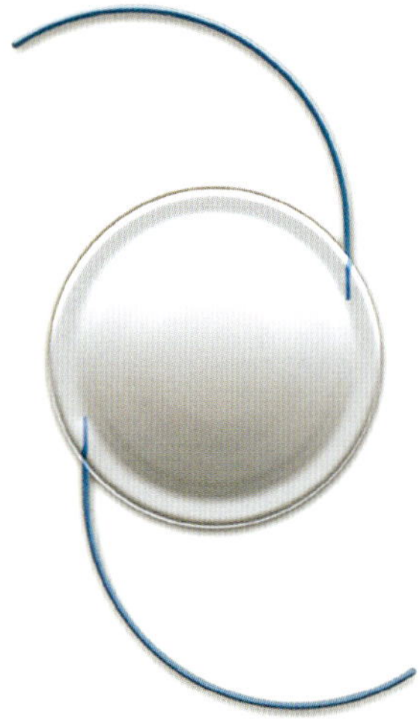

Figure 8-41 AMO ReZoom lens. *(Courtesy of Advanced Medical Optics, Inc.)*

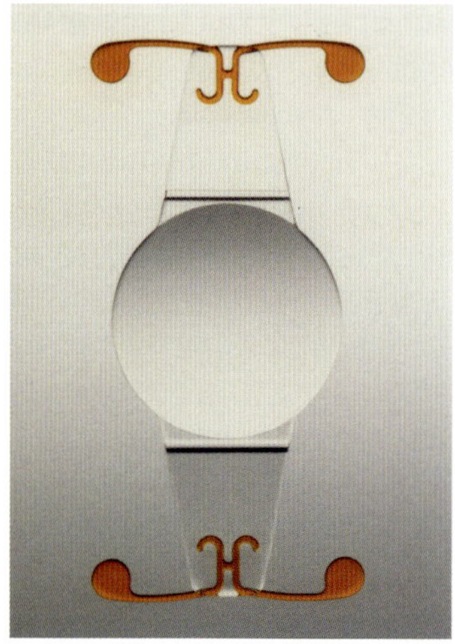

Figure 8-42 Crystalens. *(Courtesy of Eyeonics, Inc.)*

Nichamin LD. IOL update: new materials, designs, selection criteria, and insertion techniques. *Focal Points: Clinical Modules for Ophthalmologists*. San Francisco: American Academy of Ophthalmology; 1999, module 11.

Rocha KM, Chalita MR, Souza CE, et al. Postoperative wavefront analysis and contrast sensitivity of a multifocal apodized diffractive IOL (ReSTOR) and three monofocal IOLs. *J Refract Surg*. 2005;21(6):S808–812.

Other Designs

IOLs have been designed, theoretically, to limit higher-order aberrations and to improve the quality of vision in low-contrast settings. AMO offers the *TECNIS* IOL, which features an aspheric surface, a sloping side edge to reduce internal reflections, and a square edge posteriorly to limit posterior capsule opacification. This lens is available in either silicone or acrylic. Alcon (Ft Worth, TX) features its *AcrySof IQ* IOL, which is an aspheric acrylic lens with chromophores that filter both UV and blue light. Bausch & Lomb markets the *SofPort Advanced Optics (AO) Model LI61* IOL, which has prolate aspheric surfaces and is designed to reduce spherical aberrations.

Although lenses with *UV chromophores* have been standard for several decades, a blue blocker has been added to Alcon's series of acrylic posterior chamber lenses. Blue-blocking IOLs attenuate blue-wavelength light (400–460 nm). Proponents cite potential protection from blue-light exposure to the macula. Others are concerned about potential problems that these lenses might create with scotopic vision. Researchers are evaluating a light-adjustable silicone IOL that allows noninvasive postoperative adjustment of refractive power. Long-term studies will help clarify the role that these lenses may play in the future.

Schwartz DM. Light-adjustable lens. *Trans Am Ophthalmol Soc*. 2003;101:417–436.

IOL Power Determination

In the last decade, there were significant improvements in the accuracy with which the surgeon determined the IOL power required to achieve emmetropia. The development of better instrumentation for measuring the eye's axial length (AL) and the use of more precise mathematical formulas to perform the appropriate calculations contributed to these improvements. Even with this technology, the surgeon should have a basic understanding of the relationship between the patient's previous refractive state and each of the measurement parameters in order to avoid errors in calculation. To quickly calculate the approximate IOL power needed to achieve emmetropia, start with a power of 18 D, add to it the patient's refractive state before any lenticular myopia developed, and multiply by 1.6 (use negative numbers for myopia and positive numbers for hyperopia). If these calculations are very different from those obtained with ultrasonic axial biometry, the surgeon must look for an explanation (eg, posterior staphyloma).

The mathematical formulas used to calculate the appropriate IOL power are based on the refracting power of the cornea, the anticipated postoperative distance between the anterior surface of the cornea and the anterior surface of the IOL (anterior chamber depth), and the AL of the eye. The refracting power of the cornea is determined with the keratometer or by optical coherence biometry (IOLMaster; discussed later in this section). Anterior chamber depth is estimated from measurements made on eyes with implants similar to the style of IOL to be used, or it is measured with the IOLMaster. The AL is the distance between the anterior surface of the cornea and the fovea as measured by A-scan ultrasonography or optical coherence biometry. "*A* constants" for each IOL are specified by the manufacturer. The constant is a theoretical value that relates the lens power to AL and keratometry. The *A* constant is not expressed in units and is specific to the design of the IOL and its intended location and orientation within the eye.

A-scan ultrasonography is performed with either a contact applanation transducer or an immersion technique (Fig 8-43). In the immersion technique, a shell is placed on

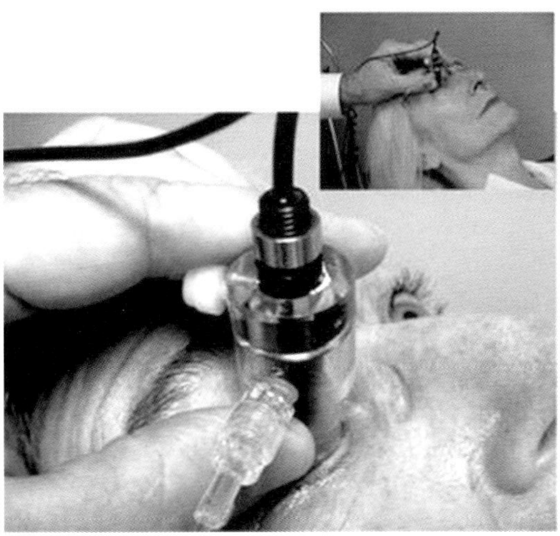

Figure 8-43 Immersion shell (Prager design). *(Courtesy of ESI, Inc.)*

the eye, between the eyelids, and provides a water bath over the cornea. The transducer is mounted in the shell. With the contact applanation method, the examiner must be careful not to compress the cornea, because corneal compression results in an artificially shortened AL measurement. Though generally not clinically significant in the patient with an "average" refraction, such errors become more important in the patient with high hyperopia, in whose short eyes (AL 20 mm or less) each millimeter of error in measured AL results in up to 3.75 D of IOL error. The immersion technique avoids this problem.

It should be remembered that ultrasonic AL measurement is actually determined by calculation. The ultrasonic biometer measures the transit time of the ultrasound pulse and, using estimated ultrasound velocities through the various media (cornea, aqueous, lens, and vitreous), calculates the distance. This concept needs to be taken into consideration in situations in which velocities differ from the norm. For example, in performing AL measurements in a patient with silicone oil in the posterior chamber, the clinician must take into account different transit times: 980 m/sec for silicone oil versus 1532 m/sec for vitreous. In addition, the index of refraction of silicone oil is significantly less than that of vitreous, and thus the refractive index of the oil (as well as the design of the IOL) must be figured into IOL calculations for these eyes. To ensure that errors have not occurred, it is helpful for the surgeon to compare measurements between both eyes of the patient. Any significant disparity in required IOL power should result in a check of the data.

The IOLMaster (Carl Zeiss Meditec, Dublin, CA) is a device that uses optical coherence biometry instead of ultrasound. It is a noncontact technology that measures the AL, keratometry, anterior chamber depth, and horizontal white-to-white distance. Although the device can yield rapid measurements with sensitivity 8 to 10 times those of ultrasound, doing so requires patience and cooperation on the part of both the patient and the technician operating the device. Because it is an optical device, the IOLMaster can be confounded by corneal scarring, mature or posterior subcapsular cataracts, or vitreous hemorrhage.

Hill WE. The IOLMaster. *Techniques in Ophthalmology*. 2003;1:62–67.

Preventing errors in IOL calculation, selection, and insertion

A technician who performs biometry should be trained on the machine he or she will use. The A-scan transducer should be calibrated before each day's use. Several scans should be done on each patient, and the measurements should cluster around a value with no more than 0.2-mm variance. Both eyes should be checked, especially if the first eye measures longer or shorter than anticipated. The intereye difference should be no greater than 0.3 mm unless there is a refractive explanation. The surgeon should make sure that the correct patient name and K readings, as well as AL and white-to-white measurements, are written on an IOL form. Also, the appropriate lens power and manufacturer's model number should be selected. In addition, lenses and powers for placement in the bag, sulcus, or anterior chamber angle should be selected and carefully distinguished on the sheet.

This sheet should be brought to surgery and a copy left with the surgeon's technician in the office in the event that any details need to be confirmed by phone from the operating room. The operating room circulator should pull the lenses before the patient enters the operating room. The surgeon should verify the correct lenses from the IOL calculation sheet and should perform a final check before opening the lens just prior to insertion.

IOL calculation

Regression formulas are empiric formulas generated by averaging large numbers of postoperative clinical results. Regression formulas are used to predict the appropriate IOL power for emmetropia. The following formula—developed by Sanders, Retzlaff, and Kraff in the 1980s (SRK formula)—will serve as illustration of IOL calculation.

$$P = A - (2.5L) - 0.9K$$

where

P = lens implant power for emmetropia (diopters)
L = axial length (mm)
K = average keratometric reading (diopters)
A = constant specific to the lens implant to be used

Newer versions of regression formulas have been developed that have been helpful in calculating lens implant power in eyes outside the range of 22–25 mm in length (eg, SRK/T, Holladay 2, Hoffer Q, Haigis).

Fang JP, Hill WE, Wang L, Chang V, Koch DD. Advanced intraocular lens power calculations. Kohnen T, Koch DD, eds. In: *Cataract and Refractive Surgery*. Berlin: Springer-Verlag; 2006: chap 4, pp 31–48.

Hill WE. Choosing the right formula. doctor-hill.com. Available at www.doctor-hill.com.

Hoffer KJ. Modern IOL power calculations: avoiding errors and planning for special circumstances. *Focal Points: Clinical Modules for Ophthalmologists*. San Francisco: American Academy of Ophthalmology; 1999, module 12.

Narváez J, Zimmerman G, Stulting RD, Chang DH. Accuracy of intraocular lens power prediction using the Hoffer Q, Holladay 1, Holladay 2, and SRK/T formulas. *J Cataract Refract Surg*. 2006;32(12):2050–2053.

Prager TC, Hardten DR, Fogal BJ. Enhancing intraocular lens outcome precision: an evaluation of axial length determinations, keratometry, and IOL formulas. *Ophthalmol Clin North Am*. 2006;19(4):435–448.

Improving outcomes

Surgeons should track their refractive outcomes and make adjustments as necessary. Are there overcorrections or undercorrections, and do they occur more often with longer eyes, shorter eyes, or both? Does the incision induce cylinder? Are the toric lenses correcting as calculated? Do the LRIs match nomogram predictions? Commercially available programs (eg, Holladay IOL Consultant) may be useful for tracking outcomes.

After the surgeon has analyzed these factors, he or she may improve outcomes by including a “surgeon factor” (a modification of the parameters used in lens calculation that reflects the surgeon’s experience), changing calculation software, or using immersion biometry or an IOLMaster. Improving outcomes is important for patient satisfaction and surgeon confidence.

IOL calculation following refractive surgery

Cataract extraction following refractive surgery poses special problems for the patient and the surgeon. These patients were initially motivated to have refractive surgery because they did not want to be dependent on glasses. They do not want to wear glasses after cataract surgery. However, the corneal change they incurred as a result of refractive surgery complicates accurate keratometry, a key element of lens implant power calculation. For example, post-cataract refractive outcomes in patients who had radial keratotomy (RK) were often fraught with undercorrections.

Neither manual keratometers nor videokeratography measures curvature directly but rather calculates the curvature of the anterior cornea. Following corneal refractive surgery, the cornea becomes aspheric and does not maintain a spherocylindrical contour. This asphericity invalidates the anterior corneal curvature measurements available by either type of device.

Compounding this problem of anterior surface measurement is the role played by the posterior corneal surface. Although RK did not change the relative positions of the anterior and posterior corneal surfaces, such is not the case following photorefractive keratectomy (PRK) or laser in situ keratomileusis (LASIK). For these reasons, different techniques must be employed to estimate accurately the anterior corneal surface curvature following refractive surgery. Technologies that measure both anterior and posterior corneal curvatures (eg, Pentacam [Oculus, Inc, Lynwood, WA]; Orbscan IIz [Bausch & Lomb Surgical, San Dimas, CA]) can improve accuracy.

Whenever several different methods are available for calculating the same value, advantages and disadvantages exist for each method. Each surgeon should use more than one technique and compare the IOL powers obtained by different methods. Selecting the highest IOL value of a tightly clustered group may avoid undercorrection.

Contact lens method The contact lens method uses a plano hard contact lens with known base curve to determine the corneal power. Corneal power is calculated as the sum of the contact lens base curve, power, and overrefraction minus the spherical equivalent of the manifest refraction without a contact lens. This method is applicable only to patients capable of at least 20/80 vision. The contact lens method, though logical, has not yet been validated through clinical studies.

Topographical method This strategy (after Maloney) uses a topography machine (Humphrey ATLAS CT System [Carl Zeiss Meditec, Dublin, CA]) to select the apical axial curvature:

$$\text{Central keratometric power} = (\text{Central topographic power} \times 376/337.5) - 4.9$$

Smith RJ, Chan WK, Maloney RK. The prediction of surgically induced refractive change from corneal topography. *Am J Ophthalmol.* 1998;125(1):44–53.

Historical methods If the patient's pre–refractive surgery data are available, the surgeon can use one of several historical methods to calculate the desired IOL power.

One historical method (after Hoffer) involves calculating the corneal power from the refractive and keratometry measurements made before and after the patient's refractive surgery. Thus, this method requires access to accurate preoperative records. The formula is

$K1$ + (sph equiv 1) – (sph equiv 2) = $K2$

where

$K1$ = average corneal power before refractive surgery
sph equiv 1 = spherical equivalent refractive error before refractive surgery
sph equiv 2 = spherical equivalent refractive error after refractive surgery but prior to cataract development
$K2$ = estimated corneal power after refractive surgery

Another historical method (after Feiz and Mannis) calculates the IOL power from the pre–refractive surgery data and then increases this power by a factor related to the amount of refractive change in the spectacle plane produced by the refractive surgery:

IOL pre–refractive surgery – (change in refraction/0.7) = IOL desired for patient

A potential problem with certain regression formulas in post–refractive surgery cases is that reduced central corneal power may be linked in the formula to an anterior chamber depth that is assumed to be less than it is, resulting in the calculation of a lower IOL power than is really required. The Holladay 2 formula includes pre-refractive corneal data that may correct for this error. Otherwise, the keratometric value may be modified so that undercorrections are reduced.

Each cataract patient who has undergone previous corneal refractive surgery should be informed of potential problems with accurate IOL selection. Overcorrections and undercorrections should be mentioned along with the possible need for IOL exchange, further corneal refractive surgery if feasible, or the need for spectacle or contact lens correction. Documenting this discussion is extremely important.

Aramberri J. Intraocular lens power calculation after corneal refractive surgery: Double-K method. *J Cataract Refract Surg*. 2003;29(11):2063–2068.

Feiz V, Mannis MJ, Garcia-Ferrer F, et al. Intraocular lens power calculation after laser in situ keratomileusis for myopia and hyperopia: a standardized approach. *Cornea*. 2001;20:792–797.

Hamed AM, Wang L, Misra M, Koch DD. A comparative analysis of five methods of determining corneal refractive power in eyes that have undergone myopic laser in situ keratomileusis. *Ophthalmology*. 2002;109:651–658.

Hill, WE. Determining corneal power following keratorefractive surgery. doctor-hill.com. Available at www.doctor-hill.com.

Seitz B, Langenbucher A, Nguyen NX, Kus MM, Küchle M. Underestimation of intraocular lens power for cataract surgery after myopic photorefractive keratectomy. *Ophthalmology*. 1999;106(4):693–702.

Wang L, Booth MA, Koch DD. Comparison of intraocular lens power calculation methods in eyes that have undergone LASIK. *Ophthalmology*. 2004;111(10):1825–1831.

Phakic IOLs

This topic is discussed in Section 13, *Refractive Surgery*.

Techniques of Lens Implantation

PMMA IOLs may be safely handled with standard fine smooth forceps for insertion. Insertion forceps often have longer tips than do tying forceps to help in positioning the lens across the anterior chamber.

Silicone and acrylic IOLs must be handled more gently than PMMA IOLs. Surgeons implanting a foldable lens use a variety of instruments to hold the IOL in its folded position during insertion. These instruments are of 2 general designs: (1) an injection tube that fits into the small incision and injects the IOL through the tube to unfold in the eye; (2) molded forceps that hold the folded IOL as it slides through the small incision.

Procedure

The microscope should be adjusted to give a full-field view of the eye. The globe is positioned so that the lens can be inserted and optimal access to and visibility of the anterior chamber, lens capsule, and incision are ensured.

The incision size must be large enough to accommodate the IOL. Larger incisions for intracapsular or extracapsular surgery are generally closed with sutures so that the appropriate opening size is obtained, whereas smaller incisions from phaco surgery may need to be enlarged if the IOL to be implanted is not folded. An OVD or air is used to stabilize the anterior chamber depth and to protect the corneal endothelium from contact with the IOL.

Posterior chamber IOL implantation

PMMA posterior chamber IOLs may be secured within the capsular bag or in front of the capsule within the ciliary sulcus. An OVD is injected either between the anterior and posterior capsules to open the capsular bag or between the iris and anterior capsular remnant for ciliary sulcus support. The IOL is advanced through the incision, with the leading haptic placed into position first. The IOL optic is then brought into the pupil, and the trailing haptic is flexed and placed into position or "dialed" with slight posterior pressure (rotated clockwise, so that the second haptic slides under the anterior capsule following the edge of the optic) under the anterior capsular rim of the CCC. With other types of capsule openings, such as a can-opener capsulotomy, visualizing the anterior capsule for precise placement of the trailing haptic may be more difficult.

Foldable IOLs with haptics are inserted in the capsular bag with insertion forceps or an injector, after OVD injection, and then allowed to open in situ. For those foldable lenses with haptics, the leading haptic is slowly pushed under the edge of the anterior capsular rim into position within the capsular bag. The optic follows and the trailing haptic is placed, with forceps or with dialing, under the rim of the anterior capsule. Similar steps are used to place the lens in the ciliary sulcus. *Plate haptic IOLs* must be inserted in a capsular bag protected by a CCC. The IOL position can be adjusted with a hook, and the lens may be rotated carefully to achieve adequate centration. Slight indentation of the sclera just posterior to the limbus should flex the plate without significantly altering centration. The surgeon then aspirates the OVD to minimize the risk of postoperative IOP rise. The anterior chamber depth is adjusted with BSS.

Several techniques have been described for securing a PCIOL behind the iris with sutures when capsular support is inadequate. Polypropylene sutures should be used instead of nylon sutures because nylon degrades over time, and lens dislocation may result. Transscleral polypropylene sutures may be used to secure the IOL haptics in the ciliary sulcus (see Chapter 9, Complications of Cataract Surgery, for a discussion of dislocation). Polypropylene sutures may also be used to attach PCIOL haptics to the overlying iris.

Sutured PCIOLs are most valuable as an alternative to ACIOL implantation in situations where an angle-supported lens might be considered problematic, such as with an angle compromised by peripheral anterior synechiae. Suture fixation techniques are more difficult than standard implantation and are associated with a greater risk of complications (such as vitreous hemorrhage, dislocation, lens tilt, or late endophthalmitis).

Osher RH, Snyder ME, Cionni RJ. Modification of the Siepser slip-knot technique. *J Cataract Refract Surg.* 2005;31(6):1098–1100.

Anterior chamber IOL implantation

Anterior chamber IOLs are supported by the chamber angle and are generally flexible. Modern 4-point fixation flexible ACIOLs are acceptable for use when posterior chamber implantation is not feasible. It is common practice to use 1 mm plus the horizontal diameter of the limbus, as measured externally with a caliper (white to white) or IOLMaster, to determine the appropriate length for the ACIOL.

A phaco incision must be enlarged with the keratome or with corneal scissors to allow ACIOL insertion. The pupil is generally constricted pharmacologically prior to IOL implantation. At least 1, and often 2, peripheral iridectomies are created to avoid pupillary block. The anterior chamber depth is stabilized, and the corneal endothelium is protected with OVD or air. A lens glide may be inserted across the anterior chamber into the distal angle to protect the iris from the advancing IOL haptic. The surgeon then inserts the IOL, placing its leading haptic into the angle while observing the iris for any indication of distortion. As the IOL is held against the distal angle stabilized with forceps, the glide is withdrawn, and the posterior lip of the incision is gently retracted to allow placement of the trailing haptic in the angle. Visual inspection should confirm the proper insertion of the trailing haptic. The surgeon can adjust IOL position by using a hook to flex the optic toward either angle for repositioning.

The pupil will peak toward any area of iris "tuck," and the IOL should be repositioned until the pupil is round and the optic is centered. Light indentation of the sclera axial to the lens position should flex the IOL haptic without significant decentration of the optic, movement of the pupil, or rotation of the lens. The OVD is aspirated and the chamber depth adjusted with BSS. The incision is carefully closed with nylon sutures.

Secondary IOL Implantation

When spectacles or contact lenses are unsatisfactory for correction of aphakia, secondary IOL implantation is indicated. The type of cataract surgery performed and the general condition of the anterior segment determine the appropriate style and technique of lens implantation.

The cornea, angle, iris, and vitreous should be studied carefully before secondary lens implantation. Pachymetry, gonioscopy, and/or endothelial cell counts may be advisable before surgery.

The pupil is constricted with preoperative miotic eyedrops or intraoperative acetylcholine (Miochol-E [Novartis Pharmaceuticals, East Hanover, NJ]) for secondary ACIOL implantation. Factors that influence selection of an incision site (superior versus temporal) include preexisting astigmatism, iris anatomy, conjunctival scarring, and corneal vascularization. An anterior vitrectomy may be needed to remove any vitreous incarcerated in the wound or adherent to the iris. Synechiae that will interfere with the positioning of the IOL may be dissected. A lens glide may be useful during insertion of anterior or posterior IOLs, and the anterior chamber depth needs to be stabilized with an OVD. The positioning of secondary IOLs is similar to that described for primary lenses but may be more difficult because of scarring from the cataract surgery.

Relative Contraindications to Lens Implantation

The surgeon must determine whether the support structures within the eye are adequate to maintain centration and stability of the IOL for the type of lens fixation anticipated. If the angle is not open and available for ACIOL implantation, a sutured PCIOL is necessary. Although proliferative diabetic retinopathy and other retinal disorders were formerly considered relative contraindications, prospective studies have shown that these conditions are not adversely affected by PCIOL implantation that maintains an intact posterior capsule.

Corneas with Fuchs dystrophy can be further assessed with endothelial cell counts and pachymetry. If the values are near normal, phacoemulsification with dispersive OVD, Balanced Salt Solution Plus (BSS+), and PCIOL implantation are strategies for minimizing further endothelial loss with surgery.

However, patients with central corneal thickness greater than 640 μm or evidence of stromal or epithelial edema may require a combined penetrating keratoplasty: penetrating keratoplasty and phacoemulsification with IOL insertion ("triple procedure"). Alternatively, cataract surgery may be followed by endothelial or penetrating keratoplasty. (See also BCSC Section 8, *External Disease and Cornea.*)

Ford JG, Karp CL. *Cataract Surgery and Intraocular Lenses: A 21st-Century Perspective.* 2nd ed. Ophthalmology Monograph 7. San Francisco: American Academy of Ophthalmology; 2001.

Outcomes of Cataract Surgery

Contemporary cataract surgery has an excellent success rate, in terms of both improving visual acuity and enhancing subjective visual function. More than 90% of otherwise healthy eyes achieve a best-corrected postoperative visual acuity of 20/40 or better. The rate of achieving a postoperative acuity of 20/40 or better for all eyes has been reported to be 85%–89% when eyes with comorbid conditions such as diabetic retinopathy, glaucoma, and age-related macular degeneration are included.

Visual acuity is but one measure of the functional success of cataract surgery. Research tools have been developed to assess how cataract progression and cataract surgery affect visual function. One of these, the VF-14 instrument, is a questionnaire administered to patients to measure functional impairment related to vision before and after cataract surgery. Another research tool, the Activities of Daily Vision Scale (ADVS), is a measure of vision-specific functional status.

Prospective studies using these tools show that patients who undergo cataract surgery have significant improvement in many quality-of-life parameters, including community and home activities, mental health, driving, and life satisfaction. Among patients with bilateral cataracts, the quality of life improves after cataract surgery on the first eye as well as the second eye. A reduction in falls and hip fractures has been documented in patients after cataract surgery.

Of course, any operation may expose patients to potential risks and complications (see Chapter 9, Complications of Cataract Surgery). However, modern cataract surgery has lessened the burden of visual loss for millions of people worldwide, and it is a remarkable story that continues to evolve.

Brenner MH, Curbow B, Javitt JC, Legro MW, Sommer A. Vision change and quality of life in the elderly. Response to cataract surgery and treatment of other chronic ocular conditions. *Arch Ophthalmol.* 1993;111:680–685.

Harwood RH, Foss AJ, Osborn F, Gregson RM, Zaman A, Masud T. Falls and health status in elderly women following first eye cataract surgery: a randomized controlled trial. *British J Ophthalmol.* 2005;89(1):53–59.

Javitt JC, Brenner MH, Curbow B, Legro MW, Street DA. Outcomes of cataract surgery. Improvement in visual acuity and subjective visual function after surgery in the first, second, and both eyes. *Arch Ophthalmol.* 1993;111(5):686–691.

Mangione CM, Phillips RS, Lawrence MG, Seddon JM, Orav EJ, Goldman L. Improved visual function and attenuation of declines in health-related quality of life after cataract extraction. *Arch Ophthalmol.* 1994;112(11):1419–1425.

Powe NR, Schein OD, Gieser SC, et al. Synthesis of the literature on visual acuity and complications following cataract extraction with intraocular lens implantation. Cataract Patient Outcome Research Team. *Arch Ophthalmol.* 1994;112:239–252.

Steinberg EP, Tielsch JM, Schein OD, et al. National study of cataract surgery outcomes. Variation in 4-month postoperative outcomes as reflected in multiple outcome measures. *Ophthalmology.* 1994;101:1131–1141.

Steinert RF, Brint SF, White SM, Fine IH. Astigmatism after small incision cataract surgery. A prospective, randomized, multicenter comparison of 4- and 6.5-mm incisions. *Ophthalmology.* 1991;98(4):417–423.

Appendix

For a more in-depth discussion of the various topics mentioned in the Appendix, please see the appropriate sections in this chapter.

The Modern Intracapsular Cataract Surgical Procedure

Patient preparation

After informed consent is obtained, the patient's pupil is maximally dilated. A local anesthetic is administered. Orbital massage by digital pressure or compressive devices may be used to decrease the pressure effect that administration of extra anesthetic can have on the eye. Some surgeons use mannitol to decrease the orbital and vitreous volume; mannitol should be used with caution in patients with congestive heart failure, diabetes mellitus, or kidney failure. The patient should have a chance to void before transport to the operating room.

Procedure

After the skin and ocular surface have been prepared and draping has been completed, an eyelid speculum is placed between the eyelids. A suture is usually required to hold the eye in a slight downward position. The surgeon can accomplish this step by placing a 6-0 silk suture beneath the superior rectus tendon or within sclera and securing the suture to the superior drape.

Incision The surgeon creates either a fornix-based or a limbal-based conjunctival flap. Battery-powered or wet-field cautery is typically used for hemostasis. A scleral support ring may be needed in young patients or in those with high myopia to avoid scleral collapse when the lens is extracted; in patients with deep-set eyes, the ring may be needed to improve exposure.

Once 160°–180° of the corneoscleral limbus has been exposed, incision placement varies according to surgeon preference and patient need. More anterior or corneal incisions may be of shorter chord length and involve less bleeding. However, their closure induces central corneal steepening in the meridian of the incision. Incisions that are more posterior heal faster and, when covered by a conjunctival flap, are more comfortable to the patient. Posterior incisions induce less astigmatism and are less damaging to the corneal endothelium, but they cause more bleeding.

Sutures are pre-placed across the incision and looped out of the way; their presence allows rapid closure of the eye in case of choroidal hemorrhage, patient valsalva, or other instances of positive posterior pressure. An additional suture may be placed through the anterior wound lip only, allowing the assistant to elevate the cornea to facilitate lens delivery.

Iridectomy and cataract delivery An iridectomy is performed at this point. If the eye has a small pupil, the surgeon can consider performing sector iridectomy, radial iridotomy, or multiple sphincterotomies or using iris hooks or pupil expanders.

α-Chymotrypsin, if available, can be injected via a cannula through the pupillary space into the posterior chamber. An iris retractor can be used to expose the superior surface of the lens. A cellulose sponge is used to dry the anterior lens capsule. The cryoprobe is positioned on the lens surface, and the foot pedal of the cryoprobe is depressed. Once an iceball has formed, gentle maneuvers are used to deliver the lens. Sometimes the iris retractor or a cellulose sponge can be used to strip the vitreous from the posterior surface of the lens during delivery (Fig 8-44). Vitreous loss, combined with the larger incision of intracapsular surgery, contributes to posterior scleral collapse. Thus, every cataract surgeon should have as a part of his or her armamentarium—especially for intracapsular surgery—strategies to manage vitreous loss. "Open sky" approach or use of automated vitrectors are two such strategies.

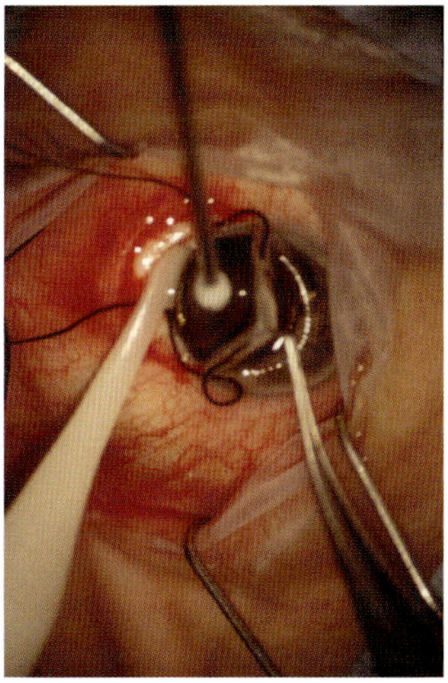

Figure 8-44 Intracapsular cataract extraction. A freezeball begins to form at the tip of the cryoprobe, which has been placed at the midperiphery of the lens. Wound edges are held clear of the cryoprobe. *(Courtesy of Lisa F. Rosenberg, MD.)*

A lens implant may be inserted at this point. An anterior chamber lens can be selected after instillation of acetylcholine (Miochol-E [Novartis]). Other lens implant options include posterior chamber lenses with either iris or scleral fixation suture support.

Fine sutures are used to close the incision while OVDs or BSS is used to keep the anterior chamber formed. The conjunctival flap is secured. Subconjunctival or sub-Tenon antibiotics or steroids can be used at this point. A patch and shield can be applied.

Postoperative course

On the first postoperative day, visual acuity should be consistent with the refractive state of the eye, the clarity of the cornea and media, and the visual potential of the retina and optic nerve. If the eye has been left aphakic, visual acuity can be estimated with a +10 to +12 D lens, or a +4 D lens can be used as a telescope. The surgeon should evaluate the cornea, the security of the incision, the depth of the anterior chamber, the degree of inflammatory reaction, and the IOP. The posterior segment should be visualized so that vitreous clarity and position can be judged and any retinal or optic nerve pathology noted.

It is not unusual to see a mild eyelid reaction with edema and erythema. The upper lid may be moderately ptotic. The conjunctiva is often mildly injected, and subconjunctival hemorrhage may be present. The cornea should be clear, but some superior edema is often present from the bending of the cornea during lens extraction. This edema generally resolves during the first postoperative week. The anterior chamber should have normal depth with mild to moderate cellular reaction. The pupil should be round, and the iridectomy patent. The anterior vitreous face location should be noted. A good red reflex should be present.

The postoperative course should be characterized by steady improvement of vision and comfort. Topical antibiotics and steroids are typically prescribed during the first postoperative weeks. The refraction generally becomes stable 6–12 weeks after intracapsular surgery, depending on the wound-closure technique employed. Because ICCE requires a larger incision, achieving a stable refraction usually takes longer than after ECCE or phaco techniques, which require smaller incisions.

The Modern Extracapsular Cataract Surgical Procedure

Patient preparation

The preparation for planned extracapsular cataract surgery is much like that for ICCE. Neither ocular massage nor hyperosmotics are as commonly used for ECCE as for ICCE. Pupillary dilation is critical to the success of ECCE.

Incision

Nucleus expression requires a limbal chord length of 8–12 mm, smaller than the incision needed for ICCE. The initial incision usually consists of a limbal groove, fashioned with a round-tipped steel blade, sharp microknife, or diamond knife. Some surgeons prefer a slightly more posterior incision with anterior dissection creating a scleral flap or tunnel. These incisions are typically placed superiorly. A stab incision is made under the flap into the anterior chamber in preparation for an anterior capsulotomy, and the cystitome is inserted to begin the procedure. The anterior chamber depth can be stabilized by OVDs, air bubble, or continuous fluid irrigation.

Anterior capsulotomy

The main function of the anterior capsulotomy is to permit removal of the cataract while leaving behind the intact capsular bag, which provides stabilization for the IOL that will be implanted. There are many techniques for opening the anterior capsule. A sharp cystitome or bent needle may be used to make a series of connected punctures or small tears in a circle to create the can-opener capsulotomy (see Fig 8-25A). Alternatively, the surgeon can create a smooth capsulorrhexis by making a puncture or small tear. The edge of this tear is then grasped with the cystitome tip or with forceps and pulled around smoothly, removing a circular portion of anterior capsule (see Fig 8-25B). This technique provides greater structural integrity for the lens capsule to maintain implant stability and centration. If a small capsulorrhexis is created and manual expression is planned, relaxing incisions are often made in the superior aspect of the capsulorrhexis to allow the nucleus adequate room to exit the capsule during expression. After the capsulotomy is completed, the incision is widened to allow safe passage of the nucleus through the incision. Anterior capsulotomy is discussed in greater detail in the section on phacoemulsification.

Nucleus removal Manual expression involves pressing on the inferior limbus to tip the superior pole of the nucleus up and out of the capsular bag. Additional counterpressure on the globe from an instrument holding the sclera posterior to the limbus 180° away from the incision will express the nucleus from the chamber. The surgeon removes the nucleus from the eye by loosening and elevating it from the capsule, with the use of a hook or irrigating cannula, and then supporting it on a lens loop, spoon, or vectis that will slide or irrigate it out of the chamber. Alternatively, the surgeon may fragment the nucleus while it is within the eye, using forceps or nucleus splitters to deliver it for removal in portions through a smaller incision.

The incision is partially sutured to allow deepening of the chamber with irrigation. Using the aspiration cannula, the surgeon then aspirates the lens cortex under direct visualization in the pupillary space. The posterior capsule may be polished with an abrasive-tipped irrigation cannula, wiped with a silicone-lined "squeegee," or vacuumed clean using low aspiration to remove epithelial and cortical particles from the capsule surface.

IOL insertion

Prior to IOL insertion, the anterior chamber is usually filled with an OVD. OVDs provide the most reliable anterior chamber maintenance along with protection of the corneal endothelium. A PCIOL may be inserted in the sulcus or in the capsular bag. Sulcus fixation usually requires an IOL with a larger overall diameter (at least 12.5 mm) and a large diameter optic (at least 6.0 mm), which is more forgiving in case of postoperative decentration.

If the surgeon wishes to insert the IOL in the capsular bag, an OVD is usually injected into the bag, with care being taken to separate the anterior capsule flap completely from the posterior capsule. Direct visualization of haptic insertion is critical.

Closure

The ECCE incision is typically closed with either multiple interrupted sutures of 10-0 nylon or with one long running suture. Proper suture tension helps reduce postoperative astigmatism; loose sutures cause astigmatism perpendicular to the axis of the suture, whereas tight sutures create astigmatism in the axis of the suture.

Postoperative course

As with ICCE, visual acuity on the first postoperative day should be consistent with the refractive state of the eye, the clarity of the cornea and media, and the visual potential of the retina and optic nerve. A mild eyelid reaction with edema and erythema may occur. The conjunctival flap may be injected and boggy, but it should not be elevated by fluid. The cornea may have some mild degree of edema. The anterior chamber should have normal depth, and a mild cellular reaction is typical. The posterior capsule should be clear and intact, and the implant should be well positioned and stable. The red reflex should be bright and clear. IOP elevations may be associated with retained OVD. Topical antibiotic and corticosteroid eyedrops are generally prescribed postoperatively.

The postoperative course should be characterized by steady improvement of vision and comfort, as the inflammatory reaction subsides during the first 2 weeks. The refraction is typically stable by the sixth to eighth postoperative week, and spectacles may then be prescribed. If a significant amount of postoperative astigmatism results along the axis of the sutures, the clinician can selectively remove the sutures as guided by wound stability, keratometry, or corneal topography.

CHAPTER 9

Complications of Cataract Surgery

Complications of cataract surgery are varied in timing as well as scope. They may occur intraoperatively or in the immediate or late postoperative period (Table 9-1). Therefore, it is necessary to observe the postoperative cataract patient at periodic intervals. A typical postoperative regimen consists of examining the patient 1 day, 1 week, about 1 month, and 3 months following cataract surgery. In case of complications or unusual clinical findings, more frequent examinations are indicated.

Jaffe NS, Jaffe MS, Jaffe GF. *Cataract Surgery and Its Complications*. 6th ed. St Louis: Mosby; 1997.

Krupin T, Kolker AE, eds. *Atlas of Complications in Ophthalmic Surgery*. London: Mosby–Year Book Europe, Ltd; 1993.

Corneal Edema

Stromal and/or epithelial edema may occur in the immediate postoperative period. The incidence is higher in eyes with preexisting corneal endothelial dysfunction such as Fuchs dystrophy. Edema is most often caused by a combination of mechanical trauma, prolonged surgery, inflammation, and elevated intraocular pressure (IOP), resulting in acute endothelial decompensation with an increase in corneal thickness. Toxic substances inadvertently introduced into the anterior chamber can also cause acute endothelial dysfunction. Small nuclear fragments retained in the anterior chamber angle may contribute to persistent focal corneal edema. Removing retained nuclear material may allow the corneal edema to resolve.

Edema from surgical trauma generally resolves completely within 4–6 weeks of surgery. If epithelial edema is present in the face of a compact stroma immediately after surgery, it is likely due to elevated IOP with an intact endothelium. Decreasing IOP via aqueous release from the paracentesis site often results in immediate resolution of epithelial edema in these cases. As a rule, if the corneal periphery is clear, the corneal edema will usually resolve with time. Corneal edema persisting after 3 months usually does not clear. Significant chronic corneal edema from loss of endothelial cells results in bullous keratopathy (Fig 9-1), which is associated with reduced visual acuity, irritation, foreign-body sensation, epiphora, and occasional infectious keratitis.

Table 9-1 Proportion of Eyes Experiencing Complications Following Cataract Surgery and Intraocular Lens Implantation

Complication	No. of Studies	Range of Complications Results (% of Eyes)	Total No. of Eyes	Pooled Result (% of Eyes)*
Major, early				
Endophthalmitis	16	0–1.9	30,656	0.13 (0.06–0.17)
Major, late				
Bullous keratopathy	27	0–6.0	15,971	0.3 (0.2–0.4)
Malposition/ dislocation of IOLs	40	0–7.8	17,944	1.1 (0.9–1.2)
Clinical cystoid macular edema	43	0–7.6	20,671	1.4 (1.2–1.6)†
Retinal detachment	42	0–2.0	33,603	0.7 (0.6–0.8)
Other, early				
Wound gape/iris prolapse	17	0–3.0	7499	0.6 (0.4–0.8)
Anterior chamber hemorrhage	19	0–4.0	7765	0.5 (0.4–0.7)
Hypopyon	10	0–2.0	3864	0.2 (0.1–0.2)
Iris trauma	8	0–9.1	5147	1.3 (1.0–1.6)
Zonular/posterior capsule rupture	38	0–9.9	19,052	3.1 (2.9–3.4)
Vitreous loss	26	0–4.0	14,622	0.8 (0.6–1.0)†
Vitreous hemorrhage	5	0–8.0	4386	0.3 (0.2–0.5)
Choroidal hemorrhage	3	0–2.0	3638	0.3 (0.1–0.5)
Other, late				
Uveitis	30	0–13.3	11,339	1.8 (1.5–2.1)†
Increased IOP (closed angle)	11	0–1.6	4391	0.2 (0.1–0.3)
Increased IOP (open angle)	34	0–19.7	11,376	1.2 (1.0–1.4)
Posterior capsular opacification	41	0.7–47.6	14,677	19.7 (19.1–20.3)

Note: This table is based on a synthesis of the literature and does not account for variation in follow-up intervals.

*Pooled result and 95% confidence interval (CI) weighted by sample size of studies.

†Pooled result and 95% CI weighted by quality score and sample size.

Reprinted from *Cataract in the Adult Eye.* Preferred Practice Patterns. San Francisco: American Academy of Ophthalmology; 1996. Original source: Powe NR, Schein OD, Gieser SC, et al. Synthesis of the literature on visual acuity and complications following cataract extraction with intraocular lens implantation. *Arch Ophthalmol.* 1994;112:239–252.

In its early stages, corneal edema after cataract surgery can be controlled by the use of topical hyperosmotic agents, topical corticosteroids, and, occasionally, bandage (therapeutic) contact lenses. Over time, subepithelial scarring may develop, resulting in a decrease in bulla formation and discomfort. Decreased visual acuity, recurrent infectious keratitis, and symptoms of pain are possible indications for penetrating or endothelial keratoplasty. The likelihood of obtaining a clear graft is high, but coexisting cystoid

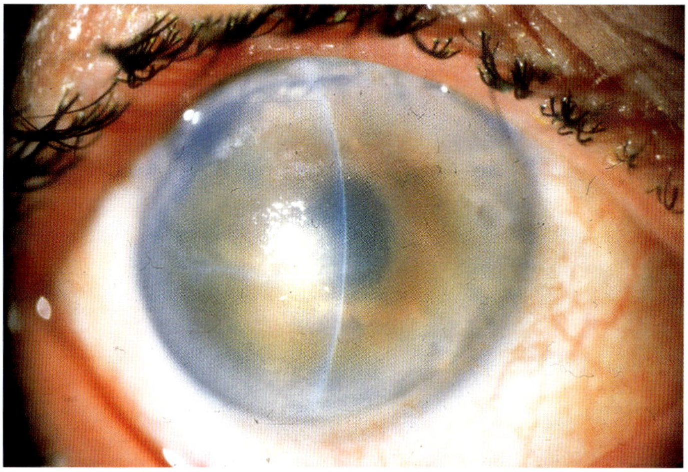

Figure 9-1 Pseudophakic bullous keratopathy. *(Courtesy of Karla J. Johns, MD.)*

macular edema (CME) may limit full recovery of visual acuity. Bulla formation and pain associated with bullous keratopathy may be alleviated with phototherapeutic keratectomy or anterior stromal micropuncture, but they may recur. Cautery of the corneal epithelium and anterior stroma can also reduce formation of bullae but could lead to bacterial keratitis or stromal melting. In the case of an eye with little or no visual potential, a Gundersen conjunctival flap or an amniotic membrane graft is an option that does not carry the greater risks of penetrating keratoplasty. (See also BCSC Section 8, *External Disease and Cornea.*)

Brown-McLean Syndrome

Brown-McLean syndrome, a clinical condition that may occur after cataract surgery, consists of peripheral corneal edema with a clear central cornea. This condition occurs most frequently following intracapsular cataract surgery, but it has also been reported following extracapsular and phacoemulsification surgery. The edema typically starts inferiorly and progresses circumferentially but spares the central cornea. Central corneal guttae (cornea guttata) frequently appear, and punctate brown pigment often underlies the edematous areas. In rare cases, Brown-McLean syndrome progresses to clinically significant central corneal edema. The etiology of this syndrome is unknown.

Brown SI, McLean JM. Peripheral corneal edema after cataract extraction. A new clinical entity. *Trans Am Acad Ophthalmol Otolaryngol.* 1969;73:465–470.

Gothard TW, Hardten DR, Lane SS, Doughman DJ, Krachmer JH, Holland EJ. Clinical findings in Brown-McLean syndrome. *Am J Ophthalmol.* 1993;115:729–737.

Vitreocorneal Adherence and Persistent Corneal Edema

Vitreocorneal adherence and persistent corneal edema can occur early or late after uncomplicated intracapsular cataract extraction (ICCE) or after complicated extracapsular cataract extraction (ECCE) or phacoemulsification. A vitrectomy may be indicated if corneal thickening or edema develops. In more advanced cases with prolonged corneal edema, penetrating or endothelial keratoplasty combined with vitrectomy may be indicated.

Corneal Complications of Ultrasound

During phacoemulsification, heat may be transferred from the probe to the cornea. The cause of such heat transfer can be an incision that is too tight to allow adequate irrigation fluid flow along the vibrating probe, or it can be irrigation or aspiration tubing that is occluded by an ophthalmic viscosurgical device (OVD) or lens material. The risk of this complication may be reduced by the use of higher aspiration flow rates and vacuum, lower ultrasound energy levels, burst or pulse modes, and cohesive OVDs during the parts of the procedure when occlusion is likely to occur. If the cornea clouds during the phacoemulsification procedure and reduces the visibility of the nucleus, the surgeon can convert to a nuclear expression technique if necessary.

When corneal burns occur, the heat causes contraction of the corneal collagen, with subsequent distortion of the incision. If the distortion is significant, incision gape may occur with associated leakage. These types of incisions will not be self-sealing and require suturing for adequate closure. The first priority is closing the incision with sutures, even if this maneuver induces astigmatism. After approximately 6 weeks, the sutures can be selectively removed based on keratometry or corneal topography and an assessment of the integrity of the incision.

Holding the phaco tip too close to the corneal endothelium during surgery increases the risk of endothelial cell injury and cell loss. Performing phacoemulsification or allowing lens fragments to circulate in the anterior chamber without adequate OVD protection can contribute to endothelial cell loss. In these cases, corneal edema may appear on the first postoperative day or may be delayed months to years following surgery.

Detachment of Descemet's Membrane

Detachment of Descemet's membrane results in stromal swelling and epithelial bullae localized in the area of detachment. This complication can occur when an instrument or IOL is introduced through the cataract incision or when fluid is inadvertently injected between Descemet's membrane and the corneal stroma. Small detachments may resolve spontaneously. Otherwise, they may be reattached with air or expansile gas (eg, sulfur hexafluoride [SF_6] or perfluoropropane [C_3F_8]) tamponade in the anterior chamber. Larger detachments can be sutured back into place. Gas may help position the detached area of Descemet's membrane prior to suture placement. An OVD can facilitate chamber maintenance during the procedure, but the surgeon must take great care not to introduce it between Descemet's membrane and corneal stroma. One or more 10-0 nylon sutures armed with long, curved cutting needles on both ends may be used. The needles are first passed through the incision or peripheral cornea distant to the area of Descemet's detachment. They are then passed from the anterior chamber and through the detached area of

Descemet's membrane, stroma, and epithelium. The ends are tied on the external surface of the cornea, and the knots are buried.

Induced Astigmatism

Postoperative astigmatism may be caused by tight radial sutures, which steepen corneal curvature in the axis of the suture. Following ECCE through a superior incision, up to 2 D of with-the-rule astigmatism will usually diminish with time and may make suture removal unnecessary. Removing one or more sutures 6–8 weeks postoperatively can reduce excessive astigmatism. If more than one suture is to be removed, it may be preferable to remove adjacent sutures in a series of visits rather than all at once. Removal of too many sutures too early in the postoperative course may result in either significant corneal flattening in the axis of the incision or a leaking incision, with an attendant increased risk of secondary intraocular infection as a result of surface organisms' entry into the eye through a suture track. Postoperative astigmatism may also be induced by corneal burns from the phaco tip; suture removal 6–8 weeks after surgery generally reduces astigmatism in this setting.

For further discussion of incision construction and astigmatism, see Chapter 8, Surgery for Cataract.

Corneal Melting

Keratolysis, or sterile melting of the cornea, may occur following cataract extraction. It is most frequently associated with preexisting tear-film abnormalities resulting from keratoconjunctivitis sicca, Sjögren syndrome, or collagen vascular diseases such as rheumatoid arthritis. Preoperative recognition of these predisposing factors is valuable because the frequent perioperative use of topical lubricants can lessen morbidity. Punctum plug placement or lateral tarsorrhaphy may also be performed at the time of surgery.

Severe stromal melting with the postoperative use of topical nonsteroidal anti-inflammatory drugs has also been reported. The melting is due in part to the epithelial toxicity and hypoesthesia induced by these drugs. A generic form of diclofenac was most frequently implicated, presumably because of matrix metalloproteinase expression induced by a solubilizer in the topical formulation.

Persistent epithelial defects accompanied by stromal dissolution require intensive treatment with nonpreserved topical lubricants. Use of topical medications, particularly preserved medications, should be minimized so that epithelial toxicity is reduced. Additional treatment modalities to encourage epithelialization and arrest stromal melting include punctal occlusion, bandage contact lenses, tarsorrhaphy, serum eyedrops (containing epithelial growth factor), and systemic tetracyclines. The prophylactic use of topical antibiotics must be monitored closely. After a week's application, many topical antibiotics begin to cause secondary toxic effects that may inhibit epithelial healing. For the treatment of any underlying collagen vascular disease, systemic immunosuppressive therapy such as methotrexate, cyclophosphamide, cyclosporine, or anti-TNF agents may be needed.

If the disease continues to progress in spite of medical therapy, the surgeon may undertake placement of amniotic membrane or lamellar or penetrating keratoplasty. Because corneal melting may recur even with grafted tissue, the physician must maintain intensive lubrication and consider management of any underlying systemic diseases in these cases.

Incision Leak or Inadvertent Filtering Bleb

Inadvertent filtration of aqueous fluid through the incision may be noted postoperatively. The filtration tends to be self-limited and may respond to observation accompanied by patching and the use of topical and systemic drugs to reduce aqueous production. Reducing or discontinuing postoperative corticosteroids is a way to encourage inflammation and more prompt healing of the incision.

If filtration persists, a bleb may develop. In the absence of symptoms, observation only is indicated. If irritation, tearing, contact lens intolerance, infection, a shallow anterior chamber, or significant hypotony occurs, the physician may consider intervention. Techniques vary considerably and consist of procedures to enhance inflammation and thus seal the leak by cicatrization of the bleb. They include light cautery, penetrating diathermy, cryotherapy, and injection of autologous blood directly into the bleb ("blood patch"), as well as the application of cyanoacrylate glue and the application of a saturated solution of trichloroacetic acid directly to the surface of the bleb. Alternatively, the surgeon may consider revising the incision in the early phase, when healing is not yet complete. In chronic cases, simple suturing may not be sufficient, and a lamellar or patch keratoplasty may be necessary.

Epithelial Downgrowth

Epithelial downgrowth is a rare complication of intraocular surgery, occurring even less frequently with today's cataract surgery techniques. The condition is characterized by a sheet of epithelium growing down from the surgical incision and covering the corneal endothelium and/or iris surfaces. One possible explanation for this condition is that epithelial cells are introduced into the anterior chamber during surgery, and they adhere to intraocular structures and begin to proliferate as a cellular membrane. Another theory is that a sheet of epithelium from the ocular surface grows into the incision (possibly because the incision is not watertight), and this cellular membrane proliferates onto the posterior corneal and iris surfaces.

The clinical signs of epithelial downgrowth include elevated IOP, clumps of cells floating in the anterior chamber, a visible retrocorneal membrane (usually with overlying corneal edema), an abnormal iris surface, and pupillary distortion. The mechanism for elevated IOP is outflow obstruction caused by the growth of the epithelial membrane over the trabecular meshwork or by epithelial cells clogging the meshwork. Diagnosis of epithelial downgrowth is confirmed with the argon laser; argon laser burns applied to the membrane or the iris surface will appear white if epithelial cells are present.

Many complex surgical procedures have been suggested for treating this condition. Local application of cryotherapy or of 5-fluorouracil has been reported to be effective. Neither of these interventions has been uniformly successful. In some patients, palliative surgery with glaucoma valve implants for IOP control and comfort is indicated.

Toxic Solutions

Certain solutions, either irrigated or inadvertently injected into the anterior chamber, can be toxic to the corneal endothelium and cause temporary or permanent corneal edema. Subconjunctival antibiotic injections have been reported to enter the anterior chamber through scleral tunnel incisions that act as 1-way valves. Skin cleansers containing chlorhexidine gluconate (eg, Hibiclens) have been reported to cause irreversible corneal edema and opacification if they unintentionally come into contact with the endothelial surface. Preservatives present in prediluted epinephrine (1:10,000) added to irrigating solutions have been implicated in corneal decompensation. Unpreserved 1:1000 epinephrine is preferred. Substitution of sterile water for balanced salt solution, intraocular use of preserved medications, or inadvertent intraocular injection of residual toxic materials, which may be present in reusable cannulas or irrigation tubing, may cause severe endothelial damage. The clinician may reduce the patient's risk of developing a toxic reaction by carefully rinsing and air-drying reusable cannulas or by using disposable cannulas, and by taking care to avoid the intraocular use of any topical antibiotics or anesthetics containing preservatives.

If a toxic solution enters the anterior chamber, it may produce severe intraocular inflammation as well as corneal edema. This syndrome has been dubbed *Toxic Anterior Segment Syndrome (TASS)* and is a form of sterile, noninfectious endophthalmitis. The symptoms and signs of TASS may mimic those of infectious endophthalmitis and include pain, photophobia, severe reduction in visual acuity, and marked anterior chamber reaction, occasionally with hypopyon. TASS presents within 12–24 hours, whereas acute infectious endophthalmitis typically develops 2–7 days after surgery. Other potentially distinguishing features of TASS include diffuse, limbus-to-limbus corneal edema; anterior chamber opacification; a dilated, irregular, or nonreactive pupil; and elevated IOP. The pathologic changes are limited to the anterior chamber. If endophthalmitis is suspected, diagnostic and therapeutic interventions as described later in this chapter should be undertaken. Treatment of TASS consists of intensive topical corticosteroids until the inflammation subsides. A brief course of systemic corticosteroids may be beneficial. Frequent follow-up is necessary to monitor IOP and to reassess for signs of bacterial infection.

Hejny C, Edelhauser HF. Surgical pharmacology: intraocular solutions and drugs used for cataract surgery. In: Buratto L, Werner L, Zanini M, et al, eds. *Phacoemulsification: Principles and Techniques.* 2nd ed. Thorofare, NJ: Slack; 2003:chap 12.

Mamalis N, Edelhauser HF, Dawson DG, Chew J, LeBoyer RM, Werner L. Toxic anterior segment syndrome. *J Cataract Refract Surg.* 2006;32:324–333.

Monson MC, Mamalis N, Olson RJ. Toxic anterior segment inflammation following cataract surgery. *J Cataract Refract Surg.* 1992;18:184–189.

Conjunctival Ballooning

In cases with a conjunctival incision or peritomy, externally misdirected irrigating solution may accumulate underneath the conjunctiva and Tenon's capsule during phacoemulsification or irrigation/aspiration, resulting in ballooning of the conjunctiva. This ballooning may interfere with access to the incisions, cause pooling of irrigating solution on the surface of the eye, and produce unwanted reflections from the operating microscope light. Several small stab incisions through the conjunctiva and Tenon's capsule allow the fluid to drain.

Shallow or Flat Anterior Chamber

Intraoperative

During ECCE or phacoemulsification, the anterior chamber may become shallow because of inadequate infusion of balanced salt solution into the anterior chamber, leakage through an oversized incision, external pressure on the globe, positive vitreous pressure, or suprachoroidal hemorrhage. If the reason for loss of normal chamber depth is not apparent, the surgeon should first raise the infusion bottle height and then check the incision. If the incision is too large and a significant volume of irrigation fluid flows out of the anterior chamber, the surgeon can place a suture across the incision in order to reduce the incision size and ultimately help keep the chamber formed. External pressure on the globe can be relieved by readjustment of the surgical drapes or the eyelid speculum. Positive vitreous pressure occurs more commonly in obese, thick-necked patients; in those with pulmonary disease such as chronic obstructive pulmonary disease (COPD); and in anxious patients or those with full bladders who perform a Valsalva maneuver. Placing obese patients in a reverse Trendelenburg position may be useful. Intravenous mannitol can often reduce the elevated vitreous pressure and allow the case to continue uneventfully.

If the reason for the loss of anterior chamber depth is still unknown, the surgeon should check the red reflex to evaluate the possibility of a suprachoroidal hemorrhage or effusion. In the presence of a suprachoroidal hemorrhage or effusion, typically the eye becomes very firm and the patient becomes agitated and complains of pain. To confirm this diagnosis, the surgeon needs to examine the fundus with an indirect ophthalmoscope. If a hemorrhage or effusion is significant, the incisions should be closed and the case postponed until the pressure has decreased.

Posterior misdirection of irrigation fluid

In rare cases, the fluid infused into the anterior chamber may be misdirected into the vitreous cavity, causing an increase in the vitreous volume, with subsequent forward displacement of the lens and shallowing of the anterior chamber. The fluid may accumulate in the retrolenticular space or dissect posteriorly along the vitreoretinal interface. This complication, termed *posterior infusion syndrome,* is most likely to occur during hydrodissection, when fluid is forcefully injected into the capsular bag. A shallow anterior chamber resulting from posterior infusion syndrome may indicate loss of integrity of the capsular bag, damaged zonular fibers, or misplacement of the irrigating tip. If gentle posterior pressure on the lens does not alleviate the situation, infusing intravenous mannitol and waiting several minutes may allow the anterior chamber to deepen. In addition, the surgeon can insert a 19-gauge needle through the pars plana into the retrolenticular space and gently aspirate to try to remove the fluid and deepen the anterior chamber. The surgeon must exercise care in placing the needle in order to avoid a retinal tear or detachment. Alternatively, a pars plana vitrectomy may be performed.

Postoperative

A flat anterior chamber during the postoperative period may cause permanent damage to ocular structures. Prolonged apposition of the iris to angle structures can cause permanent peripheral anterior synechiae and chronic angle-closure glaucoma. Following either ICCE or ECCE, iridovitreal or iridocapsular synechiae can also lead to pupillary block. Corneal contact with vitreous or an IOL can result in endothelial cell loss and chronic corneal edema.

Flat anterior chambers can be classified according to etiology and level of IOP. Classification by etiology includes the following:

- leaking incision
- choroidal detachment
- pupillary block
- ciliary block
- suprachoroidal hemorrhage

Cases associated with ocular hypotension (IOP below 10 mm Hg) are usually secondary to leakage of aqueous at the incision site or to choroidal detachment. Patients may be asymptomatic, especially if a leaking incision is plugged by iris incarceration, allowing re-formation of the anterior chamber. Even without iris incarceration, slow or intermittent leaks may coexist with a formed anterior chamber. Carefully comparing the chamber depth of the surgical eye with that of the fellow eye may be helpful for identification of these cases.

To detect an area of leakage, the clinician will usually find it sufficient to paint the surface of the incision, using a fluorescein strip, or to instill 1 or 2 drops of 2% fluorescein and then examine the entire incision, using the cobalt blue filter on the slit lamp (Seidel test). Aqueous dilution of fluorescein at the site of the leakage will produce a contrasting area of green stain. Occasionally, aqueous flow is so slight that gentle pressure on the globe is necessary for confirmation of the leakage site.

The physician managing a leaking incision can consider several options:

- Some eyes with leaking incisions may respond within hours to cycloplegia and pressure patching.
- Carbonic anhydrase inhibitors and topical beta-blockers may decrease aqueous flow through the incision.
- Avoiding the use of steroids enhances the local inflammatory reaction to facilitate spontaneous closure.

- Therapeutic soft contact lenses have been successful in reducing aqueous flow through the incision.
- Tissue adhesive may seal the incision and allow it to heal in selected cases.

These methods are appropriate both for the management of minor incision leaks with adequate and secure apposition and as temporary measures until more secure incision closure can be accomplished surgically. Patients may develop an associated ciliochoroidal detachment that resolves spontaneously after incision closure. Surgical exploration, with re-formation of the anterior chamber and repair of the incision, is indicated if no improvement occurs within 24–48 hours, if obvious incision gape is present, if the iris is prolapsed out of the incision, or if intraocular structures such as the IOL are in contact with the corneal endothelium.

Late hypotony without obvious leakage from the incision is uncommon after cataract surgery. It may result from retinal detachment, cyclodialysis, filtering bleb formation, or persistent uveitis.

Cases of a shallow anterior chamber with normal or high IOP are usually the result of pupillary block, ciliary block, or suprachoroidal hemorrhage. Pupillary block that occurs in the early postoperative period may follow a resolved incision leak. Postoperative uveitis with iridovitreal or iridocapsular synechiae may cause relatively late pupillary block. Failure to perform a peripheral iridectomy after placement of an anterior chamber IOL may also be associated with early or late postoperative pupillary block. If initial attempts at pupillary dilation fail to deepen the anterior chamber and lower the pressure, a laser peripheral iridotomy is usually effective.

Aqueous sequestration within the vitreous body may be the cause of ciliary block glaucoma, with a flat anterior chamber and high IOP that is unresponsive to medical therapy or peripheral iridectomy. Nd:YAG laser rupture of the vitreous face may correct the aqueous misdirection. If a capsulotomy is not curative, vitrectomy is the preferred treatment of this rare condition.

Elevated Intraocular Pressure

A rise in IOP is common following cataract surgery. It is generally mild and self-limited and does not require prolonged antiglaucoma therapy. However, a significant and sustained rise in IOP following cataract surgery may necessitate timely and specific management in several circumstances.

OVDs such as hyaluronate retained in the eye after cataract surgery are frequently responsible for postoperative IOP elevation. Even when it is removed from the anterior chamber at the conclusion of surgery, OVD can be sequestered in the posterior chamber or behind the lens implant. Mixtures of chondroitin and hyaluronate have been advocated to reduce the risk of this occurrence; however, even these combinations are associated with elevated IOP in certain patients. IOP elevation usually does not last more than a few days and is amenable to medical treatment. The clinician may expeditiously manage marked IOP elevation in the early postoperative period by applying gentle pressure on the posterior lip of a preexisting paracentesis and subsequently releasing a small amount of aqueous humor. Use of topical antibiotics or povidone-iodine for preparation of the ocular surface is desirable. Topical and/or systemic pressure-lowering agents should also be administered, as pressure reduction after aqueous release is short-lived, with the pressure likely to rise again within 1–2 hours of release.

Other causes of elevated IOP after cataract surgery include pupillary block, hyphema, ciliary block, endophthalmitis, retained lens material (phacolytic or phacoanaphylactic reactions), iris pigment release, preexisting glaucoma, corticosteroid usage, or peripheral anterior synechiae. The latter may result from a flat anterior chamber in the early postoperative period when the eye is inflamed. It may produce severe secondary glaucoma at a later time. Treating the underlying cause of the IOP elevation should be curative.

Intraoperative Floppy Iris Syndrome

In patients who take tamsulosin (Flomax) or other systemic α_{1a}-adrenergic antagonists for the treatment of benign prostatic hypertrophy, pupil dilation before surgery may be poor. These patients are also likely to demonstrate a flaccid iris stroma that undulates and billows in response to intraocular irrigation. In addition, they are prone to develop progressive intraoperative miosis and iris prolapse. This trio of findings characterizes intraoperative floppy iris syndrome (IFIS). The abnormal iris behavior is believed to be due to the combination of anterior chamber turbulence and unopposed sphincter constriction in the absence of countertraction from iris dilators. The risk of posterior capsule rupture and elevated IOP may be increased in these patients.

Patients with poor pupillary dilation should be questioned about the use of α_{1a}-adrenergic antagonists. Cessation of the drug before surgery may reduce the risk of IFIS. However, IFIS may still develop 1 month or longer after patients discontinue systemic α_{1a}-adrenergic antagonists. Numerous intraoperative interventions have been proposed to reduce the effects of IFIS, including maximal dilation regimens; intraocular injection of dilating agents (with an attendant risk of toxicity); bimanual microincision surgical techniques; employment of highly retentive OVDs to "viscodilate" the pupil and maintain a concave iris near the incisions without preventing egress of irrigating fluid; and use of low-flow settings and lens removal techniques that minimize anterior chamber turbulence. In addition, careful attention to incision construction has been advised.

Despite these interventions, some patients go on to develop miosis and/or iris prolapse intraoperatively. In these cases, use of iris retractors or pupil expansion rings can maintain adequate dilation and iris stability to complete the procedure safely. If iris retractors are placed after initiation of the capsulorrhexis, the pupil margin must be carefully engaged so that the edge of the anterior capsule is not captured. OVDs can be placed between the iris and the anterior capsule to facilitate placement of the retention hooks. An alternative is to prolapse the lens nucleus and emulsify it in the anterior chamber, with OVD used to protect the endothelium. Mechanical pupil-stretching techniques are ineffective in treating IFIS.

Chang DF, Campbell JR. Intraoperative floppy iris syndrome associated with tamsulosin. *J Cataract Refract Surg.* 2005;31:664–673.

Iridodialysis

Iridodialysis, the tearing of the iris at its root or insertion, may occur intraoperatively as a result of the manipulation of intraocular tissues. Insertion of the phaco tip or IOL can sometimes damage the iris. If the iridodialysis is optically and cosmetically insignificant, it can be left alone. More extensive iridodialysis that could cause optical problems or that could be cosmetically significant may require attaching the iris root to the incision surgically with permanent monofilament suture.

Cyclodialysis

Cyclodialysis, the separation of the ciliary body from its insertion at the scleral spur, also may occur as a result of surgical manipulation of intraocular tissue. Gonioscopic observation shows a deep angle recess with a gap between the sclera and the ciliary body. Repair of a cyclodialysis cleft is often indicated to relieve prolonged hypotony. The ophthalmologist may achieve closure by applying argon laser photocoagulation to the cleft. If laser is ineffective, it may be necessary to reattach the ciliary body with sutures.

Ciliary Block Glaucoma

Ciliary block glaucoma, or *aqueous misdirection* (formerly known as *malignant glaucoma*), results from the posterior misdirection of aqueous into the vitreous body. This misdirection displaces the lens–iris diaphragm anteriorly, causing the central and peripheral portions of the anterior chamber to become very shallow, and leads to a secondary elevation of IOP as a consequence of angle obstruction. This condition occurs most commonly after intraocular surgery in eyes with prior angle-closure glaucoma, but it can also occur after cataract surgery or various laser procedures in eyes with open angles. Ciliary block glaucoma is characterized by a shallow anterior chamber and elevated IOP. It must be differentiated from pupillary block, suprachoroidal hemorrhage, and choroidal detachment.

This posterior diversion of aqueous into the vitreous body after ocular surgery can elevate the IOP despite the presence of a patent iridectomy or iridotomy. Thus, ciliary block glaucoma is not relieved by simple iridectomy but requires either intense medical therapy or surgical therapy. *Medical treatment* consists of intensive cycloplegia and mydriasis with agents such as atropine 1% and phenylephrine 10% 4 times a day to attempt to move the lens–iris diaphragm posteriorly. This therapy is coupled with the use of aqueous suppressants (such as beta-blockers, alpha agonists, and/or oral carbonic anhydrase inhibitors) and hyperosmotic agents (such as oral glycerin or intravenous mannitol) to reduce aqueous production and lower the IOP. Miotics should be avoided because they make ciliary block glaucoma worse by exacerbating the anterior displacement of the lens–iris diaphragm. Medical therapy is successful in 50% of these cases. *Surgical intervention* consists of maneuvers to disrupt the anterior vitreous face and vitreous in order to reestablish a channel for aqueous to come forward. Techniques include mechanical disruption with a knife, use of the Nd:YAG laser, or pars plana vitrectomy. (See also BCSC Section 10, *Glaucoma.*)

Lundy DM. Ciliary block glaucoma. *Focal Points: Clinical Modules for Ophthalmologists.* San Francisco: American Academy of Ophthalmology; 1999, module 3.

Chronic Uveitis

Chronic uveitis following cataract surgery has been reported in association with low-grade bacterial pathogens, including *Propionibacterium acnes* and *Staphylococcus epidermidis.* These patients may have an unremarkable early postoperative course and lack the classic findings of acute endophthalmitis. Weeks or months after surgery, however, they develop chronic uveitis that is variably responsive to topical corticosteroids. This condition is usually associated with granulomatous keratic precipitates and less commonly with hypopyon. A localized focus of infection sequestered within the capsular bag may occasionally be observed, most often within the remaining lens capsule. Diagnosis requires a high level of clinical suspicion, coupled with examination and cultures of appropriate specimens of aqueous, vitreous, and, where applicable, retained lens material that may harbor a nidus of infection. Appropriate intravitreal antibiotic therapy is indicated. If this treatment fails, the clinician may need to search for and remove any visible focus of potentially infectious material in order to sterilize the eye. In some cases, total removal of the residual capsule and IOL is necessary.

The possibility of microbial endophthalmitis should be investigated in patients who have persistent uveitis without a previous inflammatory history. (For a more comprehensive discussion of endophthalmitis, see BCSC Section 9, *Intraocular Inflammation and Uveitis.*)

Meisler DM. Intraocular inflammation and extracapsular cataract surgery. *Focal Points: Clinical Modules for Ophthalmologists.* San Francisco: American Academy of Ophthalmology; 1990, module 7.

Retained Lens Material

During lens removal, lens fragments may remain in the anterior chamber angle or in the posterior chamber behind the iris, or they may migrate into the vitreous cavity if zonular dehiscence or posterior capsule rupture occurs. Lens material is thought to be left more frequently with phacoemulsification than with ECCE, and some experts believe the incidence is approximately 0.3%. (For a discussion of the surgical management of this intraoperative complication, see Capsular Rupture section later in this chapter.)

Patients with retained lens fragments present with varying degrees of inflammation, depending on the size of the lens fragment, the type of lens material, the amount of time elapsed since surgery, and the patient's individual response. The clinical signs of retained lens material may include uveitis, glaucoma, corneal edema, and vitreous opacities causing profound visual loss.

Retained cortical lens material does not necessarily require surgical intervention. In general, cortical material is better tolerated and more likely to reabsorb over time than is nuclear material, which, even in small amounts, persists longer and is more likely to incite a significant inflammatory reaction and elevated IOP. In addition, smaller fragments of lens material are better tolerated than larger pieces, for the same reasons.

Observation is warranted for patients with small amounts of retained cortical lens material in the hope that this material will be reabsorbed. Inflammation should be controlled with corticosteroid and nonsteroidal anti-inflammatory drops and cycloplegics. IOP can be controlled with topical agents and with carbonic anhydrase inhibitors given systemically. Surgical intervention may be necessary to remove residual lens material in the following situations:

- presence of a large or visually significant amount of lens material
- increased inflammation not readily controlled with topical medications
- medically unresponsive elevated IOP resulting from the inflammation
- associated retinal detachment or retinal tears
- associated endophthalmitis

If the posterior capsule is intact, simple aspiration of residual cortex through an anterior incision may be carried out with the use of an irrigation/aspiration instrument. If there is a defect in the posterior capsule, pars plana vitrectomy and removal of lens material are indicated. When such major intervention is necessary, the retained lens material should be removed from the vitreous by a surgeon skilled in pars plana vitrectomy techniques. The vitreoretinal surgeon can delay intervention up to 7–14 days following the initial cataract surgery without jeopardizing the successful outcome. Chronic glaucoma and CME may be more likely when intervention is delayed more than 3 weeks after the cataract surgery.

Monshizadeh E, Samiy N, Haimovici R. Management of retained intravitreal lens fragments after cataract surgery. *Surv Ophthalmol.* 1999;43:397–404.

Vilar NF, Flynn HW Jr, Smiddy WE, Murray TG, Davis JL, Rubsamen PE. Removal of retained lens fragments after phacomulsification reverses secondary glaucoma and restores visual acuity. *Ophthalmology.* 1997;104:787–792.

Capsular Rupture

If capsular rupture occurs during phacoemulsification, nuclear material may enter the posterior segment. The high-fluid-flow state in the anterior chamber increases this risk. The first signs of capsular rupture may be a sudden deepening of the anterior chamber. A radial tear in an anterior curvilinear capsulorrhexis may extend through the capsular fornix into the posterior capsule. A small rupture in the posterior capsule during emulsification of the nucleus can be managed by alteration of the surgical technique. If the majority of the nucleus remains and the capsular tear is large, further attempts at phacoemulsification should be abandoned. To extract the remaining nuclear fragments mechanically, the surgeon should enlarge the incision and remove the nucleus with a lens loop or spoon in a manner that minimizes vitreous traction or further damage to the capsule.

If only a small portion of the nucleus remains to be aspirated or the rent in the capsule is small, the surgeon, by lowering the infusion bottle, may be able to use the phaco tip to remove the remaining nuclear material. Full occlusion of the aspiration port and minimal phaco power will reduce the risk of further damage to the capsule and of aspiration of vitreous. Insertion of a second instrument or lens glide behind the nuclear remnant may help prevent the remnant from being dislocated into the vitreous. Alternatively, OVD can be introduced posterior to the fragment in an effort to float it anteriorly. If the nuclear material drops posteriorly but is still visible, and if the surgeon is familiar with pars plana techniques, a posterior assisted levitation maneuver may be attempted. A spatula or OVD cannula is placed through a stab incision in the pars plana and used to elevate the nuclear fragment into the anterior segment. Retrieval of nuclear fragments from the deep vitreous is not recommended.

If the nuclear fragment is not visible or if the surgeon is not experienced with pars plana incisions, an anterior vitrectomy should be performed with an aspirating guillotine cutter, and the peripheral cortical material should be removed. A 2-port anterior vitrectomy, separating infusion from the aspiration/cutting instrument, facilitates the removal of vitreous from the anterior segment of the eye. If the surgeon is familiar with vitreoretinal techniques, the aspiration/cutting instrument may be placed through a pars plana incision and directly visualized in the posterior segment through the pupil while irrigation is continued through the limbus or cornea. This directs flow posteriorly and reduces the amount of vitreous that migrates into the anterior segment. Alternatively, both the irrigation instrument and the aspiration/cutting instrument may be placed through 2 separate limbal or corneal incisions. An IOL with a total diameter greater than 12.5 mm may be inserted in the ciliary sulcus after confirmation of anterior capsule integrity. If capsular integrity is insufficient, an anterior chamber lens of appropriate power and size may be substituted. The incision should then be sutured closed. If posteriorly dislocated nuclear material remains, it should be approached within 1–2 weeks by a vitreoretinal surgeon via a pars plana vitrectomy route. Retained lens material, especially nuclear material, is often associated with elevated IOP, significant inflammation, and corneal edema. Following are some guidelines for the anterior segment surgeon faced with managing posteriorly dislocated lens fragments:

- Attempt retrieval of the fragments only if they are visible and easily accessible.
- Perform anterior vitrectomy to avoid vitreous prolapse.
- Insert IOL when safe and indicated; insert preferably by capsular fixation, but in the ciliary sulcus or anterior chamber as necessary.
- Perform watertight incision closure and OVD removal.
- Prescribe frequent postoperative topical corticosteroids, NSAIDs, and IOP-lowering agents.
- Provide referral for prompt vitreoretinal consultation.

If a small rent appears in the posterior capsule during aspiration of cortex and the vitreous face remains intact, the surgeon should attempt to remove the residual cortex without expanding the tear. After stabilizing the anterior chamber with the use of an OVD, some surgeons use forceps to convert the tear into a round capsulorrhexis that will not spread equatorially. Using low irrigation and aspiration flow to avoid disruption of the vitreous face, the surgeon can then remove residual cortex from the peripheral lens capsule. Some surgeons prefer a manual technique, using a cannula attached to a handheld syringe to remove residual cortex after capsular rupture, thereby avoiding any pressure from irrigation.

If larger posterior capsule tears occur or when the anterior vitreous face is broken, a vitrectomy is recommended to facilitate the removal of residual cortex and subsequent placement of an IOL. In addition, a vitrectomy can prevent the development of vitreomacular traction from the IOL or the incision. Vitreous loss during cataract surgery is associated with an increased risk of retinal detachment and endophthalmitis.

Chang DF, Packard RB. Posterior assisted levitation for nucleus retrieval using Viscoat after posterior capsule rupture. *J Cataract Refract Surg*. 2003;29:1860–1865.

Fishkind WJ. The torn posterior capsule: prevention, recognition, and management. *Focal Points: Clinical Modules for Ophthalmologists*. San Francisco: American Academy of Ophthalmology; 1999, module 4.

Monshizadeh E, Samiy N, Haimovici R. Management of retained intravitreal lens fragments after cataract surgery. *Surv Ophthalmol*. 1999;43:397–404.

Vitreous Prolapse

Vitreous prolapse through the pupil, resulting from rupture of the anterior vitreous face during surgery, can occur as a complication of cataract extraction by any technique; prolapse can occur with or without incarceration in the incision. Resultant vitreous traction can lead to retinal breaks and subsequent detachment. Appropriate intraoperative management involves cutting vitreous strands into short segments for removal by a suction cutter or by cellulose sponges. The surgeon, using a cellulose sponge or spatula, may detect the presence of vitreous by touching or manipulating the incision or iris. Adherent vitreous will become apparent or will cause movement of the pupil. All vitreous anterior to the posterior capsule should be removed at the time of surgery.

Vitreous in the anterior chamber may lead to chronic ocular inflammation with or without associated CME. The pupil may also be distorted, exposing the edge of the IOL, producing glare. If there is significant glare from a distorted pupil or if symptomatic uveitis or CME is unresponsive to topical anti-inflammatory therapy, the clinician may consider disruption of the vitreous incarcerated in the incision, using Nd:YAG laser or vitrectomy techniques. If the vitreous extends through the incision to the ocular surface, a vitrectomy should be performed, because the exposed vitreous may act like a wick, enabling bacteria to gain entrance into the eye and increasing the risk of endophthalmitis (vitreous wick syndrome). In cases showing considerable corneal compromise, a posterior, rather than an anterior, vitrectomy approach may be preferable to reduce surgical trauma to the cornea.

Complications of IOL Implantation

Decentration and Dislocation

An IOL may become decentered in the following situations:

- asymmetric haptic placement, with one haptic in the bag and the other in the sulcus
- insufficient zonular or capsular support

- the presence of irregular fibrosis of the posterior capsule
- capsular phimosis

Decentration can produce unwanted glare and reflections or multiple images if the edge of the lens is within the pupillary space. An IOL that is designed for intracapsular fixation is prone to decentration or dislocation when one or both haptics are placed in the sulcus. If zonular support is inadequate, the surgeon should attempt to rotate the IOL to a position where clinical evidence shows sufficient capsule and zonular fibers to support the implant. The use of transcorneal iris fixation sutures (McCannel sutures) to secure the IOL may also be considered (Fig 9-2). After a paracentesis is created and an OVD is placed in the anterior chamber, the IOL optic is subluxed into the pupil by means of a positioning instrument. Nondegradable sutures (eg, 10-0 or 9-0 polypropylene) on a long curved needle are then passed through the cornea, through the iris anteriorly to posteriorly, behind the IOL haptics, through the iris posteriorly to anteriorly, and out through the cornea. A positioning instrument placed behind the IOL may be used to push it anteriorly to highlight the position of the lens loops behind the iris as the needle is passed through the iris and behind the loops. The surgeon can minimize pupil distortion by placing the sutures between the midperiphery and the chamber angle. Then, a second paracentesis is made in peripheral cornea adjacent to the area of suture fixation. The suture ends can be retrieved through this paracentesis and tied externally. By using a Siepser slipknot technique, the surgeon can minimize iris traction when tying the suture ends. The knots are trimmed, and the iris is repositioned. Alternatively, special micro tying instruments may be placed through paracentesis incisions in order to tie the suture in the anterior chamber. After the sutures have been tied and the knots trimmed, the IOL optic is repositioned posterior to the iris.

Irregular posterior capsule fibrosis gradually decenters the IOL. Deformation of the haptics may render simple rotation insufficient to center the IOL properly. It may become necessary in these cases to move the IOL haptics into the ciliary sulcus or replace the capsule-fixated IOL with a posterior chamber sulcus-fixated IOL. If dislocation of the IOL is complete, the surgeon can sublux the optic of the implant into the pupil by means of vitrectomy techniques and use transcorneal iris-fixation sutures to fix the 2 haptics of the implant. Alternatively, the implant may be removed altogether and replaced with

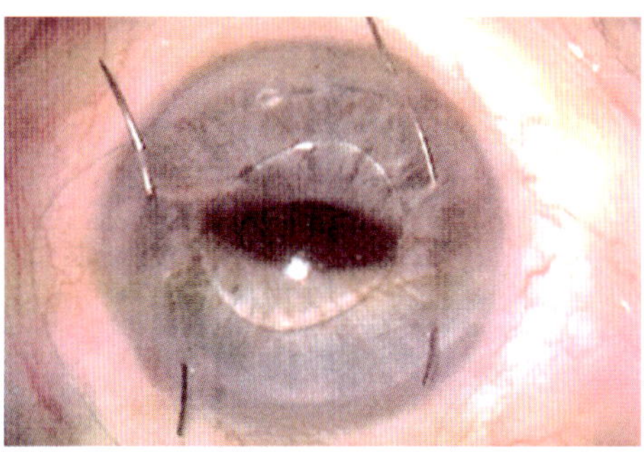

Figure 9-2 McCannel suture. The lens optic is repositioned posterior to the iris after the suture ends are retrieved and tied through a paracentesis.

either an anterior chamber IOL or a transscleral or iris-sutured posterior chamber IOL. Subluxation of scleral-fixated sutured IOLs has been reported 3–9 years after implantation with 10-0 polypropylene fixation sutures. Double-fixation techniques and thicker 9-0 polypropylene sutures are currently recommended for scleral fixation of IOLs.

Assia EI, Nemet A, Sachs D. Bilateral spontaneous subluxation of scleral-fixated intraocular lenses. *J Cataract Refract Surg.* 2002;28:2214–2216.

Chang DF. Siepser slipknot for McCannel iris-suture fixation of subluxated intraocular lenses. *J Cataract Refract Surg.* 2004;30:1170–1176.

Pupillary Capture

Postoperative pupillary capture of the IOL optic can occur for a variety of reasons, including formation of synechiae between the iris and underlying posterior capsule, improper placement of the IOL haptics, shallowing of the anterior chamber, or anterior displacement of the posterior chamber IOL optic. The latter is associated with placement of nonangulated IOLs in the ciliary sulcus, upside-down placement of an angulated IOL so that the IOL angles anteriorly, or positive vitreous pressure behind the lens optic. Placement of a posteriorly angulated posterior chamber IOL in the capsular bag decreases the likelihood of pupillary capture.

Usually, pupillary capture is purely a cosmetic issue; the patient is otherwise asymptomatic and can be left untreated. Occasionally, pupillary capture can cause problems with glare, photophobia, chronic uveitis, unintended myopia, or even monocular diplopia. Mydriatics can sometimes be used successfully to free the iris through pharmacologic manipulation of the pupil. If conservative management fails, surgical intervention may be required to free the iris, break the synechiae, or reposition the lens (Figs 9-3, 9-4).

Capsular Block Syndrome

Capsular block syndrome is an uncommon postoperative complication of capsular bag–fixated posterior chamber IOLs. Aqueous becomes trapped within the capsular bag, between the posterior capsule and the posterior surface of the IOL. There is forward dis-

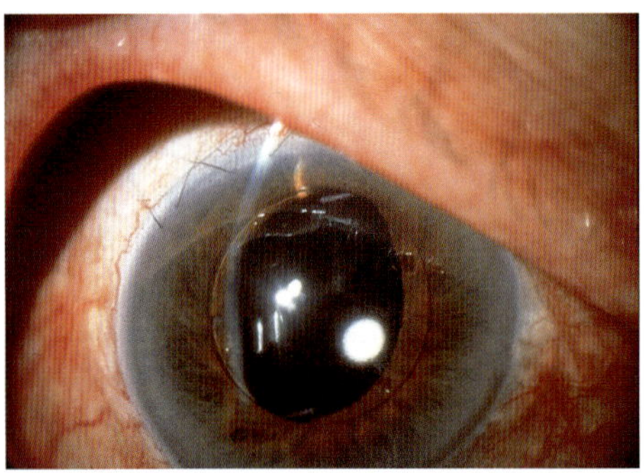

Figure 9-3 Pupillary capture. *(Courtesy of Karla J. Johns, MD.)*

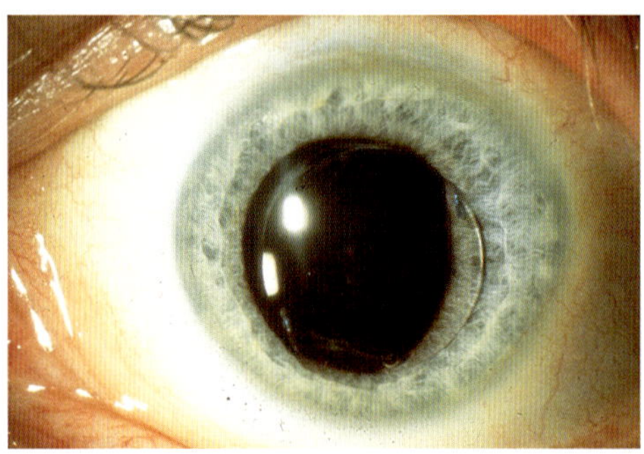

Figure 9-4 Pupillary capture by angled posterior chamber IOL in patient assaulted 2 months after surgery. *(Courtesy of Steven I. Rosenfeld, MD.)*

placement of the lens optic, with a resultant myopic shift. The fluid behind the IOL may have a turbid or milky appearance. Nd:YAG laser posterior capsulotomy results in release of the fluid, posterior movement of the IOL optic to its original position, and resolution of the myopic shift.

Uveitis-Glaucoma-Hyphema Syndrome

The syndrome of uveitis, glaucoma, and hyphema (UGH) was first described in the context of rigid anterior chamber and closed-loop IOLs. The classic triad or individual elements may occur as a result of inappropriate IOL sizing, contact between the implant and vascular structures or the corneal endothelium, or defects in implant manufacturing. UGH can also be seen in patients with posterior chamber lenses, owing to contact between lens loops and uveal tissue in the posterior chamber. Uveitis, glaucoma, and/or hyphema may respond to treatment with topical anti-inflammatory medications or antiglaucoma medications. If the symptoms are not alleviated sufficiently by medical therapy or if inflammation threatens either retinal or corneal function, IOL removal must be considered. This procedure may be very complicated because of inflammatory scars, particularly in the angle. If such scarring is present, the surgeon may need to amputate the haptics from the optic and remove the lens piecemeal, rotating the haptic material out of the synechial tunnels to minimize trauma to the eye. In some cases it is safer to leave portions of the haptics in place. Early lens explantation may reduce the risk of corneal decompensation and CME.

Pseudophakic Bullous Keratopathy

Certain IOL designs, particularly iris-clip lenses (iris-fixated lenses with the optic anterior to the iris) and closed-loop flexible anterior chamber lenses, are associated with increased risk of corneal decompensation. Iris-clip lenses have been shown to contact the corneal endothelium during eye movement. Chronic endothelial cell loss associated with closed-loop IOLs is thought to be due to chronic inflammation and contact between the lens and peripheral corneal endothelial cells. Both types of lenses are no longer in clinical use. Patients with underlying corneal endothelial dysfunction such as Fuchs corneal dystrophy are at greater risk for developing postoperative corneal edema. Progressive stromal edema eventually leads to bullous keratopathy, which is discussed earlier in this chapter.

Incorrect IOL Power

Placement of an incorrect power IOL is usually the result of a preoperative error in axial length measurement or keratometry readings. Choosing the correct power IOL is more difficult in patients undergoing simultaneous penetrating keratoplasty, in those with silicone oil in the vitreous cavity, and in those who have had prior refractive surgery. The ophthalmologist should take special care in selecting an IOL in these cases (see the section IOL Power Determination in Chapter 8, Surgery for Cataract). Inverting the IOL upon insertion so that the angulation of the optic is anterior rather than posterior changes the effective power of the IOL. Mislabeling or manufacturing defects are rarely the cause. Incorrect lens power should be suspected early in the postoperative course when the uncorrected visual acuity is less than expected and is confirmed by refraction.

If the magnitude of the implant error is likely to produce symptomatic anisometropia, the surgeon can consider several options: replacing the IOL with one of the appropriate power, inserting a piggyback IOL, or performing a secondary keratorefractive procedure.

Removal of an incorrect IOL involves separating the anterior capsule from the posterior capsule with an OVD, "dialing" the haptics into the anterior chamber, transecting the lens optic with specially designed scissors, and removing the lens halves through a 3-mm incision. Referral to a surgeon experienced in these techniques may be appropriate.

Jin GJ, Crandall AS, Jones JJ. Intraocular lens exchange due to incorrect lens power. *Ophthalmology.* 2007;114(3):417–424.

IOL Design, Glare, and Opacification

In addition to lens decentration and capsular opacification, glare can result when the diameter of the IOL optic is smaller than the diameter of the scotopic pupil. Optics with a square-edge design and multifocal IOLs are more prone to producing glare and halos. Spherical aberration may produce some degree of distortion or glare under scotopic conditions when the pupil is dilated, even if the iris covers the edge of the lens optic. Aspheric IOLs may reduce some of these phenomena and improve contrast sensitivity. *Temporal dysphotopsias,* described as a dark or dim region or other subjective distortion in the temporal visual field, may be more common with square-edge IOLs and those manufactured from high-index materials. A number of IOLs have developed intralenticular opacities after implantation. "Glistenings" visible in some early acrylic lenses were occasionally visually significant. Calcium deposition within or on the surface of hydrophilic acrylic lenses has produced significant visual symptoms, leading in some cases to lens explantation.

Werner L, Apple DJ, Escobar-Gomez M, et al. Postoperative deposition of calcium on the surfaces of a hydrogel intraocular lens. *Ophthalmology*. 2000;107:2179–2185.

Capsular Opacification and Contraction

Posterior Capsule Opacification

Overall, the most common complication of cataract surgery by means of ECCE or phacoemulsification is opacification of the intact posterior capsule. In addition, the introduction of continuous curvilinear capsulorrhexis has been accompanied in some cases by anterior capsule contraction and fibrosis (see the following subsection). Fortunately, posterior capsule opacification is amenable to treatment by means of Nd:YAG posterior capsulotomy.

Capsular opacification stems from the continued viability of lens epithelial cells remaining after removal of the nucleus and cortex. These cells proliferate in several patterns. Where the edges of the anterior capsule adhere to the posterior capsule, a closed space will be reestablished consisting of nucleated bladder cells *(Wedl cells),* resulting in a *Soemmering ring.* If the epithelial cells migrate outward, *Elschnig pearls,* which resemble fish eggs, are formed on the posterior capsule. These pearls can fill the pupil or remain hidden behind the iris. Histopathology shows that each "fish egg" is a nucleated bladder cell, identical to those proliferating within the capsule of a Soemmering ring but lying outside the capsule and usually lacking a basement membrane. If the epithelial cells migrate across the anterior or posterior capsule, they may cause capsular wrinkling and opacification. Significantly, the lens epithelial cells are capable of undergoing metaplasia with conversion to myofibroblasts. A matrix of fibrous and basement membrane collagen can be produced by these cells, and contraction of this collagen matrix will cause wrinkles in the posterior capsule, with resultant distortion of vision and glare. Meticulous hydrodissection and attention to complete cortical cleanup are important preventive measures for reducing the likelihood of these events.

Apple DJ, Auffarth GU, Peng A, et al. *Foldable Intraocular Lenses: Evolution, Clinicopathologic Correlations, and Complications.* Thorofare, NJ: Slack; 2000.

Apple DJ, Solomon KD, Tetz MR, et al. Posterior capsule opacification. *Surv Ophthalmol.* 1992;37:73–116.

Caporossi A, Casprini F, Tosi GM, Balestrazzi A, Stumpo M, Toti P. Histology of anterior capsule fibrosis following phacoemulsification. *J Cataract Refract Surg.* 1998;24:1343–1346.

The reported incidence of posterior capsule opacification varies widely. Factors known to influence this rate include the age of the patient, history of intraocular inflammation, presence of exfoliation syndrome, size of the capsulorrhexis, quality of cortical cleanup, capsular fixation of the implant, design of the lens implant (particularly a square-edge optic design), modification of the lens surface, and time elapsed since surgery. In addition, the presence of intraocular silicone oil may dramatically speed the progression of opacity. Anterior capsule opacity appears to be influenced by these same circumstances but is also more likely to occur in cases of a small capsulorrhexis or in the presence of weakened zonules.

Analysis of pooled multiple reports has found the visually significant posterior capsule opacification rate overall to be approximately 28% at 5 years. Quantitatively measured opacification incidence at 3 years has been reported at 56% for polymethylmethacrylate, 40% for silicone, and 10% for acrylic material, although the Nd:YAG rate is lower. In a large postmortem review, the prevalence of Nd:YAG capsulotomy was 0.9% for acrylic IOLs, 12%–21% for various silicone IOLs, and 27%–33% for polymethylmethacrylate IOLs. Newer generations of silicone materials appear to have a lower rate of opacification. It is now believed that this variation may be due not to the lens material but rather to the lens design and the quality of the capsular bend where the capsule overlaps the lens optic.

Apple DJ, Peng Q, Visessook N, et al. Eradication of posterior capsule opacification: documentation of a marked decrease in Nd:YAG laser posterior capsulotomy rates noted in an analysis of 5416 pseudophakic human eyes obtained postmortem. *Ophthalmology.* 2001;108:505–518.

Daynes T, Spencer TS, Doan K, Mamalis N, Olson RJ. Three-year clinical comparison of 3-piece AcrySof and SI-40 silicone intraocular lenses. *J Cataract Refract Surg.* 2002;28:1124–1129.

Dewey S. Posterior capsule opacification. *Curr Opinion Ophthalmol.* 2006;17:45–53.

Hollick EJ, Spalton DJ, Ursell PG, et al. The effect of polymethylmethacrylate, silicone, and polyacrylic intraocular lenses on posterior capsular opacification 3 years after cataract surgery. *Ophthalmology.* 1999;106:49–55.

Nishi O. Posterior capsule opacification. Part 1: Experimental investigations. *J Cataract Refract Surg.* 1999;25:106–117.

Schaumberg DA, Dana MR, Christen WG, Glynn RJ. A systematic overview of the incidence of posterior capsule opacification. *Ophthalmology.* 1998;105:1213–1221.

Anterior Capsule Fibrosis and Phimosis

Capsular fibrosis is associated with clouding of the anterior capsule. If a substantial portion of the IOL optic is covered by the anterior capsule, including portions exposed through the undilated pupil, the patient may become symptomatic when fibrosis occurs. Symptoms may include glare, especially at night owing to natural mydriasis in darkness, or the sensation of a peripheral cloud or haze.

Capsular phimosis is a term used to describe the postoperative contraction of the anterior capsule opening as a result of fibrosis, such that the rim of capsular tissue is also visible through the undilated pupil. Phimosis produces symptoms similar to, and often more pronounced than, fibrosis itself and may cause decentration of an IOL optic. Phimosis occurs more frequently with smaller capsulorrhexis openings, in patients with underlying exfoliation syndrome of the lens, in other situations with abnormal or asymmetric zonular support (eg, penetrating or blunt trauma, Marfan syndrome, or surgical trauma), and with plate haptic posterior chamber IOLs.

Treatment, which should be reserved for symptomatic patients, usually consists of a Nd:YAG laser anterior capsulotomy to enlarge the anterior capsule opening. This procedure is performed in a fashion similar to a Nd:YAG laser posterior capsulotomy, with care taken not to defocus too far posteriorly and damage the underlying IOL with laser pitting. In general, the anterior capsule tissue is tougher and requires more laser power than does the posterior capsule.

Nd:YAG Capsulotomy

Use of the Nd:YAG laser is now a standard procedure for treating secondary opacification of the posterior capsule or contraction of the anterior capsule, although a discission knife can be used through an ab externo corneal incision to open an opacified capsule in special cases.

Indications

The following are indications for Nd:YAG capsulotomy:

- best-corrected visual acuity symptomatically decreased as a result of a hazy posterior capsule
- a hazy posterior capsule preventing the clear view of the ocular fundus required for diagnostic or therapeutic purposes
- monocular diplopia or glare caused by posterior capsule wrinkling or by encroachment of a partially opened posterior capsule into the visual axis of a patient with otherwise clear media and good acuity
- contraction of anterior capsulotomy margins *(capsular phimosis)*, causing encroachment on the visual axis or alteration of the lens optic position; requires relaxing incisions

Contraindications

The following are contraindications to Nd:YAG capsulotomy:

- inadequate visualization of the posterior capsule

- an uncooperative patient who is unable to remain still or hold fixation during the procedure (use of a contact lens or retrobulbar anesthesia may enhance the feasibility of a capsulotomy in some of these patients)

Procedure

Nd:YAG laser discission is usually painless and is performed as an outpatient procedure. The surgeon should first adjust the oculars of the microscope-laser delivery system so that the focal point of the helium-neon aiming beam is clearly brought into focus. The pulse energy threshold for puncture of the posterior capsule is generally 0.8–2.0 mJ with either Q-switched (5–30 ns pulse length) or mode-locked (30–200 ps pulse length) systems. To puncture the posterior capsule, the surgeon should use the lowest effective energy output setting. Higher energy levels may be required for areas of dense fibrosis. The Nd:YAG laser emits radiation at a wavelength of 1064 nm.

Observation of the posterior capsule through an undilated pupil can help the surgeon pinpoint the location of the visual axis. The center of the visual axis is the desired site for the opening, which is usually adequate at 3–4 mm in diameter. In some circumstances, larger diameter openings may be required for more complete visualization of the fundus. Dilation is not always necessary for the procedure, but it may be helpful in producing a larger opening in the posterior capsule. When viewing the posterior capsule, the examiner should note *before* dilation any specific landmarks near the visual axis, because the location of the visual axis may not be obvious through the dilated pupil.

A high-plus-power anterior segment laser lens, used with topical anesthesia, improves ocular stability and enlarges the cone angle of the beam, reducing the depth of focus. The smaller-focus diameter facilitates the laser pulse puncture of the capsule, and structures in front of and behind the point of focus are less likely to be damaged (Fig 9-5). If light reflections from the slit-lamp illumination or the aiming beam obscure the area to be treated, the position of the biomicroscope may be adjusted, or the patient can shift fixation slightly.

Occasional reports of IOL dislocation into the vitreous following capsulotomy have been of concern, particularly with silicone plate haptic lenses. Constructing the capsulotomy in a spiraling circular pattern, rather than in a cruciate pattern, creates an opening less likely to extend radially (Fig 9-6) and reduces the risk of dislocation.

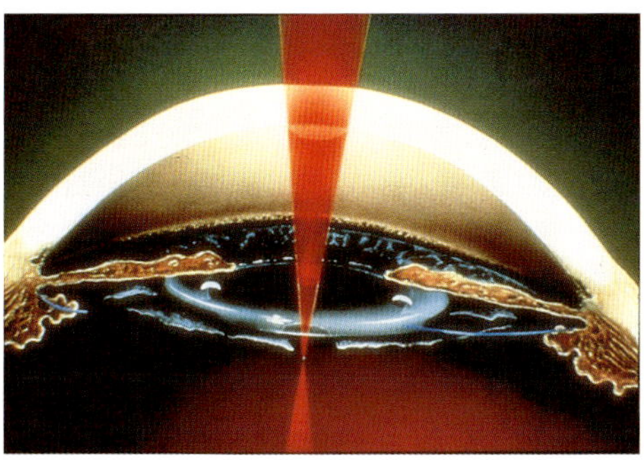

Figure 9-5 Enlarged cone angle of laser beam produces a narrower depth of field, facilitating laser pulse puncture of the capsule. *(Courtesy of Woodford S. Van Meter, MD.)*

If the energy output applied is minimal, the anterior vitreous face may remain intact. A ruptured anterior vitreous face will often be kept in check by the presence of a posterior chamber IOL, although vitreous strands occasionally migrate around the lens through the pupil.

Any posterior chamber IOL can be damaged by laser capsulotomy, but the threshold for lens damage appears to be lower for silicone than for other materials. The laser pulse should be focused just behind the posterior capsule, but pulses too far behind the IOL will be ineffective. The safest approach is to focus the laser beam slightly behind the posterior surface of the capsule for the initial application and then move subsequent applications anteriorly until the desired puncture is achieved. The surgeon should also search for sites where the capsule might have dropped more posterior to the IOL, because these sites can be treated more safely.

In cases of anterior capsule contraction, multiple relaxing incisions of the fibrotic ring are applied to relieve the contracting force and create a larger optical opening. Cycloplegic and anti-inflammatory drugs are not routinely necessary. Preoperative and postoperative application of topical apraclonidine hydrochloride (Iopidine) or brimonidine tartrate (Alphagan) is recommended to prevent postoperative IOP elevation.

The success rate of Nd:YAG laser discission for opening the capsule appears to exceed 95%. Occasionally, opacification that is exceptionally thick and dense is not affected by the Nd:YAG laser; these patients may require an invasive surgical procedure using a discission knife or scissors.

Newland TJ, McDermott ML, Eliott D, et al. Experimental neodymium:YAG laser damage to acrylic, poly(methyl methacrylate), and silicone intraocular lens material. *J Cataract Refract Surg.* 1999;25:72–76.

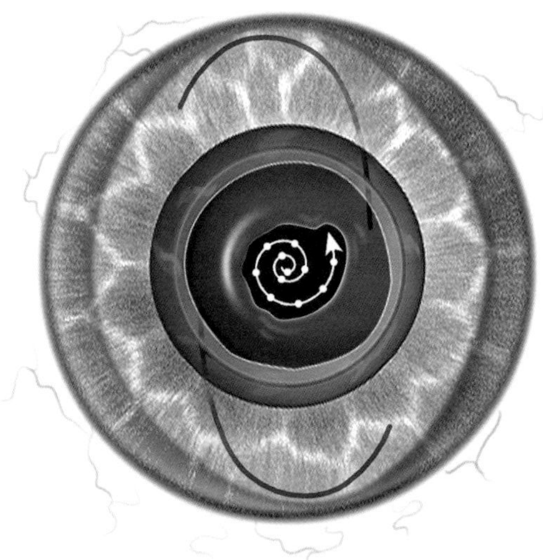

Figure 9-6 Making the series of laser punctures in a spiraling, rather than cruciate, pattern decreases the risk of radial tears. *(Illustration by Christine Gralapp.)*

Complications

Transient elevation of IOP can appear in a significant number of patients and may be treated prophylactically with a topical alpha-adrenergic agent, with monitoring of postdiscission IOP. Pressure levels peak within 2–3 hours. This elevation appears to be a consequence of obstruction of the outflow pathways by debris or macromolecules scattered by the laser treatment. Elevations respond quickly to topical glaucoma medications, which can be continued for 3–5 days following the procedure. Special precautions should be taken to observe and treat patients with preexisting glaucoma.

Nd:YAG capsulotomy increases the risk of retinal detachment. Approximately half of the retinal detachments following cataract extraction occur within 1 year of surgery, often associated with a posterior vitreous detachment. In many cases, it is difficult to ascertain whether the retinal detachment is related to the capsulotomy or to the cataract surgery itself. High myopia, vitreous trauma, a family history of retinal detachment, and preexisting pathology are risk factors that increase the risk of retinal detachment following Nd:YAG capsulotomy.

CME can occur following Nd:YAG capsulotomy. In patients with a history of CME, or in high-risk patients such as those with diabetic retinopathy, the use of topical steroids and nonsteroidal anti-inflammatory agents (pretreatment and posttreatment) may be beneficial. The risk of retinal detachment and CME may be greater when Nd:YAG capsulotomy is performed within 6 months of cataract surgery.

It is possible for an implant to dislocate into the vitreous cavity following capsulotomy. This complication is more likely to occur with plate haptic silicone implants (especially those with smaller fenestrations) than with any other type of IOL. Nd:YAG capsulotomy should be delayed for 3 months when a plate haptic silicone lens is present to increase the likelihood of capsular fixation.

Future improvements in surgical technique, new modifications in lens design and materials, and someday perhaps pharmacologic intervention all offer increasing opportunity for further reduction of posterior capsule opacification. Although the incidence of complications with modern Nd:YAG capsulotomy is small, a zero percent opacification rate is the ultimate surgical goal.

Javitt JC, Tielsch JM, Canner JK, Kolb MM, Sommer A, Steinberg EP. National outcomes of cataract extraction. Increased risk of retinal complications associated with Nd:YAG laser capsulotomy. The Cataract Patient Outcomes Research Team. *Ophthalmology.* 1992;99:1487–1498.

Hemorrhage

A large prospective cohort study was unable to demonstrate an increased risk of hemorrhagic complications in patients on anticoagulant or antiplatelet therapy during cataract surgery. In addition, no increase in the risk of medical complications was observed when such therapy was temporarily discontinued for surgery. This result is in contrast to earlier reports, which suggested that anticoagulation increases the risk of suprachoroidal effusion and suprachoroidal hemorrhage, and to more recent reports that cessation of anticoagulation carries significant risks of thromboembolic complications.

Katz J, Feldman MA, Bass EB, et al. Risks and benefits of anticoagulant and antiplatelet medication use before cataract surgery. *Ophthalmology*. 2003;110:1784–1788.

Retrobulbar Hemorrhage

Retrobulbar hemorrhages are more common with retrobulbar anesthetic injections than with peribulbar injections, and they may vary in intensity. Reports estimate the incidence of significant retrobulbar hemorrhage to be 1%–3%. *Venous* retrobulbar hemorrhages are usually self-limited and tend to spread slowly. They often do not require treatment.

Arterial retrobulbar hemorrhages occur more rapidly and are associated with taut orbital swelling, marked proptosis, elevated IOP, reduced mobility of the globe, inability to separate the eyelids, and massive ecchymosis of the lids and conjunctiva. This type of retrobulbar hemorrhage causes an increase in orbital volume and associated orbital pressure, which can restrict the vascular supply to the globe. Large orbital vessels may be occluded, or tamponade of the smaller nutrient vessels in the optic nerve may occur, resulting in severe visual loss and subsequent optic atrophy despite the absence of obvious retinal vascular occlusion.

Ophthalmologists can often make the diagnosis of retrobulbar hemorrhage by observing the rapid onset of lid and conjunctival ecchymosis and tightening of the orbit. The diagnosis can be confirmed by tonometry revealing elevated IOP. A simple handheld tonometer kept in a sterile pack in the operating room is ideal for this situation. Direct ophthalmoscopy may reveal pulsation or occlusion of the central retinal artery in severe cases.

Treatment of acute retrobulbar hemorrhage consists of maneuvers to lower the orbital and intraocular pressure as quickly as possible. These may include digital massage; intravenous osmotic agents or topical aqueous suppressants; and lateral canthotomy and cantholysis, localized conjunctival peritomy (to allow egress of blood), and, occasionally, even anterior chamber paracentesis. Serial tonometry demonstrating a reduction in IOP will help confirm the success of the treatment. Without demonstration of normalization of IOP and mobility of the globe, surgery should be postponed even in the presence of a red reflex. In general, cataract surgery should not be performed when a serious retrobulbar hemorrhage occurs, as the risk of iris prolapse or even an expulsive choroidal hemorrhage is far greater than usual. The surgery can be rescheduled for several days later. To reduce the risk of a recurrent retrobulbar hemorrhage, many surgeons would consider using peribulbar, sub-Tenon, topical, or general anesthesia for the second attempt at surgery.

Cionni R, Osher RH. Retrobulbar hemorrhage. *Ophthalmology*. 1991;98:1153–1155.
Feibel RM. Current concepts in retrobulbar anesthesia. *Surv Ophthalmol*. 1985;30:102–110.
Morgan CM, Schatz H, Vine AK, et al. Ocular complications associated with retrobulbar injections. *Ophthalmology*. 1988;95:660–665.

Suprachoroidal Effusion or Hemorrhage

Suprachoroidal effusion with or without suprachoroidal hemorrhage generally occurs intraoperatively. Secure incision closure to prevent hypotony can significantly reduce the postoperative risk of this complication. Typically, a forward prolapse of posterior ocular structures including iris and vitreous occurs, generally accompanied by a change in the red reflex. Clinically, suprachoroidal effusion may be difficult to differentiate from suprachoroidal hemorrhage. Patient agitation and pain followed by an extremely firm globe suggest suprachoroidal hemorrhage. Both complications are more common in the presence of underlying hypertension, tachycardia, obesity, high myopia, anticoagulation, glaucoma, advanced age, or chronic ocular inflammation. Fortunately, both complications are much less likely with modern phacoemulsification because of the relatively closed system formed by the architecture of the small, self-sealing incision and the relatively tight fit of the phaco tip in the incision.

Suprachoroidal effusion may be a precursor to suprachoroidal hemorrhage. Exudation of fluid from choroidal vasculature ultimately tents veins or arteries that supply the choroid after coursing through the sclera. If suprachoroidal hemorrhage occurs in this situation, it is presumably a result of disruption of one or more of these tented blood vessels. Alternatively, suprachoroidal hemorrhage may represent a spontaneous rupture of choroidal vasculature, particularly in patients with underlying systemic vascular disease.

Expulsive Suprachoroidal Hemorrhage

Expulsive suprachoroidal hemorrhage, a rare but serious problem, generally occurs intraoperatively. It requires immediate action. This condition usually presents as a sudden increase in IOP, with darkening of the red reflex; incision gape; iris prolapse; expulsion of the lens, vitreous, and bright red blood; accompanied by the sudden onset of pain. The instant this condition is recognized, the incision must be closed with sutures or digital pressure. Posterior sclerotomies allow the escape of suprachoroidal blood, which may help decompress the globe; allow the repositioning of prolapsed intraocular tissue; and facilitate permanent closure of the cataract incision. If the incision can be closed without posterior sclerotomies, more rapid tamponade of the bleeding vessel is achieved.

Treatment of both suprachoroidal and expulsive suprachoroidal hemorrhage consists of rapid closure of the incision. Subsequent elevation of IOP will tamponade the bleeding. Having closed the globe, the surgeon may wish to drain the suprachoroidal blood by performing a sclerotomy in one or more quadrants, 5–7 mm posterior to the limbus, if a hemorrhagic component can be seen. If the involved quadrants cannot be readily identified, posterior sclerotomies can empirically be placed in the inferotemporal quadrant. If this attempt fails to adequately drain the suprachoroidal hemorrhage, additional sclerotomies can be placed in the other quadrants. The sclerotomy can be created with either a blade or a small (Elliot) trephine. Hemorrhagic fluid is drained, while the elevated IOP serves both to stop bleeding and to expel suprachoroidal blood. Once optimal clearance of blood from the suprachoroidal space has occurred, the surgeon may wish to leave the sclerotomies open to allow further drainage postoperatively. In addition, the surgeon may consider repeating the drainage procedure 7 days or more after an expulsive hemorrhage in case of residual suprachoroidal blood that could threaten ocular integrity or visual acuity. These procedures may lower dangerously elevated IOPs and restore appropriate anatomic relationships within the eye, but they carry some risk that bleeding will recur. Because this condition is rare, there is no consensus, thus far, about whether visual outcomes are superior with or without posterior sclerotomies. Some surgeons prefer to close the incision and refer the patient to a vitreoretinal specialist.

Delayed Suprachoroidal Hemorrhage

Less commonly, suprachoroidal hemorrhage may occur in the early postoperative period, presenting with sudden onset of pain, loss of vision, and shallowing of the anterior chamber. If the incision remains intact and the IOP can be controlled medically, limited suprachoroidal hemorrhage may be observed and frequently will resolve spontaneously. If the incision is not intact, surgical revision alone may be sufficient to allow the hemorrhage to resolve. Surgical drainage of the suprachoroidal space is indicated with persistent flat anterior chamber, medically uncontrolled glaucoma, adherent (kissing) choroidals, or persistent choroidal detachment. Medical management consists of empiric corticosteroids given systemically, topical and oral ocular hypotensive agents, topical cycloplegia, and close observation.

Hyphema

Hyphema in the immediate postoperative period usually originates in the incision or the iris; it is commonly mild and resolves spontaneously. The risk of hyphema is greater in patients with pseudoexfoliation syndrome. Resolution may take longer if vitreous is mixed with the blood. The 2 major complications from prolonged hyphema are elevated IOP and corneal blood staining. IOP should be monitored closely and treated in the usual medical fashion, although it may be difficult to control if the blood is mixed with the OVD used during the procedure.

Hyphema that occurs months to years after surgery usually comes from incision vascularization or erosion of vascular tissue by an IOL. Argon laser photocoagulation of the bleeding vessel, often performed through a goniolens, will usually stop the bleeding or prevent rebleeding. To reduce the risk of continued or recurrent bleeding, antiplatelet or anticoagulation therapy may be withheld, if medically possible, until the hyphema resolves.

Endophthalmitis

Endophthalmitis may present in an acute form or in a more indolent or chronic form; the latter is associated with organisms of lower pathogenicity. The symptoms of endophthalmitis include mild to severe ocular pain, loss of vision, floaters, and photophobia. The hallmark of endophthalmitis is vitreous inflammation, but other signs include eyelid or periorbital edema, ciliary injection, chemosis, anterior chamber reaction, hypopyon, decreased visual acuity, corneal edema, and retinal hemorrhages (Fig 9-7).

Commonly employed methods to reduce the risk of endophthalmitis include placing povidone-iodine 5% drops in the conjunctival sac as part of the preoperative preparation of the eye; using adhesive incise drapes to isolate the lashes and lid margins from the operative field; and maintaining appropriate intraoperative aseptic technique. Meticulous attention to watertight incision closure is an important element of endophthalmitis prevention, particularly when clear corneal incisions are employed. The effectiveness of antibiotics in the prevention of endophthalmitis has been controversial. Topical therapy for 3 days prior to surgery can reduce bacterial counts but has not been shown to reduce

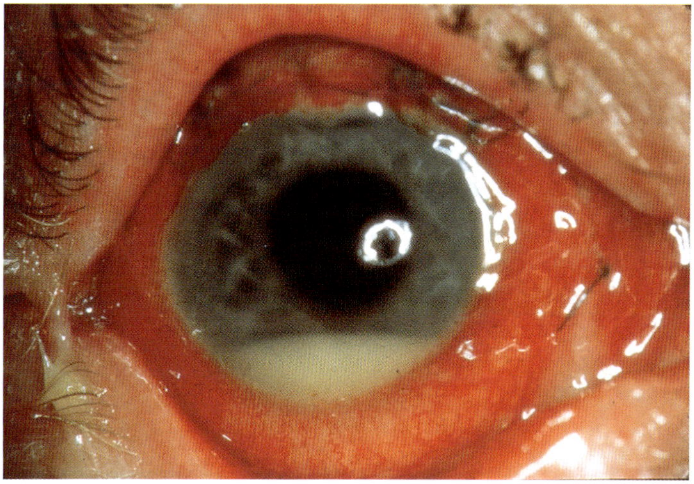

Figure 9-7 Endophthalmitis. *(Courtesy of Karla J. Johns, MD.)*

the incidence of infection. In 2006, a preliminary report from a large European prospective multicenter randomized clinical trial indicated that injection of 1 mg cefuroxime into the anterior chamber at the conclusion of cataract surgery can reduce the incidence of endophthalmitis fivefold. The validity of generalizing these results to all cataract procedures awaits publication of the final report. Given the difficulty of obtaining preservative-free antibiotics that are commercially available in doses appropriate for intracameral prophylaxis, surgeons need to weigh these results against the risk of dilutional errors or preservative toxicity.

Diagnosis

Acute endophthalmitis typically develops 2–5 days postoperatively and runs a fulminant course. Decreasing vision and increasing pain and inflammation are hallmarks. Early diagnosis is extremely important, as delay of treatment can substantially alter the visual prognosis. *Chronic endophthalmitis,* in contrast, may have its onset weeks or months after surgery. It may be characterized by chronic iritis or granulomatous uveitis and is often associated with decreased visual acuity, little or no pain, and the presence of a nidus of the infectious agent within the eye. (See also BCSC Section 9, *Intraocular Inflammation and Uveitis*, and BCSC Section 12, *Retina and Vitreous.*)

Noninfectious (sterile) endophthalmitis is a rare complication of cataract surgery. It is often associated with the introduction of toxic materials into the eye via contaminants on an IOL, inadvertent intracameral injection of a toxin, or a severe inflammatory reaction to retained lens material. The clinician can diagnose sterile endophthalmitis by excluding possible infectious causes by means of appropriate aqueous and vitreous cultures.

Treatment

The recommended approach to the diagnosis and management of postoperative endophthalmitis is based on the results of the Endophthalmitis Vitrectomy Study (EVS).

In this study, patients were randomized to receive either an immediate 3-port pars plana vitrectomy (VIT) or a tap/biopsy of the vitreous (TAP). Patients were further randomized either to receive or not to receive intravenous antibiotics. All study patients received a standard antibiotic regimen consisting of 0.4 mg/0.1 mL intravitreal amikacin and 1.0 mg/0.1 mL intravitreal vancomycin, along with subconjunctival injections of 25 mg vancomycin, 100 mg ceftazidime, and 6 mg dexamethasone. Topical antibiotics included 50 mg/mL vancomycin and 14 mg/mL amikacin, which were administered frequently, along with topical cycloplegics and corticosteroids. Patients assigned to intravenous antibiotics received ceftazidime and amikacin.

Results of vitreous cultures were positive in 69% of cases, with 70% of culture-positive cases yielding gram-positive, coagulase-negative staphylococcal species (especially *Staphylococcus epidermidis*). The remaining culture-positive cases grew other gram-positive organisms (15%), gram-negative species (6%), or multiple organisms (9%).

Final posttreatment visual acuity of 20/40 or better was achieved by 53% of all patients in the EVS, with 74% attaining 20/100 or better. For all study patients presenting with better than light perception (LP) vision (ie, hand motions or better), the visual results were equal in both groups; there were no benefits with either VIT or TAP in the final visual outcome. Vitrectomy was found to be of benefit only for those patients presenting with LP vision, as VIT patients achieved better visual acuity than did TAP patients. No benefit was found with the use of intravenous antibiotics. This result is not surprising given the poor penetration of most intravenous antibiotics into the vitreous cavity.

As soon as endophthalmitis is recognized, assessment of visual acuity will help direct the management decisions. Fortified topical antibiotics may be started if doing so does not delay referral to a vitreoretinal specialist. Immediate 3-port pars plana vitrectomy is indicated when vision has been reduced to light perception, whereas less invasive vitreous biopsy or needle aspiration is adequate when the vision is hand motions or better. Because there are no reliable clinical features to distinguish between gram-positive and gram-negative organisms, the mainstay of treatment for both remains broad-spectrum intravitreal antibiotics. Fortified topical and subconjunctival antibiotics are administered in the period following antibiotic injection into the vitreous while waiting for culture results. Intravenous antibiotics are of no benefit. Although intravitreal corticosteroids are frequently used because of their theoretical role in reducing inflammation and scarring, their benefit has yet to be demonstrated in a controlled study. Oral fluoroquinolones have been shown to achieve significant levels in the aqueous and vitreous fluids.

Barry P, Seal DV, Gettinby G, et al. ESCRS study of prophylaxis of postoperative endophthalmitis after cataract surgery: preliminary report of principal results from a European multicenter study. *J Cataract Refract Surgery*. 2006;32:407–410.

Doft BH. Managing infectious endophthalmitis: results of the Endophthalmitis Vitrectomy Study. *Focal Points: Clinical Modules for Ophthalmologists*. San Francisco: American Academy of Ophthalmology; 1997, module 3.

Endophthalmitis Vitrectomy Study Group. A randomized trial of immediate vitrectomy and of intravenous antibiotics for the treatment of postoperative bacterial endophthalmitis. *Arch Ophthalmol*. 1995;113:1479–1496.

Cystoid Macular Edema

Cystoid macular edema is a common cause of decreased vision after both complicated and uncomplicated cataract surgery (it is also known as *Irvine-Gass syndrome*). Although the pathogenesis of CME is unknown, the final common pathway appears to be increased perifoveal capillary permeability, possibly associated with generalized intraocular vascular instability. Associated factors include inflammation with release of prostaglandins, vitreomacular traction, excessive UV light exposure, posterior capsule rupture, vitreous loss, iris prolapse, and transient or prolonged hypotony.

CME can be recognized by an otherwise unexplained reduction in visual acuity, by the characteristic petaloid appearance of cystic spaces in the macula on ophthalmoscopy or fluorescein angiography (Fig 9-8), or by retinal thickening on optical coherence tomography (OCT). *Angiographic* CME occurs in 40%–70% of eyes following ICCE and in approximately 1%–19% of eyes following ECCE via nuclear expression or phacoemulsification. Most of the affected patients are visually asymptomatic.

If the diagnosis of *clinical* CME is based on visual loss to the 20/40 level or worse, the incidence is 2%–10% following intracapsular surgery and 1%–2% following extracapsular surgery with an intact posterior capsule. The risk of clinical CME after phacoemulsification with an intact posterior capsule is believed to be even lower. However, patients with *angiographic* CME after phacoemulsification demonstrate significantly lower logMAR visual acuity scores than do patients with no CME, even though their Snellen visual acuities remain better than 20/40. Macular edema after cataract surgery may be associated with some loss of contrast sensitivity even in the absence of reduced Snellen acuity. The peak incidence of both angiographic and clinical CME occurs 6–10 weeks after surgery. Spontaneous resolution occurs in approximately 95% of uncomplicated cases, usually within 6 months. Rarely, CME may develop many years after ICCE, especially in association with delayed postoperative rupture of the anterior vitreous face. It is also associated with the

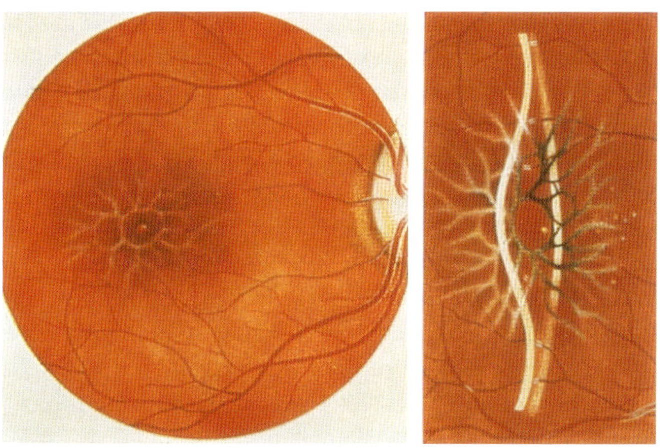

Figure 9-8 Artist's rendering of cystic spaces in macula associated with cystoid macular edema. *(Reprinted from Gass JD, Norton EW. Cystoid macular edema and papilledema following cataract extraction. A fluorescein fundoscopic and angiographic study.* Arch Ophthalmol. *1966;76:647.)*

use of epinephrine and dipivefrin topically for the treatment of aphakic glaucoma. Prostaglandin analogs have been associated with reversible CME in eyes that have undergone recent intraocular surgery, although a cause-and-effect relationship has not been established. The risk is believed to be greater in the absence of an intact posterior capsule. Other risk factors for CME include poorly controlled postoperative inflammation, preexisting epiretinal membrane, diabetes mellitus, and a previous occurrence of CME.

The relationship between IOLs and both clinical and angiographic CME is not completely understood. Some retrospective studies suggest a higher incidence and later onset, as well as a poorer prognosis, in eyes with iris-supported IOLs. Closed-loop anterior chamber IOLs are associated with a high incidence of uveitis, CME, glaucoma, hyphema, and corneal decompensation. Quiet postoperative eyes with evidence of malpositioned implants (iris tuck, intermittent corneal touch, pupillary capture, short anterior chamber lens), as well as eyes with implant-related uveitis show a higher incidence of chronic CME. The presence of a well-positioned posterior chamber or open-loop anterior chamber IOL does not appear to increase the risk of CME. A UV-filtering IOL may reduce the incidence of angiographic CME after cataract surgery.

CME with visual loss occurs more commonly in eyes with surgical complications and in eyes with vitreous adhering to the incision, the iris, or the IOL. The risk of CME can be reduced with preoperative and postoperative prophylactic use of topical or systemic indomethacin or topical ketorolac. Other topical NSAIDs may have similar effects, but they have not been as extensively studied. Because most cases of postoperative CME resolve spontaneously, it is difficult to assess the effect of therapeutic agents. In a prospective randomized controlled clinical trial, topical ketorolac 0.5% or prednisolone acetate 1% was demonstrated to be effective therapy for chronic CME, but greater improvement in acuity was obtained with a combination of topical ketorolac 0.5% and prednisolone 1% 4 times a day than with either medication alone.

If topical medications fail, some surgeons will try sub-Tenon injections of corticosteroids. Intravitreal triamcinolone acetonide appears to be effective, but in commercially available formulations of this agent, the vehicle and the preservatives, which include benzyl alcohol, are potentially toxic. The risk of toxicity can be mitigated by the use of nonpreserved triamcinolone for intravitreal injection. Despite the lack of controlled clinical studies, it is believed that pretreatment with any one of several topical nonsteroidal anti-inflammatory drops will be of benefit in CME prophylaxis and treatment. In an uncontrolled pilot study, treatment with topical ketorolac for 3 days prior to cataract surgery reduced the incidence of CME detectable by OCT, but no significant effect on clinical CME was detectable.

Surgical therapy may be indicated when the inciting source of chronic clinical CME can be defined, but the edema fails to respond to medical therapy. Nd:YAG laser treatment or vitrectomy surgery can be used to remove vitreous adhering to the cataract incision, thus relieving vitreomacular traction. This approach has been shown to be of value in patients with chronic CME, especially when medically unresponsive, low-grade uveitis is present. IOL exchange may be helpful if the IOL is malpositioned, has vitreous adherent to it, or contributes to chronic uveitis (For further discussion of CME, see BCSC Section 12, *Retina and Vitreous.*)

Conway MD, Canakis C, Livir-Rallatos C, Peyman GA. Intravitreal triamcinolone acetonide for refractory chronic pseudophakic cystoid macular edema. *J Cataract Refract Surg.* 2003;29:27–33.

Donnenfeld ED, Perry HD, Wittpenn JR, Solomon R, Nattis A, Chou T. Preoperative ketorolac tromethamine 0.4% in phacoemulsification outcomes: pharmacokinetic-response curve. *J Cataract Refract Surg.* 2006;32:1474–1482.

Heier JS, Topping TM, Baumann W, Dirks MS, Chern S. Ketorolac versus prednisolone versus combination therapy in the treatment of acute pseudophakic cystoid macular edema. *Ophthalmology.* 2000;107:2034–2038.

Ursell PG, Spalton DJ, Whitcup SM, Nussenblatt RB. Cystoid macular edema after phacoemulsification: relationship to blood–aqueous barrier damage and visual acuity. *J Cataract Refract Surg.* 1999;25:1492–1497.

Wand M, Shields BM. Cystoid macular edema in the era of ocular hypotensive lipids. *Am J Ophthalmol.* 2002;133:393–397.

Retinal Light Toxicity

Prolonged exposure to the illuminating filament of the operating microscope can result in an increased risk of CME or a burn to the retinal pigment epithelium (RPE). The risk of an RPE burn is particularly high during cataract surgery, when the filtering effects of the natural lens (cataract) are removed, exposing the vulnerable RPE to unfiltered blue light and near-UV radiation. If the burn occurs in the fovea, visual acuity may be reduced. If the burn is extrafoveal, the patient may complain of a paracentral scotoma. Minimizing retinal exposure to the operating microscope light is the key to avoiding this complication.

Actions to reduce the risk of retinal photic injury include the following:

- Use the minimum light intensity needed to safely perform the procedure.
- Replace lamps with manufacturer-approved products.
- Add a filter to exclude light below 515 nm.
- Use oblique lighting, when possible.
- Use pupillary shields, either built into the microscope or placed on the cornea.
- Minimize direct exposure of the fovea.

Retinal photic injuries from operating microscopes during cataract surgery. FDA Public Health Advisory. Rockville, MD: US Dept Health and Human Services; 1995.

Macular Infarction

Extensive retinal nonperfusion and macular infarction, clinically similar in appearance to central retinal artery occlusion, may occur after uncomplicated subconjunctival injection of aminoglycosides for endophthalmitis prophylaxis at the conclusion of cataract surgery. This complication appears to be uncommon, but the incidence is unknown. The risk may be greatest with injection of gentamicin, but amikacin and tobramycin can cause a similar clinical picture. Aminoglycosides are not the agent of choice in any case, given the EVS findings that gram-positive organisms are the etiologic agent in 70% of cases of postoperative endophthalmitis. Endophthalmitis is treatable, whereas macular infarction is not. Therefore, routine subconjunctival aminoglycoside prophylaxis at the conclusion of cataract surgery is no longer recommended.

Campochiaro PA, Conway BP. Aminoglycoside toxicity—a survey of retinal specialists. *Arch Ophthalmol.* 1991;109:946–950.

Retinal Detachment

Retinal detachment occurs in 2%–3% of eyes following ICCE, in 0.5%–2.0% of eyes following ECCE, and in approximately 1% of eyes following phacoemulsification. Retinal detachment occurs most frequently within 6 months of cataract surgery or following posterior capsulotomy (Fig 9-9).

Predisposing factors include axial myopia (>25 mm), age under 50, lattice degeneration of the retina, a previous retinal tear or detachment in the surgical eye, a history of retinal detachment in the fellow eye, or a family history of retinal detachment. The presence of any of these factors should make the surgeon more vigilant in examining the peripheral fundus in these patients before and after surgery and should be considered in the decision to treat asymptomatic retinal breaks preoperatively.

The presence of an intact posterior capsule reduces the incidence of retinal detachment. Conversely, complicated cataract surgery with a broken posterior capsule and vitreous loss increases the postoperative risk of retinal detachment. Evidence suggests that the risk of retinal detachment increases fourfold following Nd:YAG laser posterior capsulotomy. Anecdotal reports have suggested that delaying the Nd:YAG laser posterior capsulotomy may reduce the risk of subsequent retinal detachment. Although no prospective randomized controlled studies confirm this belief, delaying capsulotomy for at least

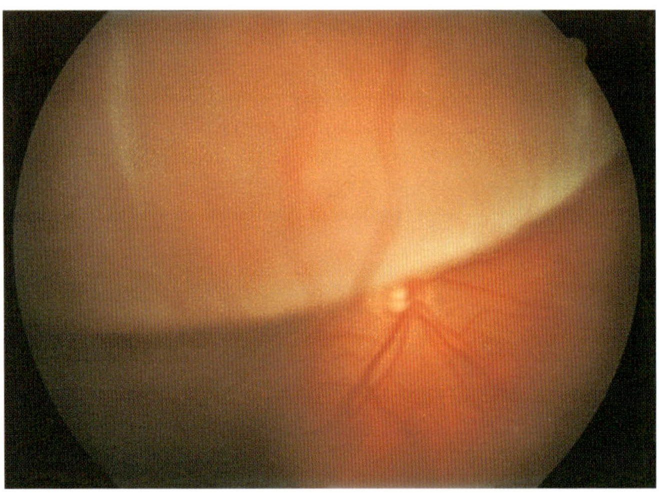

Figure 9-9 Bullous superior rhegmatogenous retinal detachment following extracapsular cataract extraction and posterior chamber lens implantation. *(Reproduced with permission from Wilkinson CP. Retinal complications following cataract surgery.* Focal Points: Clinical Modules for Ophthalmologists. *San Francisco: American Academy of Ophthalmology; 1992, module 12.)*

3–6 months after cataract surgery may allow for posterior vitreous separation and be less disruptive to the vitreoretinal interface. The successful repair of retinal detachment is not influenced by the presence or absence of either an anterior or a posterior chamber IOL.

Boberg-Ans G, Henning V, Villumsen J, la Cour M. Long-term incidence of rhegmatogenous retinal detachment and survival in a defined population undergoing standardized phacoemulsification surgery. *Acta Ophthalmol Scand*. 2006;84:613–618.

Haller JA. Retinal detachment. *Focal Points: Clinical Modules for Ophthalmologists*. San Francisco: American Academy of Ophthalmology; 1998, module 5.

CHAPTER 10

Cataract Surgery in Special Situations

Cataract in Children

Surgical Planning

The surgical management of cataracts in the pediatric age group requires consideration of a wide range of factors unique to this population. The risk of amblyopia has an impact on the timing of surgery and the method of aphakic correction. The patient's parents play a critical role in the postoperative care of the eye and the treatment of amblyopia. They must understand that a successful visual result depends on more than the surgical procedure; it also depends on their ability to follow through with amblyopia therapy. The surgeon must be certain that the parents' expectations of a successful visual result are realistic, given the child's age and type of cataract.

The child may have to undergo repeated general anesthesia for surgery and for some postoperative examinations. Optimal management often requires the coordinated efforts of several physicians: the ophthalmologist who will perform the surgery and direct the postoperative amblyopia therapy, the pediatrician, and the anesthesiologist.

Bilateral congenital cataracts

The management of bilateral congenital cataracts depends on the etiology and the degree to which the cataracts interfere with vision. Patients with small axial cataracts often maintain good vision if their pupils are continuously dilated with mydriatic drops. Severe bilateral cataracts must be removed if the patient is to develop functional vision. Current concepts of amblyopia and the normal development of the fixation reflex necessitate timely cataract removal when the visual axis is significantly obstructed. Children with profound bilateral amblyopia from cataracts develop nystagmus at approximately 3 months of age because the fixation reflex normally develops by that time. Once nystagmus has developed, it is likely to persist even if the cataracts are subsequently removed. Visual acuity in eyes with nystagmus and infantile cataracts is rarely better than 20/200 after cataract surgery. The only way to obtain a better visual result is to perform the surgery as early as possible and provide appropriate aphakic correction, which today most surgeons would agree requires primary intraocular lens (IOL) placement. Thus, in bilateral, severe cataracts, surgery is recommended on the first eye as soon as possible after diagnosis—ideally, before 3 months of age. If all goes well with the first eye, removal of the cataract from the fellow eye should follow promptly. It has been suggested that surgeries be separated by 2 weeks for children younger than 2 years and by 1 month for children older than 2 years.

Peterseim MW, Wilson ME. Bilateral intraocular lens implantation in the pediatric population. *Ophthalmology*. 2000;107:1261–1266.

Unilateral congenital cataract

With a unilateral congenital or infantile cataract, the prognosis for useful vision in the affected eye depends on prompt restoration of a clear visual axis, correction of aphakia, and aggressive treatment of amblyopia. Studies have suggested that intervention before 6 weeks of age may minimize the effects of congenital unilateral deprivation on the visual system and provide for optimal rehabilitation of vision. Although excellent results have been reported when such children have received optimal care, the overall prognosis is guarded, regardless of amblyopia therapy and the technique used for refractive correction. Before agreeing to early surgery, parents must understand the hardships that occlusion therapy will cause during the first decade of the child's life. In addition, they must realize that multiple surgeries may be required to maintain a clear visual axis and that despite sometimes heroic efforts, the overall visual results may be disappointing.

Birch EE, Stager DR. The critical period for surgical treatment of dense congenital unilateral cataract. *Invest Ophthalmol Vis Sci*. 1996;37:1532–1538.

Surgical Technique

Cataract surgery in children is similar in many respects to that in adults, although significant differences exist. Features unique to a child's eye include changing axial length, corneal curvature, and lenticular refracting power; increased tissue reactivity; less scleral rigidity; more elastic capsule; smaller size; and potential for amblyopia. Parents should be informed that these children will require follow-up care for their entire lives. Also, compared with adults, children have an enhanced inflammatory and fibrotic response to cataract surgery.

Over the past decade, advances in adult cataract surgery techniques have been transferred to pediatric cataract removal. Although a temporal approach is possible in children, just as in adults, a superior incision beneath a scleral tunnel is thought to provide the child with a more secure incision, at less risk from a subsequent traumatic injury. Scleral tunnel incisions help maintain the anterior chamber during the procedure. Scleral incisions should be closed with suture. Incisions that self-seal in adults require suture in pediatric patients. High-viscosity ophthalmic viscosurgical devices (OVDs) facilitate the anterior capsulotomy. Because the capsule is more elastic in a child's eye and expansion of the capsulotomy is predictable, the surgeon should aim for a smaller opening. Several variations of pediatric anterior capsulorrhexis have been described, including mechanized anterior capsulotomy using a vitrector. If an IOL is to be implanted, it is important to avoid radial tears that ultimately could result in IOL displacement. The anterior capsulotomy should be large enough not to contract and reduce the effective pupil size but not so large that peripheral anterior synechiae form between the iris and edge of the capsule and exposed lens.

Congenital cataracts are removed by simple aspiration or lensectomy. The nucleus and cortex in a young child's eye tend to be gummy and do not aspirate in the same manner as the adult lens cortex. Cannulas with a 0.3-mm port, which are commonly used in adult irrigation/aspiration systems, are less effective in this situation than the larger aspiration port of a vitrectomy instrument or phaco tip.

In cataracts with associated blood vessel anomalies, such as persistent fetal vasculature (PFV, previously known as *persistent hyperplastic primary vitreous*), intraoperative bleeding may occur. Vitrectomy instrumentation is often used in such cases to assist with hemostasis and to remove the posterior lens capsule, abnormal membranes, and anterior vitreous.

Use of IOL implants is common practice today in the treatment of aphakia in the pediatric population, in the absence of congenital anomalies that preclude their placement. Although to date, the FDA has not given any IOL premarket approval as being safe and effective for use in children, the literature contains an increasing number of articles regarding the efficacy and safety of IOL use in the pediatric group.

A physician may follow the *good medical practice rule* and decide to implant a commercially available IOL in a child after determining the FDA status of the implant and obtaining appropriate, informed consent from the adult responsible for the child. This rule states that good medical practice and patient interests require physicians to use commercially available drugs, devices, and biologics according to their best knowledge and judgment. A physician who uses a product in the practice of medicine for an indication not in the approved labeling has the responsibility to be well informed about the product and to base its use on firm scientific evidence. This usage does not require an investigational device exemption or a review by an institutional review board unless such review is otherwise needed.

In the past, complete or large posterior capsulectomy and limited anterior vitrectomy were recommended because of the high incidence of lens capsule opacification and secondary membrane formation across the intact hyaloid face and capsule remnants, which contribute to sensory deprivation amblyopia. In the 1990s, Gimbel and colleagues demonstrated that posterior capsulorrhexis with posterior capture of the IOL optic decreased the incidence of secondary membrane formation and provided for a stable implant. The decision whether to perform a limited anterior vitrectomy in addition to the capsulectomy is thought to be best determined by the patient's age, with patients younger than 5 years benefiting from the additional vitrectomy. In one study, even though both a posterior capsulorrhexis and an anterior vitrectomy were performed, secondary membrane formation necessitating a pars plana vitrectomy at a later date occurred in almost all infants younger than 1 month and in most infants up to 6 months of age.

If a secondary opacification occurs, an alternative approach to its treatment is the Nd:YAG laser posterior capsulotomy; however, this procedure is more easily performed in children older than 6 years. If an IOL is present, poor patient cooperation during the laser procedure may result in lens pitting. The posterior capsule in children is often thick and may require higher laser energy levels for discission than those used in adults.

Enyedi LB, Peterseim MW, Freedman SF, Buckley EG. Refractive changes after pediatric intraocular lens implantation. *Am J Ophthalmol.* 1998;126:772–781.

Forbes BJ, Guo S. Update on the surgical management of pediatric cataracts. *J Pediatr Ophthalmol Strabismus.* 2006;43:143–151.

Gimbel HV, DeBroff BM. Posterior capsulorrhexis with optic capture: maintaining a clear visual axis after pediatric cataract surgery. *J Cataract Refract Surg.* 1994;20:658–664.

Kohnen T. Visual axis opacification after pediatric intraocular lens implantation. *J Cataract Refract Surg.* 2001;27:1141–1142.

Kugelberg M, Zetterstrom C. Pediatric cataract surgery with or without anterior vitrectomy. *J Cataract Refract Surg.* 2002;28:1770–1773.

Lundvall A, Zetterstrom C. Primary intraocular lens implantation in infants: complications and visual results. *J Cataract Refract Surg.* 2006;32:1672–1677.

O'Keefe M, Fenton S, Lanigan B. Visual outcomes and complications of posterior chamber intraocular lens implantation in the first year of life. *J Cataract Refract Surg.* 2001;27:2006–2011.

Pandey SK, Wilson ME, Trivedi RH, et al. Pediatric cataract surgery and intraocular lens implantation: current techniques, complications, and management. *Int Ophthalmol Clin.* 2001;41:175–196.

Stager DR Jr, Weakley DR Jr, Hunter JS. Long-term rates of PCO following small incision foldable acrylic intraocular lens implantation in children. *J Pediatr Ophthalmol Strabismus.* 2002;39:73–76.

Tsao K, Kazlas M. The pediatric cataract. In: Pineda R, Espaillat A, Perez VL, et al, eds. *The Complicated Cataract: The Massachusetts Eye and Ear Infirmary Phacoemulsification Practice Handbook.* Thorofare, NJ: Slack; 2001:129–140.

Postoperative Care

To reduce the inflammatory reaction to surgery, infants and young children require a more aggressive course of topical corticosteroids than do adults. Cycloplegia with cyclopentolate 1% or 2%, scopolamine 0.25%, or atropine 1% drops for about 1 month postoperatively is advised.

Complications

Although any of the complications discussed in Chapter 9 can occur in children, glaucoma, retinal detachment, and opacification of retained posterior capsule are the more frequent late complications of congenital cataract surgery. Glaucoma has been reported to occur in 13%–24% of the eyes of children with pediatric cataracts. There have been reports, however, of a reduced incidence of glaucoma in children receiving an IOL. Some surgeons recommend that, at the time of surgery, a peripheral iridectomy be performed for angle-closure glaucoma prophylaxis. Parents should be informed that these children will require follow-up care for their entire lives. There is also a high prevalence of ocular hypertension after pediatric cataract surgery.

Egbert JE, Wright MM, Dahlhauser KF, Keithahn MA, Letson RD, Summers CG. A prospective study of ocular hypertension and glaucoma after pediatric cataract surgery. *Ophthalmology.* 1995;102:1098–1101.

Prognosis

The visual prognosis for congenital cataract depends on the age of the child at the time of surgery, the severity of the opacity, and the degree of adherence to aphakic correction and amblyopia therapy. It also depends on whether the cataract is unilateral or bilateral. Visually significant cataracts virtually always result in deprivation amblyopia if left untreated.

Advances in surgical technique and the increasing use of IOLs, along with early diagnosis and treatment, have resulted in significant improvements in the prognosis for children with unilateral cataract. A child whose unilateral congenital cataract is removed within the first 4 months of life may achieve visual acuity of 20/40 or better. When the surgery is performed between 4 and 12 months, best visual acuity is reported to be between 20/50 and 20/100. A child up to 5 years old with a unilateral cataract of undetermined age may achieve a visual acuity outcome as good as 20/50, as long as the child has had some normal visual experience before the development of the cataract. Associated ocular abnormalities, such as persistent fetal vasculature or microphthalmos, often limit the postoperative visual results, even when the patient receives optimal treatment.

Ruttum MS. Childhood cataracts. *Focal Points: Clinical Modules for Ophthalmologists.* San Francisco: American Academy of Ophthalmology; 1996, module 1.

Correction of Aphakia

Prompt restoration of a focused image is necessary to prevent amblyopia in young children. Retinoscopic refraction is often stable within 1 week of cataract surgery, because of the small incision length and rapid wound healing in children. (For a discussion of the treatment of amblyopia, see BCSC Section 6, *Pediatric Ophthalmology and Strabismus.*)

Aphakic spectacles

Children older than 1 year (and some younger than 1 year) with bilateral aphakia may tolerate aphakic spectacles well. Children adapt more easily to the various distortions of spectacles than do adults. Lens size and weight should be minimized to avoid discomfort to the ears and bridge of the nose. Fitting aphakic glasses properly and ensuring compliance in wearing them is usually difficult in children younger than 1 year old. For infants, the lenses of these glasses often require more than 25 D of hyperopic correction. Single-vision near correction may be adequate in very young children, as most of their activities are generally within arm's length. As children grow older, distance correction and near add are more appropriate.

Contact lenses

Contact lens correction can be used for monocular or binocular aphakia. It is a well-established method of optical correction for unilateral aphakia in infants. Children can be sedated for lens fittings and examination, and parents can generally be taught to handle lens insertion and removal for a small child. Soft hydrophilic contact lenses are approved for daily wear and are relatively easy to fit and handle. Silicone hydrogel lenses are approved for extended wear and are available in powers from +20 to –20 D in a range of base curves from 7.4 to 9.2 and diameters from 13.2 to 14.8 mm. Removal on a weekly basis is typical, although the risk of infectious keratitis and other complications increases with overnight lens wear. Rigid gas-permeable lenses are less costly, but they are more complicated to fit and must be removed each day. Visual results in aphakia corrected with a contact lens can be quite good, but a significant physical, emotional, and economic commitment is required from the parents.

Intraocular lens implantation

The advent of improved microsurgical techniques and instrumentation, high-quality posterior chamber lens implants, and OVDs has moved IOL implantation in children from a purely investigational procedure to a mainstream approach. Studies that have compared the use of contact lenses to IOLs for the correction of aphakia in this setting have shown improved binocularity with IOLs.

Ocular measurements used to calculate the IOL power in the pediatric patient may need to be done with the patient under general anesthesia at the time of surgery. Some surgeons select an IOL power with a refractive goal of emmetropia in patients older than 4 years; others aim for hyperopia of varying amounts to allow for growth of the eye and resultant refractive power changes. Choosing the correct IOL power in pediatric patients can be challenging because the corneal curvature and axial length change with age. The amount of residual hyperopia should be adjusted to the patient's age. However, most of the formulas commonly used to calculate IOL power appear to be less accurate for children's eyes than for adult eyes.

Posterior chamber lenses are the preferred IOLs for children. The lens material of choice is acrylic, because of its low inflammatory potential, although heparin-coated lenses are also used. While sulcus fixation can be successful, fixation in the capsular bag, or "in the bag" placement, with or without posterior optic capture is the preferred technique.

Secondary lens implantation can also be used in unilaterally aphakic children who are unable to tolerate contact lenses, provided that there is sufficient visual potential to justify the surgery and enough capsular support to allow for adequate lens stability. Anterior chamber IOLs in children are generally not recommended.

Tromans C, Haigh PM, Biswas S, Lloyd IC. Accuracy of intraocular lens power calculation in pediatric cataract surgery. *Br J Ophthalmol.* 2001;85:939–941.

Wilson ME. Management of aphakia in children. *Focal Points: Clinical Modules for Ophthalmologists.* San Francisco: American Academy of Ophthalmology; 1999, module 1.

Wilson ME, Bluestein EC, Wang XH. Current trends in the use of intraocular lenses in children. *J Cataract Refract Surg.* 1994;20:579–583.

Psychosocial Considerations

Claustrophobia

All surgical candidates should be questioned preoperatively about their ability to tolerate having their face covered or being confined to a small space. Patients who are claustrophobic often do better with general anesthesia. Hypercarbia, which can occur if exhaled carbon dioxide accumulates under the surgical drapes, can cause even cooperative patients to suddenly become quite anxious. Placing a suction catheter under the drape or venting the carbon dioxide by some other means are ways to avoid this situation.

Dementia or Other Mental Disabilities

It may be difficult to evaluate the functional deficit caused by cataract in patients with dementia or other mental disability. Questioning the patient's caregiver may provide valuable insight into the patient's functional visual impairment. The surgeon frequently gets the best clinical impression of the significance of the cataract based on retinoscopy, slit-lamp, and fundus examinations. The potential for improvement in visual function and the visual needs of the patient should both be carefully considered preoperatively. In some cases, improvement in visual status increases the patient's mental functioning.

Prior to surgery, the surgeon must determine whether the patient can cooperate if local anesthesia is used. Sedating a patient with a mental disability may cause confusion and increased agitation. If the patient cannot cooperate and is otherwise in good health, general anesthesia should be used. In patients with dementia, regression in mental status following general anesthesia is not uncommon. If the patient seems susceptible to ocular trauma postoperatively, small-incision surgery is preferred.

Inability to Communicate With the Patient

Good communication with the patient is a definite advantage, especially during eye surgery with local anesthesia. A patient with hearing loss should be reminded to wear a hearing aid into the operating room. Before surgery, the surgeon and patient should determine how best to communicate. In cases of profound hearing loss, for example, simple hand signals between the patient and anesthesiologist can be helpful. If the surgeon and patient do not speak the same language, an interpreter or a family member can be brought into the operating room.

Systemic Conditions

Anticoagulation Therapy or Bleeding Disorders

Cataract surgery with IOL implantation in patients receiving long-term anticoagulation therapy is not associated with additional risk of intraoperative or perioperative bleeding in the eye, but anticoagulants can potentiate bleeding should it occur. Retrobulbar and peribulbar anesthetic injections carry an increased risk of retrobulbar hemorrhage. (See Hemorrhage in Chapter 9.) Contact between the implant and vascular intraocular tissues increases the risk of late postoperative hemorrhage within the eye.

The 3 most common indications for anticoagulation therapy are atrial fibrillation, prosthetic heart valves, and deep vein thrombosis (DVT). In deciding how to handle a patient on long-term anticoagulation therapy, the surgeon and the primary care physician must weigh the potential systemic risks of stopping anticoagulation, which include transient ischemic attack, cerebrovascular accident, myocardial infarction, recurrent DVT, pulmonary embolus, or failure of coronary or peripheral bypass grafts, against the localized ocular surgical risks of maintaining the therapy. Although no prospective controlled studies have yet been reported, many retrospective reports have shown that maintenance of anticoagulation is relatively safe in intracapsular cataract extraction (ICCE), extracapsular cataract extraction (ECCE), and clear corneal surgery. The main reported complications include subconjunctival hemorrhage, eyelid ecchymosis, incisional bleeding, and rare hyphema. The incidence of retrobulbar or choroidal hemorrhage is rare in this population.

The anticoagulation effects of warfarin sodium (Coumadin) and heparin are far greater than those of platelet-inhibiting medications such as aspirin, dipyridamole (Persantine), clopidogrel (Plavix), and vitamin E. The decision to discontinue anticoagulation therapy before surgery should be made on an individual basis. Whereas it takes 3–5 days to restore normal coagulation after stopping warfarin, it takes at least 10 days to restore normal platelet function after stopping antiplatelet therapy. Patients should be questioned about the use of all medications, including nonprescription items that could affect their coagulation status.

If the patient requires a retrobulbar or peribulbar injection, or if the surgery requires an approach through vascular tissue, the clinician should talk to the patient's primary care physician about adjustment of the anticoagulation therapy. Although patients with atrial fibrillation or a single episode of DVT can usually have their anticoagulation medication temporarily discontinued, patients with prosthetic heart valves and recurrent DVT often must maintain their anticoagulation. In these and similar cases, decreasing the warfarin dose and lowering the international normalized ratio (INR) may be sufficient.

Evaluation of the coagulation status prior to surgery should be considered for any patient with a condition that might affect clotting ability—for example, chronic liver disease, bone marrow suppression, malabsorption syndrome, or debilitation. A hematology consult is advised in the presence of these conditions or a known bleeding diathesis. Preoperative transfusion of platelets or fresh frozen plasma may reduce the risk of hemorrhage.

Use of topical anesthesia or a sub-Tenon infusion, along with a clear corneal incision and IOL placement in the capsular bag, is an effective way to minimize the risk of hemorrhage. Many surgeons who routinely use this approach do not require their patients to discontinue anticoagulation therapy before surgery. If the surgeon is not comfortable or experienced with these techniques for cataract surgery, he or she may consider referring the patient to an appropriately qualified surgeon.

The reverse Trendelenburg position reduces venous congestion and may lessen the risk of hemorrhage associated with anesthetic injection. Patients can undergo cataract surgery with peribulbar or retrobulbar anesthetic injections, but surgeons should apprise such patients of the increased risk of periocular hemorrhage and advise them to call immediately if the signs or symptoms of a retrobulbar hemorrhage develop.

Carter K, Miller KM. Phacoemulsification and lens implantation in patients treated with aspirin or warfarin. *J Cataract Refract Surg.* 1998;24:1361–1364.

Kearon C, Hirsh J. Management of anticoagulation before and after elective surgery. *N Engl J Med.* 1997;336:1506–1511.

McMahan LB. Anticoagulants and cataract surgery. *J Cataract Refract Surg.* 1988;14:569–571.

Arthritis

Because of discomfort, a patient with severe arthritis may be less able to cooperate during surgery, but adjusting the position to optimize patient comfort may create technical difficulties for the surgeon. Often, a compromise position can be found, one that allows the patient to lie still and also gives the surgeon adequate access to the eye. When such a compromise cannot be reached, general anesthesia should be considered. (Patients with marked kyphosis may be poor candidates for general anesthesia because of associated pulmonary disease.) Adjusting the table for optimal surgical access may compromise respiratory function and may increase periorbital venous congestion. A patient who has ankylosing spondylitis, along with the cervical spine frozen in the face-down position, offers a challenge in surgical positioning. This situation may require the surgeon to operate with the patient's head in a vertical position (Fig 10-1). Medications used to treat arthritis, such as aspirin, nonsteroidal anti-inflammatory drugs (NSAIDs), and systemic steroids, may increase the risk of intraoperative and perioperative hemorrhage. Systemic steroids and antimetabolite medications may slow postoperative wound healing.

Chronic Obstructive Pulmonary Disease

Nuclear sclerotic cataracts are commonly seen in older patients, but posterior subcapsular cataracts may occur at a younger age in persons who have chronic obstructive pulmonary disease (COPD) and who are steroid dependent. Medical evaluation should always be part of the preoperative planning process, and efforts should be made to assess and maximize pulmonary function before the proposed surgery date. Patients should be encouraged to bring their inhalers into the operating room.

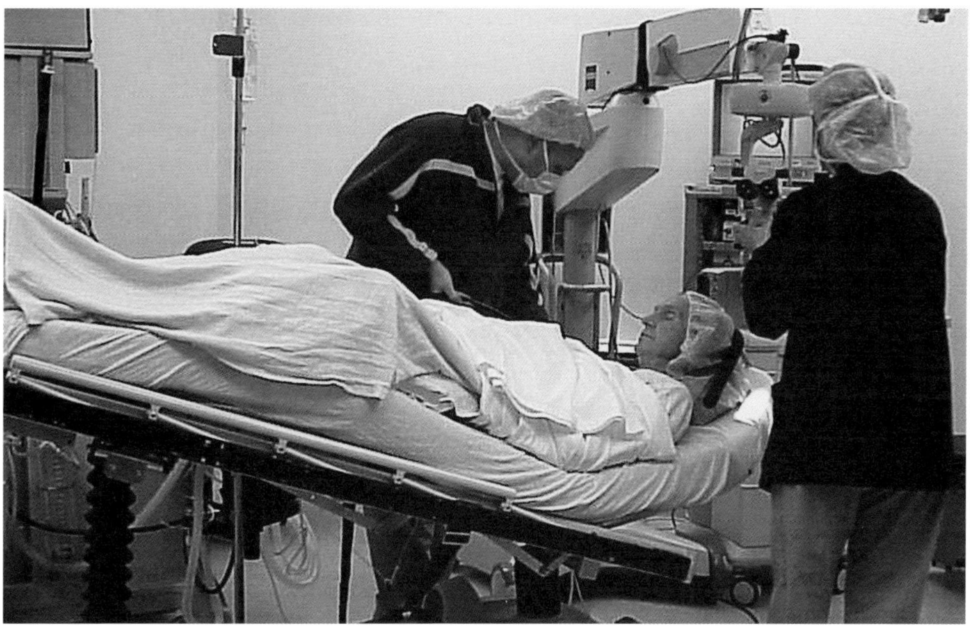

Figure 10-1 Patients with ankylosing spondylitis often have their necks frozen in flexion. So that the surgeon can gain surgical access, the operating room bed needs to have flexion capabilities and may need to be tilted. In spite of these maneuvers, the surgeon may be required to operate with the patient's head in a vertical position. A floor-mounted microscope can be maximally tilted to allow adequate visualization.

Patients with COPD, bronchitis, or congestive heart failure may have increased venous pressure, which may increase vitreous pressure and make the surgery riskier. Retrobulbar hemorrhage associated with local anesthetic and bleeding during surgery may be more likely. Patients with more severe disease may not be able to lie flat for the procedure without becoming short of breath. A surgical microscope with forward tilt may be helpful. Unfortunately, the operating table adjustment that is optimal for the patient may be awkward for the surgeon.

Monitored local anesthesia is preferred in these patients. General anesthesia may be considered when the patient cannot endure the required table position but can tolerate this form of anesthesia.

Coughing, both during the procedure and in the immediate postoperative period, is hazardous, particularly with large-incision surgery, and must be anticipated as a significant risk in this patient group. Although narcotics can be used judiciously to suppress coughing during surgery, and although intravenous lidocaine may also be effective as a cough suppressant, care must be taken to avoid respiratory depression. Many anesthesiologists prefer to have control of the airway through intubation. Patients with severe pulmonary disease may require long-term oxygen therapy. As the oxygen delivery system may harbor pathogenic bacteria, these patients may be at increased risk of endophthalmitis in the perioperative period.

Small-incision surgery can offer a distinct advantage for wound security in patients with COPD. The small incision reduces the risk of intraoperative hemorrhage and of complications related to coughing. Further, a smaller incision is less affected by the poor wound healing that can occur in the patient with steroid dependency or chronic debilitation.

Rosenfeld SI, Litinsky SM, Snyder DA, Plosker H, Astrove AW, Schiffman J. Effectiveness of monitored anesthesia care in cataract surgery. *Ophthalmology.* 1999;106:1256–1261.

Diabetes Mellitus

Patients with diabetes develop lens opacities at an earlier age than do individuals without diabetes. Cataract surgery is indicated when the visual function is significantly reduced as a result of the lenticular opacity or if the cataract reduces the view of the retina, thus impeding the diagnosis and treatment of diabetic retinopathy. Cortical cataracts commonly associated with diabetes can greatly reduce the view of the retina before they significantly affect visual function.

Macular function tests, such as the macular photostress test or the potential acuity test described in Chapter 7, may be needed to help determine visual potential. Fluorescein angiography may help detect the presence of retinopathy and the degree of leakage into the foveal area, while optical coherence tomography (OCT) can also help identify macular edema. If diabetic macular edema is present and the view of the retina is adequate, focal laser treatment should be done preoperatively, as nonproliferative diabetic retinopathy can progress following cataract surgery. (See also BCSC Section 12, *Retina and Vitreous.*)

After cataract surgery, patients with proliferative retinopathy are more likely to develop increasing retinopathy, including iris neovascularization. Panretinal photocoagulation reduces considerably the risk of iris neovascularization. The risk is greatest for the patient who undergoes ICCE without further treatment. The risk is lower with ECCE with an intact posterior capsule. The risk is even lower with small-incision surgery.

Preoperative consultation with the primary care physician regarding local or general anesthesia is recommended in cases of long-standing diabetes, because these patients have an increased incidence of associated renal and cardiac disease. In general, if a patient with diabetes is required to fast after midnight on the day of surgery, the oral hypoglycemic agent should be withheld on that day. Insulin-dependent patients should have their insulin dose adjusted after consultation with the physician regulating their diabetes care. Surgery on any diabetic patient should be performed as early in the day as possible. It is essential to have intravenous access to the diabetic patient prior to, during, and immediately after surgery in order to treat a potential hypoglycemic reaction. (For a fuller discussion of ocular surgery in patients with diabetes, see BCSC Section 1, *Update on General Medicine.*) Recent studies have shown that preoperative administration of topical NSAIDs can decrease the incidence of postoperative cystoid macular edema and that NSAIDs are particularly appropriate to use in patients with diabetes.

The surgeon should take extra care to protect the corneal epithelium during surgery. Corneal abrasions occurring during or after surgery may be slow to heal in diabetic patients and can lead to recurrent corneal erosions. Corneal hypoesthesia is not uncommon in a patient with diabetes. Small-incision surgery can minimize any further decrease in corneal sensation. If the pupil is small preoperatively, it may be enlarged during cataract surgery through the use of multiple sphincterotomies, pupil-stretching techniques, or mechanical iris retractors. A generous anterior capsulotomy and complete cortical cleanup will enhance the view of the retinal periphery.

Patients with diabetes are poor candidates for long-term aphakic contact lens wear, and aphakic spectacles limit visual function. Thus, when possible, a posterior chamber IOL should be inserted. Silicone IOLs can develop condensation during pars plana vitrectomy with or without silicone oil and thus may be a relative contraindication for individuals who may be at risk for vitrectomy. An optic with 6.0-mm diameter or larger will facilitate the diagnosis and treatment of peripheral retinal pathology following cataract surgery. If a posterior capsulotomy becomes necessary, the posterior chamber lens will act as a barrier to the anterior movement of vitreous. Anterior chamber lenses should generally not be used in diabetic patients who are at risk for iris neovascularization.

Obesity

A patient with severe obesity should be evaluated by the primary care physician prior to cataract surgery. The evaluation may reveal associated diseases such as diabetes mellitus, hypertension, or sleep apnea that can affect the intraoperative status of the patient. A large blood pressure cuff should be used; also, extenders (with elbow pads) should be added to the sides of the operating table if the patient does not fit properly on the table. The reverse Trendelenburg position is advantageous because it reduces venous congestion. Positioning the patient's head in the neck-flexed position should be avoided because this position can cause airway obstruction. Intraoperative continuous positive airway pressure is a useful technique to prevent airway obstruction. Topical or sub-Tenon anesthesia is preferable to avoid posterior pressure on the globe. Ocular massage may be performed prior to surgery in order to reduce orbital pressure. Small-incision cataract surgery using phacoemulsification has made surgery in the obese, bull-necked patient substantially safer, greatly reducing the risk of vitreous loss.

Ocular Conditions

External Eye Disease

Blepharitis and acne rosacea

The hallmarks of blepharitis and meibomianitis are collarettes on the lashes, increased vascularization of the eyelid margins, and plugging of the meibomian gland orifices, with frothy discharge on the lid margin. Chronic injection of the bulbar conjunctiva may also occur. Patients with acne rosacea have erythema, telangiectasias, papules, and pustules distributed over the cheeks, chin, forehead, and nose (Fig 10-2). Patients with associated inflammation of the eyelid margin are at greater risk of endophthalmitis. The patient should undertake a preoperative therapeutic regimen of hot compresses, lid scrubs, and antibiotic ointment applied to the eyelid margins at bedtime. The condition should be controlled before surgery. Systemic tetracyclines help control eyelid disease associated with acne rosacea.

Keratoconjunctivitis sicca

Patients with rheumatoid arthritis and Sjögren syndrome present a special challenge to the cataract surgeon. Although these patients do not display symptoms preoperatively, keratolysis may occur postoperatively as a result of a combination of denuded corneal

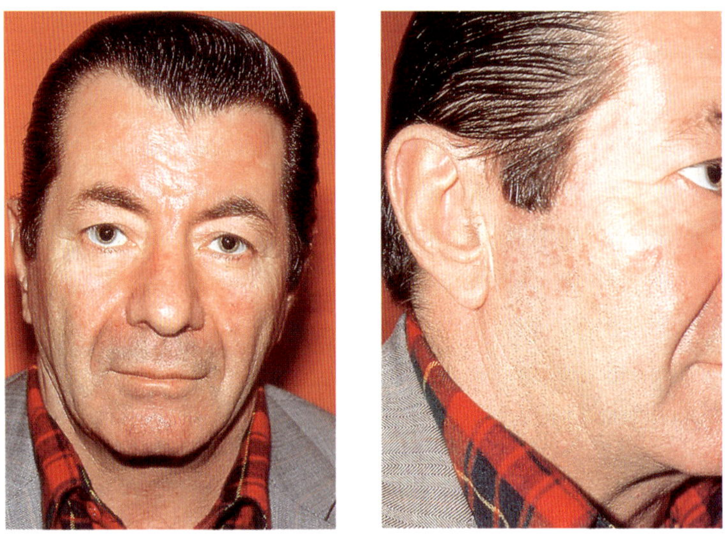

Figure 10-2 Acne rosacea is associated with erythema of the cheeks, nose, chin, and forehead. Papules and pustules are seen in the same distribution. Telangiectatic blood vessels, another common finding, are easily visible in these photographs. *(Courtesy of Mariannette Miller-Meeks, MD.)*

epithelium, corneal hypoesthesia related to transection of corneal nerves, and use of topical steroids or nonsteroidal anti-inflammatory eyedrops. The dry eye condition should be controlled before surgery through the liberal use of nonpreserved tears and, if warranted, with punctal occlusion. During the procedure, the surgeon should take meticulous care to avoid disturbance or dessication of the corneal epithelium. Small-incision surgery is advantageous.

Close observation in the weeks following surgery is necessary, and prolonged use of antibiotics and steroids should be avoided if the wound is stable and postoperative iritis has diminished. Prolonged antibiotic therapy may lead to a toxic keratoconjunctivitis, which may slow postoperative visual rehabilitation. Further, prolonged steroid use can inhibit wound healing and increase the risk of corneal ulceration associated with steroid enhancement of collagenase. Topical NSAIDs have also been associated with a significant risk of corneal melting.

Persistent corneal epithelial defects accompanied by stromal loss may require intensive treatment with topical lubricants, punctal occlusion, bandage contact lens, tarsorrhaphy, and/or amniotic membrane transplant. Before cataract surgery is planned, active scleritis associated with collagen vascular diseases such as rheumatoid arthritis should be controlled with oral steroid and/or antimetabolite therapy so that the risk of scleral or corneal necrosis is reduced.

Pemphigoid

The inflammation associated with ocular cicatricial pemphigoid should be well controlled with systemic steroid and/or antimetabolite therapy before cataract surgery is considered. Even so, the condition may reactivate several weeks after surgical trauma. Progressive conjunctival scarring induces a severe dry eye condition resulting from loss of meibomian glands and accessory lacrimal glands in the conjunctiva and scarring of the lacrimal gland orifices. These dry eyes are at risk of corneal melting following cataract surgery. Extensive symblepharon or ankyloblepharon may severely limit the surgeon's ability to position the eye and obtain exposure. Traction on the globe induced by the lid speculum may cause vitreous pressure. Corneal scarring may reduce the visibility of anterior segment structures during the procedure. If visualization is adequate, clear corneal surgery is advantageous in patients with pemphigoid. Patients should be warned that, even if their disease is controlled preoperatively, any ocular surgery may cause flare-ups.

Corneal Conditions

When evaluating the cataract patient preoperatively, the clinician should determine how much existing corneal pathology contributes to the patient's overall vision impairment. Corneal conditions that disrupt the anterior refractive surface induce irregular astigmatism that can dramatically reduce visual acuity. The status of the anterior refractive surface can be assessed with keratometry. If the mires are irregular, the ophthalmologist can determine the contribution of the irregular surface to the patient's diminished visual acuity by placing a suitable hard contact lens (which will mask the irregular astigmatism) on the cornea and performing an overrefraction. Substantial improvement in visual acuity may indicate that the role played by the cataract is relatively minor.

Epithelial basement membrane dystrophy (Fig 10-3) is a commonly encountered corneal condition that, if pronounced in the area of the visual axis, can reduce vision by disrupting the anterior surface, making accurate keratometry readings difficult. Epithelial debridement may be the preferred procedure in this situation. Stromal opacities in the presence of a pristine anterior refractive surface are less likely to affect visual acuity.

Endothelial dystrophy (Fig 10-4) presents a special challenge to the cataract surgeon, who must predict how well the cornea will survive routine cataract surgery. The best indicator of endothelial function is corneal thickness measured by ultrasonic pachymetry;

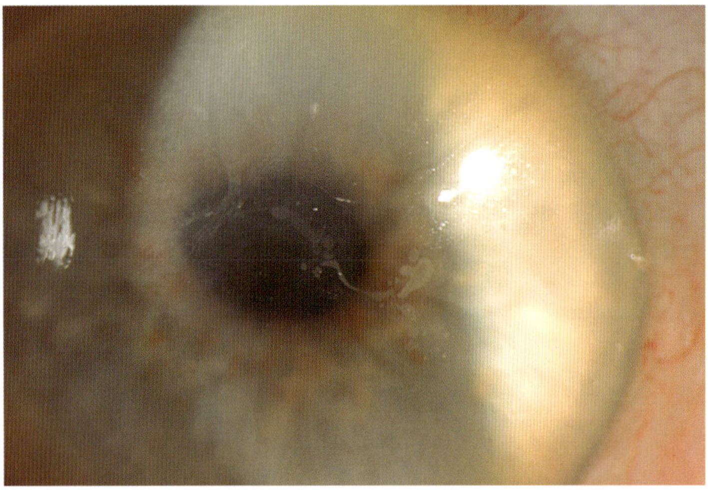

Figure 10-3 Epithelial basement membrane dystrophy. Irregular corneal astigmatism may occur in patients with epithelial basement membrane dystrophy and will appear preoperatively on keratometry as mire irregularity. These patients often have reduced visual acuity related to the abnormal anterior refractive surface. The corneal contribution to decreased acuity may be greater than that from the cataract, in which case the visual improvement after cataract surgery might be less than expected. *(Courtesy of Christopher Rapuano, MD.)*

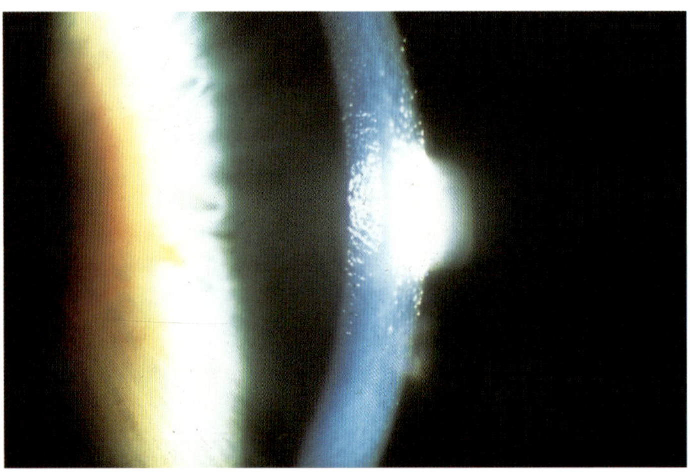

Figure 10-4 Endothelial dystrophy. *(Courtesy of George O. Waring III, MD.)*

in general, if the central corneal thickness is less than 640 µm in the early morning (when the cornea is thickest), the corneal status will probably remain stable following routine cataract surgery. A useful clinical indicator of corneal endothelial dysfunction is a history of diurnal visual fluctuations, with the patient's vision being worse each morning, because of corneal edema. Every effort should be made to minimize trauma to the endothelium in such a case. The choice of OVDs can be important, with the more-retentive type remaining in the eye to protect the cornea during lens removal.

If the cornea has already decompensated or is very likely to decompensate, there are several options:

- cataract surgery followed by endothelial or penetrating keratoplasty (PK)
- combined PK and cataract extraction with IOL implantation (triple procedure)
- penetrating keratoplasty followed by cataract extraction and IOL implantation

Endothelial keratoplasty

A recent development, endothelial keratoplasty is a surgical technique that involves stripping of Descemet's membrane in the recipient and transplanting a thin lamella of donor corneal stroma, along with Descemet's membrane and the endothelial cells, in the host. This procedure can be performed through a small (5–6 mm) limbal incision, which minimizes alterations to corneal curvature. Endothelial keratoplasty is technically easier to accomplish in pseudophakic patients than in phakic or aphakic patients. Therefore, it is often done as a separate procedure after cataract removal and lens implantation. Because the incision size is small and the corneal curvature is preserved with endothelial keratoplasty, visual rehabilitation is more rapid than with PK. However, cell loss in the graft is greater, so the risk of graft failure may be higher. Replacement of the endothelial graft is possible.

Triple procedure

When a corneal transplant is necessary and the cataract is visually significant, the cataract is generally removed concomitantly. When a corneal transplant is necessary and the cataract is *less* significant, there are several reasons for removing the cataract:

- Cataracts may progress more rapidly after keratoplasty.
- The use of topical steroids after surgery can hasten cataract development.
- Postkeratoplasty cataract surgery may traumatize the grafted endothelium.

The surgeon may perform a modern triple procedure as an ECCE through an open-sky approach, using a capsulorrhexis with capsular fixation of a posterior chamber lens implant. The capsulorrhexis should be somewhat larger than usual to accommodate nucleus removal and reduce the risk of inadvertent radial tear. Hydrodissection may facilitate separation of the nucleus from the cortex and ease nuclear expression. Cortical removal is easier when a low-flow manual aspiration technique is used rather than an automated approach.

Alternatively, if the view through the cornea is adequate, phacoemulsification of the cataract, along with posterior IOL insertion, can be done in the usual fashion followed by PK. This procedure has 2 advantages: (1) it reduces the time that the eye is open; (2) the globe is stabilized and the vitreous kept in place by the use of a posterior chamber IOL. After the IOL is inserted, the pupil is constricted and an OVD is placed on the exposed optic to protect the graft endothelium. If capsular support is not adequate, a posterior chamber IOL can be sutured to the iris or sclera. Alternatively, a flexible anterior chamber IOL can be used.

The results of the modern triple procedure are excellent. More than 90% of patients will have clear grafts at 1 year, and more than 75% will achieve a best-corrected visual acuity of 20/40 or better in the absence of other vision-limiting conditions. Choosing the correct IOL power in this setting can be challenging because the postoperative corneal contour cannot be accurately predicted preoperatively. To improve the predictability of the implant power calculation, most surgeons who perform keratoplasty develop a formula for their specific surgical technique. Patients should be warned of the potential for postoperative anisometropia and the possible need for a contact lens after keratoplasty. Refractive surgery using the excimer laser can reduce symptomatic anisometropia that may occur after all graft sutures have been removed.

Some cornea surgeons prefer a staged approach to the triple procedure. Performing the corneal transplant first allows for a more accurate IOL power calculation once the cornea has stabilized. This approach increases the stress to the endothelium, delays visual recovery when a visually significant cataract is present at the time of the keratoplasty, and may increase the risk of graft rejection.

Cataract following keratoplasty

Cataract is a well-recognized complication of corneal transplant surgery. It may be a consequence of the same pathology that disrupted the cornea. It may also result from lens trauma during the transplant procedure or from prolonged use of corticosteroids to prevent rejection. Even though a graft can remain clear with surprisingly low cell counts, it may not survive routine cataract surgery. The surgeon should also look for preoperative corneal thickening and anticipate the possibility that visualization through the graft may be reduced by swelling during the procedure or by instability of the epithelial surface. When the cornea is subjected to a surgical procedure, the surgeon can reduce the risk of graft failure by minimizing endothelial trauma and controlling postoperative inflammation.

Ideally, cataract surgery should be delayed until the PK sutures are removed so that the keratometric readings are stable. If the IOL power is chosen before the corneal contour has stabilized, a change in the refractive power of the cornea can cause significant anisometropia. Posterior chamber lenses are preferred because they minimize the risk of contact between the optic and the corneal endothelium. If capsular support is inadequate, a posterior chamber lens can be sutured to the sclera or the iris. However, the additional manipulation needed to secure the lens may have a negative impact on the graft endothelium. Insertion of a flexible open-haptic anterior chamber IOL is another option. The probability of corneal graft survival 5 years after cataract surgery is better than 80%.

Mature Cataract/Poor Red Reflex

Capsulorrhexis is more difficult and subject to errant radial tears when a poor red reflex is present, as occurs with a brunescent or mature cataract or with a vitreous opacity such as a hemorrhage. Corneal opacities that compromise the view of the capsule also make the capsulotomy more challenging. The use of a capsular dye in these situations makes visualization and manipulation of the capsule easier. Two dyes, trypan blue 0.1% and indocyanine green (ICG) 0.5%, currently used for this purpose, appear to be safe for the corneal endothelium. Trypan blue is a more effective capsular stain. It is less expensive than ICG and comes as a ready-to-use solution. Indocyanine green has to be reconstituted and is prepared as follows: combine the dye with 0.5 mL of the diluent supplied by the manufacturer and add 4.5 mL of balanced salt solution. The dye is stable for 10 hours.

At the beginning of surgery, the anterior chamber fluid is exchanged for a single air bubble through a small peripheral paracentesis. A small amount of OVD can then be placed just inside the opening to prevent the air from escaping. Several drops of capsular dye are then introduced from the syringe through a 27-gauge cannula onto the surface of the anterior capsule and wiped to distribute across the surface. OVD is then exchanged for the air and residual dye. The main cataract incision is constructed and the capsulotomy performed. In mature cataracts, the capsule is often more brittle (less elastic); thus, the surgeon must regrasp the capsular edge more frequently in order to direct the tear. It has been reported that hydrophilic acrylic lenses with a high water content can be permanently stained and discolored by some ophthalmic dyes.

Pandey SK, Werner L, Wilson ME Jr, Izak AM, Apple DJ. Anterior capsule staining. Techniques, recommendations and guidelines for surgeons. *Indian J Ophthalmol.* 2002;50:157–159.

Werner L, Apple DJ, Crema AS, et al. Permanent blue discoloration of a hydrogel intraocular lens by intraoperative trypan blue. *J Cataract Refract Surg.* 2002;28:1279–1286.

Cataract Following Refractive Surgery

The development of cataract immediately after radial keratotomy (RK) is a rare complication generally associated with perforation of the cornea during surgery. Prolonged use of topical steroids after refractive surgery may also induce cataract.

The most significant problem encountered in RK patients is the instability of the refractive result after cataract surgery. Patients may experience a significant hyperopic shift caused by early postoperative flattening, attributable to corneal edema. Even though the flattening may regress, the resulting corneal curvature cannot be predicted by preoperative keratometry readings. Fluctuating refractive error can occur, along with increased glare, similar to that experienced after the refractive procedure. Another problem encountered in RK patients is visual interference during cataract surgery. The multiple, deep RK incisions create reflections from the microscope light; the surgeon should anticipate this potential difficulty with visualization. In addition, the multiple deep incisions may increase the likelihood of anterior chamber shallowing during the procedure. If a corneal incision is used, it must not cross prior RK incisions, or the cornea will not be stable.

Intraoperative visualization of the cataract following photorefractive keratectomy (PRK) is a problem only in the setting of anterior stromal haze. The kind of progressive refractive effect seen after RK does not occur in the PRK patient. Superficial haze is not a problem after laser in situ keratomileusis (LASIK), but extensive epithelial ingrowth and scarring from postoperative infection or an inadvertent buttonhole in the flap could compromise the surgeon's view of the cataract. If a corneal incision is used, interference with the LASIK flap should be avoided.

Irregular astigmatism resulting from a refractive surgical procedure may compromise the ultimate visual outcome of cataract surgery. To counsel the patient preoperatively, the surgeon should attempt to estimate the degree to which irregular astigmatism is responsible for decreased visual function by using a hard contact lens to mask the astigmatism while performing an overrefraction. Choosing the lens implant power for a cataract patient after refractive surgery can be difficult because the effective corneal power cannot be accurately assessed from the keratometric readings. For further discussion, see Chapter 8, Intraocular Lens Implantation, IOL Power Determination.

Developmental Abnormalities

When considering surgery in an adult with an acquired cataract and a developmentally abnormal eye, the ophthalmologist must first determine the visual potential of the eye. A review of medical records may reveal the patient's visual acuity and/or visual fields before the development of cataract. After determining when the cataract developed, the clinician can question the patient specifically about visual tasks that have subsequently become more difficult. Potential acuity testing may be helpful. The clinician must be reasonably certain that the reduction in visual function is a result of the cataract and not a consequence of another ocular problem such as amblyopia or retinal disease. The presence of a significant afferent pupillary defect and/or the absence of entoptic phenomena or color discrimination suggest a poor prognosis for recovering visual function. Nevertheless, improvement in visual acuity, such as from hand motions or counting fingers to 20/200, can significantly improve the quality of life for a low vision patient. If the lens opacity interferes with the fundus examination, B-scan ultrasonography should be performed to rule out retinal detachment, staphyloma, or a mass lesion in the posterior segment. Ultrasonography can also be used to assess the size of the globe.

Next, the clinician should evaluate how well the eye will tolerate cataract surgery. A small cornea has less endothelial reserve because it has fewer endothelial cells. By performing pachymetry in the morning (when the cornea is thickest), the surgeon can identify a cornea that is likely to decompensate postoperatively.

Eyes with abnormal angle structures are at greater risk for glaucoma. Even if the patient has no history of glaucoma, elevated IOP can develop postoperatively. If the patient's elevated IOP has already been diagnosed as requiring multiple medications for control, preoperative laser trabeculoplasty or cataract surgery combined with glaucoma filtering surgery should be considered (see "Cataract surgery combined with glaucoma filtering procedure" later in this chapter). Preoperative evaluation in this setting should include a visual field, if possible. Glaucomatous optic nerve damage may be difficult to assess when the discs are anomalous.

In the presence of *iris coloboma* (Fig 10-5A), zonular dehiscence and/or congenital absence of zonules may occur in the area of the defect. Preoperative detection of iris coloboma and zonular dehiscence prepares the surgeon and the patient for an increased risk of vitreous loss. A capsular tension ring with coloboma diaphragm (Fig 10-5B) may help the surgeon maintain the capsular bag and reduce the risk of vitreous loss.

Posterior polar cataracts, which are often bilateral and inherited in an autosomal dominant pattern, increase the risk of intraoperative posterior capsule rupture and require careful

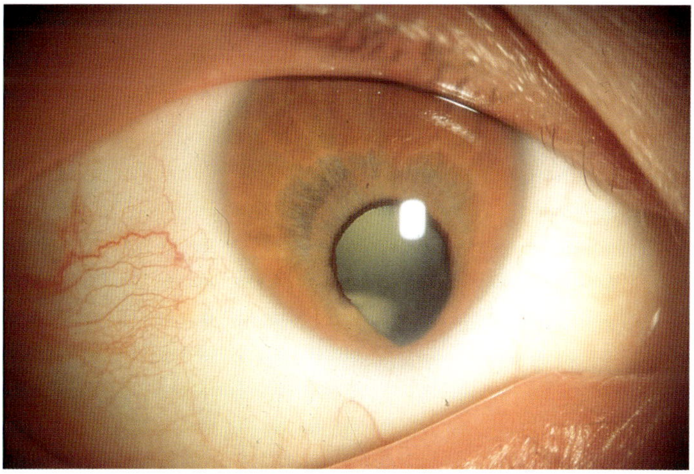

A

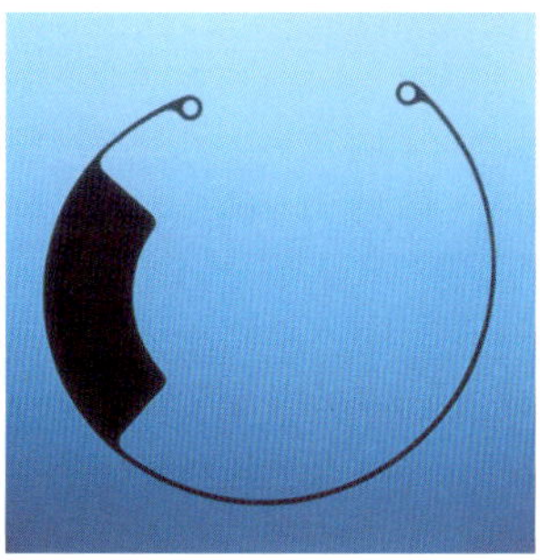

B

Figure 10-5 **A,** Coloboma of the iris with nuclear cataract. Instability of zonular support may be present in the area of the iris defect. Preoperative evaluation to identify associated posterior segment abnormalities is important in determining visual potential. **B,** A capsular tension ring with coloboma diaphragm. *(Part A courtesy of Robert S. Feder, MD; part B courtesy of Morcher GmbH, Stuttgart.)*

patient selection and preoperative counseling. To minimize the risk of this complication, the surgeon must place the least amount of stress possible on the posterior capsule. Retrobulbar or peribulbar anesthetic can be used to prevent ocular movement that could result in posterior vitreous pressure. Also, throughout the procedure, elevated IOP must be avoided so that pressure on the posterior capsule is minimized. An OVD can be used to maintain the anterior chamber. Hydrodelineation should be performed, but hydrodissection should be avoided. Endophacoemulsification helps maintain coverage over the possible posterior capsule defect. Removing the core nucleus should be done first, with removal of the peripheral epinucleus left until the end. Epinucleus removal is the most likely time for the posterior capsule to rupture. Lowering the infusion bottle will decrease the pressure on the posterior capsule. Attempts to polish the posterior capsule may result in capsular rupture.

Retinopathy of prematurity (ROP) is associated with nuclear cataracts that can be denser than anticipated for the patient's age. ROP eyes are often highly myopic but generally do not have a long axial length. If they have undergone retinal cryotreatment or retinal detachment repair, they may have associated zonular laxity.

Nanophthalmos is a rare condition in which the eye is pathologically small (Fig 10-6). The ratio of lens volume to eye volume is higher than normal in these eyes, which also have shallow anterior chambers, narrow angles, and thickened sclerae. Intraocular surgery is generally hazardous because of the risk of intraoperative or postoperative uveal effusion. Small-incision surgery minimizes these risks.

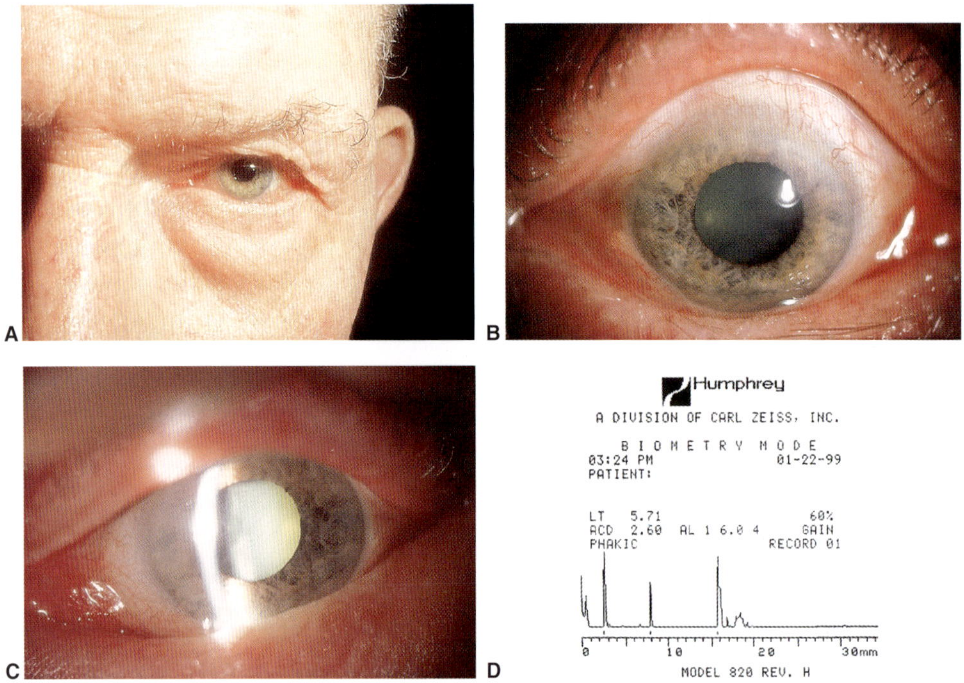

Figure 10-6 Nanophthalmos. **A,** Although this patient with nanophthalmos was phakic, he wore aphakic spectacles to correct high hyperopia. **B,** Corneal diameter was 10.5 mm. **C,** Preoperatively, the anterior chamber was somewhat shallow and a nuclear cataract was present. The best-corrected visual acuity was 20/200. **D,** Ultrasound axial length measurement was 16 mm, and biometry suggested the need for a 48 D lens implant. A 45 D PMMA lens, the highest power commercially available at the time, was implanted. A piggyback IOL approach is perhaps a less suitable alternative in such a small eye. *(Photographs courtesy of Robert S. Feder, MD.)*

The surgeon must decide if and when an IOL should be inserted in eyes whose size or proportions differ substantially from normal. For example, standard size IOLs are not suitable for use in eyes with *microphthalmos* or *congenital anterior megalophthalmos* (Fig 10-7). In the latter condition, which is usually bilateral and inherited as an X-linked recessive trait, the anterior segment is disproportionately large compared to the rest of the eye. The cornea is usually larger than 13 mm in diameter. This condition is associated with corneal arcus, pigmentary dispersion syndrome, cataract, zonular dehiscence, dislocated lens, and high myopia. IOL manufacturers may be willing to adapt a standard lens implant design to meet the needs of an individual patient with an ocular developmental abnormality, but it may take several months to obtain such a lens and may require permission from the hospital's institutional review board.

Choosing the proper lens power may be difficult if the cornea is abnormally flat—for example, in a patient with *sclerocornea* (Fig 10-8). This condition is usually sporadic. In addition to the flat corneal contour, it is characterized by opacification that can involve the entire cornea or just the periphery. Abnormalities of the iris and anterior chamber angle may also be associated.

It may also be a challenge to determine IOL power in a *keratoconus* patient, because the cornea is abnormally steep and irregular astigmatism is usually present. If the pa-

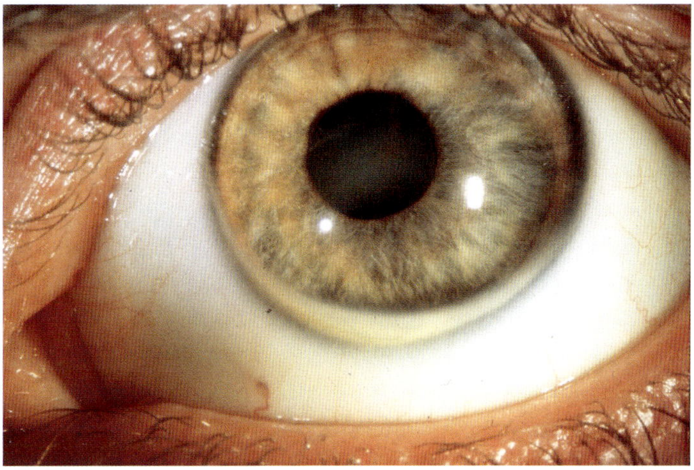

Figure 10-7 Anterior megalophthalmos. In this condition, the anterior segment is disproportionately large in proportion to the rest of the eye, and the cornea is usually greater than 13 mm in diameter. The diameter of the cornea shown here is 15 mm.

tient successfully wears a contact lens, the clinician should explain that contact lens wear will most likely still be needed postoperatively despite IOL implantation. If the patient is young, the keratoconus may continue to progress until PK is required. In that case, at the time of the PK a lens exchange or piggyback IOL procedure may be performed to adjust the refractive power to the anticipated postoperative corneal contour. A piggyback IOL can also be inserted after the cornea is stable.

An aphakic contact lens may or may not be a suitable alternative to an IOL. Its suitability depends on the contour and size of the cornea and the presence or absence of nystagmus. A binocular patient who cannot use a contact lens and whose cataractous eye is not suitable for IOL insertion may not be a candidate for cataract surgery. However, in a binocular patient with a mature cataract, even the aphakic state may provide enough improvement in peripheral vision to justify the surgery. A monocular aphakic patient could be offered aphakic spectacles.

When surgery on a developmentally abnormal eye is being planned, it is especially important for the surgeon to carefully discuss the risks and benefits of surgery and to encourage the patient to participate in the decision-making process. The surgeon should alert the operating room staff about the nature of the case so that potentially necessary equipment is readily available. In general, it is wise in this surgical situation to expect the unexpected.

Increased Risk of Expulsive Hemorrhage

Among the risk factors for expulsive choroidal hemorrhage are advanced age, uncontrolled glaucoma, myopia, choroidal sclerosis, arterial hypertension, generalized arteriosclerosis, anticoagulation therapy or bleeding diathesis, recent trauma or surgery with active inflammation, prolonged hypotony, and previous expulsive hemorrhage in the fellow eye with intraocular surgery. Although it is impossible to control all of these risk factors, preparing the patient and surgical team for the possibility of expulsive hemorrhage

A

B

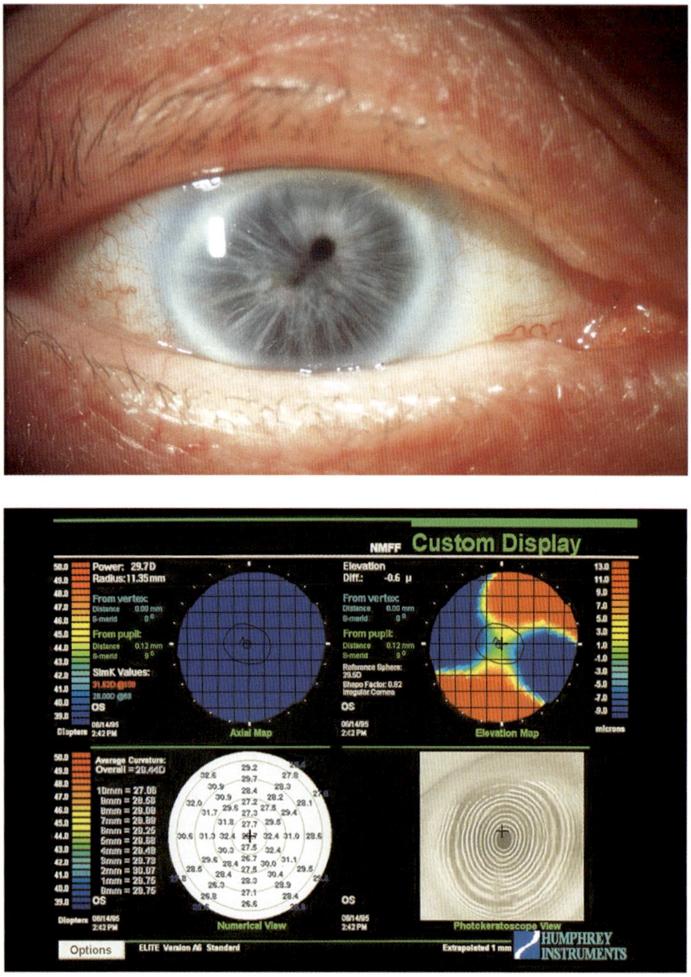

Figure 10-8 A, Sclerocornea (cornea plana). Though sometimes inherited, this condition usually occurs sporadically. It is characterized by a flat corneal contour and by opacification that may involve the periphery of, or the entire, cornea. The average keratometry value of the cornea illustrated here is 30.0 D (normal corneas average 42.5 D). Lens implant power can be difficult to determine when the cornea is flatter than the limit of measurement with the keratometer. **B,** A corneal power map from a sclerocornea patient shows markedly flat cornea with simulated keratometry readings of less than 30.0 D. *(Photographs courtesy of Robert S. Feder, MD.)*

is helpful. Expulsive choroidal hemorrhage can occur under general or local anesthesia (regardless of whether epinephrine is used with the local retrobulbar anesthetic). It may occur with general anesthesia if the level of anesthesia lightens and the patient bucks or coughs because of the endotracheal tube, although with modern anesthesia techniques this complication is less likely to occur.

Phacoemulsification surgery provides several advantages to the high-risk patient. The small incision can be closed rapidly if hemorrhage occurs. The technique minimizes the time that the eye is hypotonous and helps reduce the wide fluctuations in IOP that can occur with some irrigation/aspiration systems. In general, the overall operating time is significantly less for small-incision surgery. Nevertheless, small-incision surgery cannot entirely prevent the occurrence of choroidal hemorrhage.

A compression device such as a Honan balloon or gentle digital massage may be used to lower IOP before the eye is surgically opened. The conjunctiva can be opened more posteriorly than normal and an area of sclera prepared for a sclerostomy, if needed, in the event of a hemorrhage. If IOP is high, the surgeon should avoid rapid decompression of the eye when making the initial incision. Meticulous attention to incision closure is essential: expulsive hemorrhage can occur postoperatively as well as intraoperatively. In the perioperative period, the patient should be cautioned to avoid Valsalva maneuvers.

Glaucoma

Management

In patients with glaucoma, cataract surgery can be considered for improvement of vision, better visualization of the optic nerve, or both. In countries where miotics are still in wide use to treat glaucoma, these patients may come to surgery sooner, because compromise of visual function will occur earlier through a small pupil. Surgical options include cataract surgery alone, combined cataract/filtering surgery, or staged procedures of filtering surgery followed by cataract surgery at a later time. To lower IOP, endocyclophotocoagulation is sometimes used as an adjunct to cataract surgery. Cataract surgery alone may be appropriate if the IOP is well controlled with medical therapy, the patient is adherent and tolerates the medications, and the glaucomatous optic nerve damage is not severe. Small-incision cataract surgery with posterior chamber lens implantation has been shown to restore visual function without compromising glaucoma control. In some glaucoma patients, IOP control improves after cataract extraction, obviating the need for glaucoma surgery. This improvement may result either from correction of a phacomorphic component to the obstruction of aqueous outflow or from a change in aqueous production. Small-incision cataract surgery by the clear corneal approach is advantageous because it minimizes conjunctival damage, an important consideration if future filtering surgery may be needed.

If the glaucoma patient has a borderline cataract and could easily tolerate a second procedure, a staged approach can be considered. Patients should be advised, however, that as a result of inflammation, lens trauma, flat anterior chamber, hypotony, or corticosteroid use, their cataracts may progress more quickly after glaucoma filtering surgery. In addition, the function of the glaucoma filter may be compromised by later cataract surgery.

Cataracts and other opacities, including corneal dystrophic changes, can cause abnormalities of visual fields. The clinician who fails to consider the effect of abnormal media may underestimate the visual potential of the eye. Other factors, such as the appearance of the disc and the reactivity of the pupil, must also be evaluated when possible. (Figure 10-9 demonstrates visual fields in a glaucoma patient before and after combined cataract and PK surgery.)

Complications of cataract surgery in the glaucoma patient

Postoperative *inflammation* is frequently more severe in a glaucomatous eye, with more serious consequences. The degree of inflammation is a function of both the preoperative ocular condition and the amount of intraocular manipulation during surgery. In addition,

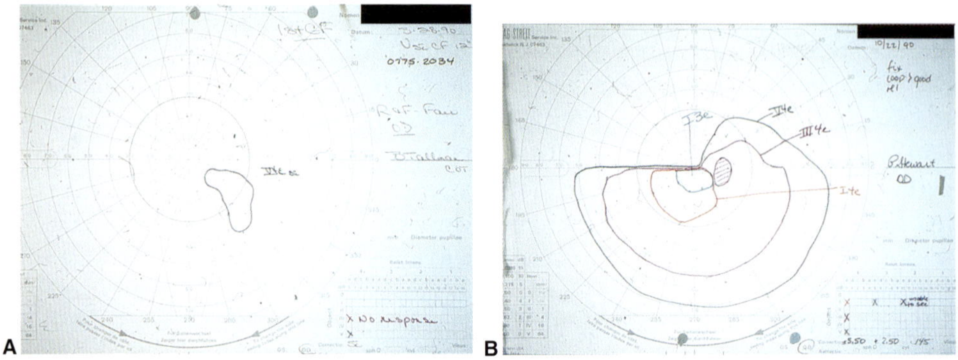

Figure 10-9 Cataracts, as well as other media opacities, can markedly reduce the visual field. **A,** The preoperative Goldmann visual field in a 78-year-old glaucoma patient with Fuchs corneal dystrophy and cataract. **B,** The Goldmann visual field following penetrating keratoplasty with ECCE and insertion of a posterior chamber lens. *(Courtesy of Robert S. Feder, MD.)*

strong miotics such as echothiophate iodide (Phospholine), which is no longer in use in the United States, can be associated with an exuberant postoperative inflammatory reaction. The use of latanoprost (Xalatan) and other topical prostaglandin preparations can also be associated with increased postoperative inflammation.

Postoperative *IOP increases* after cataract surgery occur more commonly and to higher levels in patients with glaucoma. Two-thirds of glaucomatous eyes have a pressure rise of more than 7–10 mm Hg on the first postoperative day. OVDs commonly used in cataract surgery can easily block an already compromised trabecular meshwork, even when the material is aspirated. Blood, pigment, inflammatory material, and lens cortex can also obstruct outflow and contribute to a postoperative pressure elevation. Thus, glaucoma patients should be followed closely in the immediate postsurgical period in order to detect and manage increases in IOP.

The clinician should consider combined cataract and filtering surgery if the eye will not tolerate a significant pressure elevation or if the patient will not be able to tolerate the medications needed to obtain pressure control. (For more detailed discussion, see the section "Cataract surgery combined with glaucoma filtering surgery.")

The glaucoma patient is at higher risk of postoperative *cystoid macular edema (CME).* CME may occur more frequently in glaucoma patients because of their tendency toward greater postoperative inflammation. Moreover, some of the medications used by glaucoma patients, including possibly latanoprost and related compounds, increase the risk of postoperative CME. Although CME is usually reversible, its resolution may take months. Patients should be warned that CME can slow their postoperative visual rehabilitation. Topical NSAIDs may be helpful. (For further discussion of CME and its treatment, see Cystoid Macular Edema in Chapter 9.)

Intraoperative *vitreous loss* resulting from loose zonular fibers may be more common in the glaucoma patient. Loose zonular fibers are seen in glaucoma associated with pseudoexfoliation syndrome or trauma. Therefore, zonular status should be assessed preoperatively. Signs indicating lack of zonular support include asymmetric anterior chamber depth, iridodonesis, iridodialysis, phacodonesis, or tilting of the lens. Phacoemulsification decreases the risk of vitreous loss because no external pressure is required to remove the nucleus. If ECCE is required because of a miotic pupil or lens density, care should be taken when external pressure is applied in expressing the nucleus; removing the nucleus with a lens loop can sometimes be helpful. If vitreous loss occurs in the presence of a functioning filter, the vitreous can clog the sclerostomy. A careful vitrectomy is required to ensure that such an obstruction does not occur.

Small pupils are frequently seen in patients with glaucoma and can be managed in a variety of ways. See also Chapter 8, Surgery for Cataract.

Cataract surgery following glaucoma filtering surgery

The ophthalmologist can perform cataract surgery following a glaucoma filtering procedure in several different ways. Small-incision cataract surgery using phacoemulsification should be employed in this setting unless contraindicated. Compared to ECCE, the smaller incision is more secure, the surgery is generally less traumatic, and visual rehabilitation is more rapid.

If the glaucoma filter is no longer functioning but is still needed, cataract extraction can be done at the site of the existing filter, and the bleb can be revised at the same time. Operating at a familiar position is advantageous; however, revising the bleb may be less successful than performing a combined cataract extraction and filtering surgery at a virgin site. If a new filtering site is selected, cataract surgery can be performed through the new site or through a temporal clear corneal approach.

If the glaucoma filter is still functioning, every effort should be made to protect it. It is estimated that 20%–40% of glaucoma filters fail after cataract surgery when the conjunctiva has been manipulated. Clear corneal phacoemulsification through a temporal approach is the preferred technique in the presence of a functioning bleb because it reduces conjunctival trauma and minimizes corneal astigmatism. Some surgeons inject subconjunctival 5-fluorouracil (5-FU; 50 mg/mL, 0.1 mL) at the end of cataract surgery, away from the existing bleb.

"In-the-bag" posterior chamber lens implantation is the preferred technique, as optimal lens centration is more reliably obtained. In addition, this technique reduces the following risks: capture of the optic within the pupil, postoperative inflammation, and vitreous herniation through a posterior capsulotomy. Further, in the event of a shallow or flat chamber postoperatively, the cornea is probably better protected if the IOL is behind the iris and within the capsule.

Hylton C, Congdon N, Friedman D, et al. Cataract after glaucoma filtration surgery. *Am J Ophthalmol.* 2003;135(2):231–232.

Cataract surgery combined with glaucoma filtering surgery

For the patient with glaucoma and cataract, cataract surgery combined with glaucoma filtering surgery is recommended if any of the following circumstances exist:

- visually significant cataract and maximally tolerated glaucoma medications
- visually significant cataract and poor adherence to using required glaucoma medications
- visually significant cataract with moderate to severe glaucomatous visual field loss

- visually significant cataract with severe glaucomatous damage to the optic nerve, which could not withstand a postoperative IOP increase
- visually significant cataract together with inadequate bleb function
- visually significant cataract in a glaucoma patient unable to tolerate multiple procedures
- even if not otherwise visually significant, a cataract that prevents adequate visual fields or optic disc evaluation

Many techniques have been described for combined cataract and glaucoma filtering surgery. Trabeculectomy and guarded posterior lip sclerostomy are most commonly used. Phacoemulsification is preferred over conventional extracapsular cataract surgery in this setting. The rate of bleb survival is more than 3 times higher after combined procedures using phacoemulsification than after trabeculectomy and extracapsular surgery (62% versus 20%). Finally, phacoemulsification reduces the risks of postoperative hyphema, fibrinous iritis, hypotony, and choroidal detachment.

Small-incision cataract surgery can be completed under a partial-thickness scleral flap at the site of the trabeculectomy or through a separate incision. The temporal clear corneal approach to cataract surgery combined with a superior trabeculectomy is gaining popularity, and several studies have shown that it provides better results than does single-site surgery.

Failure of the filter is more likely when the patient is young or has a darkly pigmented iris, a history of iritis, conjunctival scarring, or a previously failed filter. Such patients may require antimetabolite therapy at the time of surgery, which may reduce the likelihood of poor filtration caused by scarring of the conjunctiva or the sclerostomy. Mitomycin C is currently the preferred antiproliferative agent. (See also BCSC Section 10, *Glaucoma.*)

Balyeat HD. Cataract surgery in the glaucoma patient. Part 1: a cataract surgeon's perspective. *Focal Points: Clinical Modules for Ophthalmologists.* San Francisco: American Academy of Ophthalmology; 1998, module 3.

Shingleton BJ, Jacobson LM, Kuperwaser MC. Comparison of combined cataract and glaucoma surgery using planned extracapsular and phacoemulsification techniques. *Ophthalmic Surg Lasers.* 1995;26:414–419.

Skuta GL. Cataract surgery in the glaucoma patient. Part 2: a glaucoma surgeon's perspective. *Focal Points: Clinical Modules for Ophthalmologists.* San Francisco: American Academy of Ophthalmology; 1998, module 4.

Verges C, Cazal J, Lavin C. Surgical strategies in patients with cataract and glaucoma. *Current Opin Ophthalmol.* 2005;16(1):44–52.

High Refractive Error

The crystalline lens adds approximately 15–20 D of refractive power to the eye. Individuals with a refractive error greater than –6.00 or +6.00 D have reduced visual function. Spectacle lenses can be thick and heavy. The image size through a high-minus lens is minified and that through a high-plus lens is magnified. Peripheral vision is reduced through either a high-plus or a high-minus lens. Much of this disability can be eliminated if the patient can tolerate contact lenses. Further, when the patient with high myopia develops a significant cataract, surgery with implantation of an IOL can greatly improve visual function.

Surgical considerations in high myopia

At the start of phacoemulsification in a patient with high myopia, the anterior chamber may deepen dramatically, making nuclear sculpting difficult. Lowering the irrigation bottle and increasing the flow rate before placing the phaco tip in the eye is advisable. If surgery is performed with the patient under topical anesthesia, intracameral lidocaine can help blunt the discomfort associated with pronounced lens/iris diaphragm displacement. Alternatively, elevation of the pupillary margin with a second instrument will reduce the relative pupillary block. The patient should receive an IOL, which can act as a barrier to the forward movement of vitreous if a capsulotomy becomes necessary. A minus-power IOL is available for those patients who would have significant residual myopia with even the lowest plus-power IOL. Foldable IOLs are available in minus powers in both silicone and acrylic material. Even uncomplicated cataract surgery in patients with high myopia increases the risk of retinal detachment. If the posterior capsule is open, silicone IOLs develop condensation that compromises the retinal surgeon's view if a pars plana vitrectomy is required; therefore, their use is relatively contraindicated for these patients.

Surgical considerations in high hyperopia

The cataract patient with high hyperopia often has a shallow anterior chamber and is more prone to uveal prolapse and iris trauma than is the patient with myopia. The surgeon can facilitate phacoemulsification by deepening the anterior chamber through the use of an extra OVD and by raising the irrigation bottle prior to insertion of the phaco tip. The risk of iris prolapse can be reduced if a slightly more anterior incision is created. The hyperopic eye may have a smaller-than-average corneal diameter, which makes this eye more susceptible to complications from corneal trauma associated with cataract surgery. To protect the cornea, particularly when a more anterior incision has been created, the surgeon should minimize intraocular manipulation.

Clear lens extraction

Clear lens extraction has been advocated for the correction of high myopia and high hyperopia, given the success of phacoemulsification surgery. The purported advantages of this technique over other refractive surgery techniques include sparing the central visual axis from corneal manipulation and preserving Bowman's layer and the normal corneal contour. Another advantage is that most cataract surgeons are familiar with the technique.

However, the improvement in visual function must be weighed against the risks associated with this technique. For example, the risk of retinal detachment after clear lens extraction is estimated to be 1.1% per year in the patient with high myopia. Further, if Nd:YAG laser posterior capsulotomy becomes necessary, it may increase the risk of retinal detachment. In addition, standard IOL power formulas are less predictable when larger degrees of refractive error correction are attempted. The patient should be informed that additional procedures, including laser refractive surgery, may be needed to achieve excellent uncorrected acuity. Thus, this refractive procedure is used more often for correction of moderate hyperopia. Other potential complications of clear lens extraction include endophthalmitis, corneal decompensation, glaucoma, hemorrhage, IOL dislocation, and ptosis. Use of a consent form specific to this procedure will help the patient decide whether the potential benefits outweigh the risks. The controversy over the risk–benefit ratio of refractive lensectomy continues to be influenced by the development of alternative surgical methods for the correction of high degrees of refractive error.

Horgan N, Condon PI, Beatty S. Refractive lens exchange in high myopia: long-term follow up. *Br J Ophthalmol.* 2005;89(6):670–672.

Hypotony

In general, severe ocular hypotony (pre-phthisis) is a prognostic indicator of poor visual potential. An evaluation of the cause of the hypotony should be undertaken preoperatively. If the view of the posterior segment is inadequate, ultrasonography can be helpful. Reversible causes of hypotony, such as iritis with ciliary body hyposecretion, should be controlled before cataract surgery. The presence of a cyclodialysis cleft or retinal detachment may necessitate a separate corrective procedure or a more extensive procedure combined with cataract surgery. Chronic hypotony can result in shortened axial length and choroidal thickening, which can make IOL power selection more complicated and less predictable. Irreversible hypotony is a contraindication for cataract surgery.

Uveitis

Chronic recurring intraocular inflammation and the corticosteroid therapy used to treat it are both risk factors for the development of cataract. When the cataract becomes significant, the surgeon must determine the relative contributions of the cataract and the coexisting ocular disease to the reduction in visual function. Cystoid macular edema, when associated, can usually be seen with fluorescein angiography, angioscopy, or OCT. Patients with uveitis should be warned that their visual prognosis is guarded because of potential postoperative complications: corneal edema; exacerbation of intraocular inflammation, glaucoma, or hypotony; choroidal effusion; or macular edema. Before the physician plans the surgery, the patient should have an appropriate workup to determine the cause of the uveitis.

The risk of complications can be reduced if the inflammation is well controlled prior to the surgery and if postoperative inflammation is treated aggressively. In most cases, these patients should be pretreated with frequent topical or oral steroids and maintained on intensive therapy in the perioperative period. Topical or systemic antimetabolites or cyclosporine may be indicated in selected patients.

Historically, IOLs were strictly contraindicated in uveitis patients. Since the technique of ECCE with intracapsular posterior chamber IOL became widely adopted, however, this contraindication has become more circumscribed. The widespread use of small-incision phacoemulsification surgery has reduced still further the contraindications to IOL placement in uveitis patients. Certain types of uveitis, including Fuchs heterochromic iridocyclitis, quiescent recurrent acute iritis, and inactive posterior uveitis, may do well with IOLs. A relatively small, prospective, randomized study of IOL insertion in uveitis cases concluded that patients with chronic iridocyclitis or pars planitis do well with lens implants but that visual acuity may be better without an implant. An IOL with a polymethylmethacrylate or acrylic optic may be preferable to a flexible silicone IOL in the uveitis patient.

Foster CS. Cataract surgery in the patient with uveitis. *Focal Points: Clinical Modules for Ophthalmologists.* San Francisco: American Academy of Ophthalmology; 1994, module 4.

Kawaguchi T, Mochizuki M, Miyata K, Miyata N. Phacoemulsification cataract extraction and intraocular lens implantation in patients with uveitis. *J Cataract Refract Surg.* 2007;33(2):305–309.

Tessler HH, Farber MD. Intraocular lens implantation versus no intraocular lens implantation in patients with chronic iridocyclitis and pars planitis. A randomized prospective study. *Ophthalmology.* 1993;100:1206–1209.

Retinal Disease

Macular degeneration

The coexistence of macular degeneration and cataract can present a challenge to the surgeon attempting to predict the outcome of planned cataract surgery. A review of old records may help uncover the patient's visual acuity before the development of the cataract but after the macular disease was present. As a rule, functional testing using potential acuity evaluation techniques is a better predictor of surgical outcome than is macular appearance. Good performance on potential acuity testing is encouraging; however, a poor performance is not necessarily an accurate predictor of surgical outcome. Another test of macular function that may be helpful is a macular photostress test (see the section Tests of Macular Function in Chapter 7).

Whenever cataract surgery is planned in the presence of macular degeneration, the patient must be forewarned that the prognosis is guarded. Surgery is indicated if the cataract interferes with a detailed examination of the macula, hindering the diagnosis and treatment of a subretinal neovascular membrane or other pathology. Patients with dense cataracts are often appreciative of the improved mobility that usually results from surgery.

Retinitis pigmentosa

Retinitis pigmentosa (RP) is often associated with posterior subcapsular cataracts. Dense cataracts can constrict the already diminished visual field, and disabling glare can further reduce visual function. The assessment of visual potential in patients with RP may be difficult. Favorable results of potential acuity testing may be misleading. The clinician should examine the macula preoperatively to rule out the presence of CME or other abnormalities in this region of the retina. The patient's subjective complaints of decreased vision coinciding with cataract development, along with the surgeon's appreciation of the degree of opacity, are often good indications that surgery will improve visual function.

Cataract following pars plana vitrectomy

Cataract is a common complication of phakic pars plana vitrectomy. The cataract induced is most often nuclear, with central distortion of the red reflex. Posterior subcapsular cataract is common after the placement of silicone oil. The visual significance of the cataract may not be appreciated by slit-lamp appearance. Some affected eyes benefit from cataract extraction and IOL implantation. The lack of a stabilizing influence from the vitreous body makes the posterior capsule unusually mobile, dictating modifications in surgical technique. Zonular integrity may be diminished because of prior surgery. During phacoemulsification, the anterior chamber may become quite deep. It is recommended that the irrigation bottle be lowered and the flow rate increased prior to placing the phaco tip in the eye. Attempting phacoemulsification in an extremely deep anterior chamber places further stress on the zonular fibers, but a large capsulorrhexis will allow prolapse of the nucleus during hydrodissection for iris plane phaco chop. If an extracapsular surgical technique is selected because of a large brunescent nucleus, attempts to express the nucleus by external pressure on the inferior limbus are generally unsuccessful and may cause zonular dehiscence. Alternatively, after capsulorrhexis, the nucleus can be hydrodissected from its cortical attachments, elevated with a spatula or cannula, and removed by means of a lens loop or irrigating vectis.

Trauma

Cataract may be an early or late manifestation of ocular trauma (see Chapter 5, Pathology). Rupture of the lens capsule generally leads to rapid hydration of the lens cortex, causing a milky white cataract to form. Lens protein may leak into the aqueous and vitreous and may cause uveitis and/or glaucoma. When cortical material is noted in the anterior chamber, the cataract should be removed promptly. A mature cataract obscures the fundus and interferes with the diagnosis and treatment of injuries in the posterior segment. Release of lens material may produce a secondary glaucoma that is difficult to treat and can mask or mimic infectious endophthalmitis. Any of these conditions may necessitate the removal of a cataract acutely after ocular trauma. The ophthalmologist must take care to rule out the possibility of fibrin covering a clear lens. Children are especially likely after trauma to form fibrin in the aqueous that can masquerade as cataract.

A slowly progressive cataract should be followed while intraocular inflammation is being controlled. Slowly progressive or stationary cataracts should be removed only if visually significant for the patient. A patient with a dense cataract and a history of ocular trauma should be evaluated so that the potential for visual recovery following surgery can be determined. In addition to reviewing the complete history and available records, the surgeon should look for gross visual field defects, afferent pupillary defect, sphincter tears or angle abnormalities, elevated or abnormally low IOP, and ultrasound evidence of posterior segment pathology. The ophthalmologist must consider many factors in planning cataract extraction after recent trauma, as discussed in the following sections.

Visualization

Corneal laceration and/or edema may impair the surgeon's ability to remove lens material safely and may indicate the need for an open-sky approach. Hemorrhage can occur during lens removal and further interfere with visualization. If the hemorrhage cannot be controlled and visualization is difficult, use of OVDs and/or air may be helpful. If visualization remains insufficient, the eye should be closed to allow an adequate clot to form.

Inflammation

During the acute phase of ocular trauma, fibrin rapidly forms membranes on the iris that can cause synechiae, pupil seclusion, and distortion of intraocular structures. Gentle sweeping of the posterior synechiae may allow the pupil to dilate, but if it does not, pupilloplasty may be necessary. A peripheral iridectomy is important in this setting in order to prevent postoperative pupillary block. Inflamed uveal tissue is fragile, and bleeding frequently occurs during surgery. OVDs should be used liberally to protect damaged corneal endothelium and possibly to improve the view of anterior segment structures. Postoperative IOP elevation may occur when OVD removal has been incomplete and may require the use of topical, oral, and even intravenous agents. Use of cycloplegics and intensive topical and possibly oral steroid therapy are essential to control the perioperative inflammation.

Retained Foreign Matter

Depending on the type of injury, the ophthalmologist may suspect that an intraocular foreign body is present. If the media are sufficiently clear, indirect ophthalmoscopy is an excellent way to look for a retained foreign body; if the view is inadequate, CT scan or ultrasound can be helpful. MRI should not be used if there is a possibility of a metallic foreign body because the foreign body could be dislodged by the magnet. Significant cataract in the presence of retained foreign matter in the posterior chamber may be handled via a pars plana approach or an anterior approach (with lens implantation if indicated) followed by a pars plana vitrectomy and foreign-body removal. Intracameral foreign bodies may be easier to see when the patient is seated at the slit lamp rather than positioned horizontally under the operating microscope. In addition, irrigating solutions can dislodge a foreign body from its preoperative position.

Damage to Other Ocular Tissues

The iris is frequently disrupted when trauma to the lens occurs (Fig 10-10). Sphincter ruptures rarely need repair unless clinically significant papillary distortion has resulted. The ophthalmologist may repair dialyses by suturing the iris root to the scleral spur. Vitreous is generally disturbed by trauma that ruptures the posterior lens capsule, and careful removal of vitreous from the anterior segment improves the prognosis for the trauma surgery. Large amounts of lens material can become sequestered behind the iris; iris

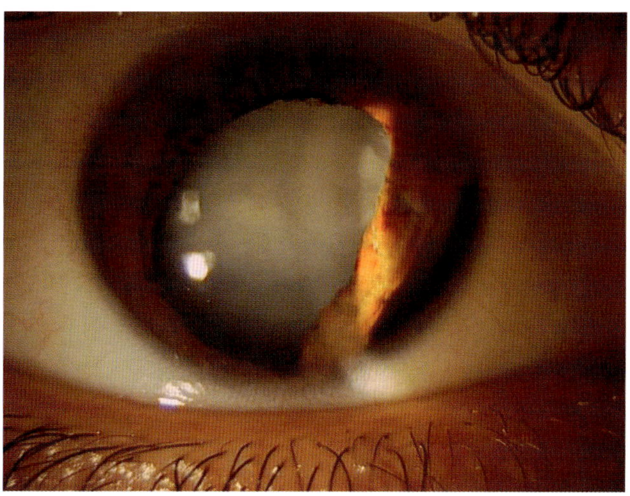

Figure 10-10 Traumatic cataract and iridodialysis secondary to a paintball injury. *(Courtesy of Mark H. Blecher, MD.)*

retraction and removal of this material should be attempted to allow a clearer view of the peripheral retina. Cataract extraction may be necessary to allow adequate visualization if a retinal detachment occurs early or late in the course.

Zonular Dehiscence With Lens Subluxation or Dislocation

Commonly encountered causes of zonular incompetence include exfoliation syndrome and trauma. Congenital and developmental disorders such as Marfan syndrome and inborn errors of metabolism are less common causes of inadequate zonular support. Iridodonesis may be the initial clinical sign indicating zonular disruption. Posterior dislocations without lens rupture may require only observation. Frequently, some zonular fibers remain intact, tethering the lens in the anterior vitreous. When the patient is examined upright at the slit lamp, the lens may seem easily accessible for extraction, but when the patient is positioned for surgery, the lens may fall back out of reach. Thus, it is helpful if the patient is in the supine position for the preoperative examination.

Zonular incompetence not suspected preoperatively may present intraoperatively by decentration of the lens and capsular bag or vitreous prolapse into the anterior chamber, with loss of efficient nuclear removal. Phacoemulsification can sometimes be used to extract a cataract in the presence of limited zonular support. A generous capsulorrhexis will facilitate nucleus extraction; however, the surgeon should be careful to avoid extending the capsular tear into the area of zonular fiber insertion on the anterior capsule. Reducing the flow rate helps decrease anterior chamber turbulence and the risk of vitreous prolapse through the zonular dehiscence. Lowering the height of the irrigating bottle reduces the risk of a very deep anterior chamber, which can further stress the zonular fibers.

A traumatic cataract is usually soft and can be aspirated through the large aspiration port of the phaco tip, especially in a young patient. OVD tamponade of vitreous can be used for areas of zonular incompetence. If a nuclear cataract was present before the trauma, sufficient ultrasound power should be used to emulsify the nucleus without moving it excessively. If vitreous has migrated into the anterior chamber, the surgeon should perform an anterior vitrectomy before starting phacoemulsification or cortical aspiration in order to avoid vitreous aspiration with resulting retinal traction.

If there is not enough capsular support to allow phacoemulsification, a *capsular tension ring* (CTR) (Fig 10-11) can be inserted into the capsular bag. This device provides adequate support for nuclear and cortical removal, as well as for in-the-bag IOL insertion. Insufficient zonular support can be addressed with a Cionni-modified CTR sutured to the scleral wall. If a CTR is not available and zonular support is sufficient for in-the-bag IOL placement, a 3-piece IOL with the haptics placed in the area of zonular weakness helps prevent capsular contraction.

When the nucleus is markedly subluxed and vitreous fills a substantial part of the anterior chamber, the surgeon should consider removing the cataract through a pars plana approach. Referral to a retina specialist is advisable if the surgeon is not skilled in this technique. An anterior chamber IOL or transclerally fixated posterior chamber lens may be necessary in case of inadequate capsular support for a posterior chamber IOL.

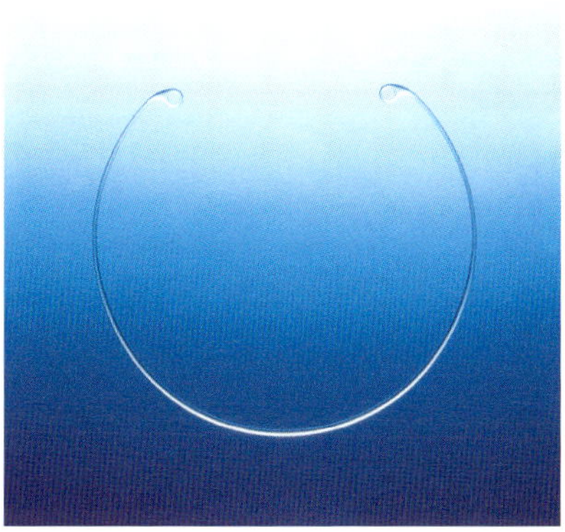

Figure 10-11 A capsular tension ring. *(Courtesy of Morcher GmbH, Stuttgart.)*

Lens Implantation

Primary IOL insertion can be considered when intraocular inflammation and hemorrhage are minimal and the view of anterior segment structures is good. Primary IOL insertion has the advantage of avoiding an additional operation, thus reducing the cost and risks associated with further intraocular surgery. The surgeon may nevertheless decide against primary IOL insertion in favor of aphakic contact lens use.

However, primary IOL insertion has some important disadvantages that should be considered preoperatively. Depending on the nature of the injury, some patients may be better served by having the IOL inserted in a secondary procedure. For example, less-than-optimal visualization may interfere with proper placement of the lens. Defects in the posterior capsule or zonular fibers that might not be recognized at the time of surgery can result in lens decentration or dislocation. The presence of an IOL may compromise a retinal surgeon's view of the peripheral retina and make repair more difficult in case of retinal detachment.

Further, if accurate biometry cannot be performed before primary IOL insertion, significant anisometropia may result. For example, corneal scarring resulting from a laceration can change the contour of the cornea at the visual axis and, ultimately, alter the IOL power required. A hard contact lens may be needed to mask irregular astigmatism, and the aphakic correction could be added to this lens. Finally, the risk of endophthalmitis increases with perforating intraocular trauma, although the presence of an IOL does not seem to affect the ultimate prognosis.

Basic Texts

Lens and Cataract

Apple DJ, Auffarth GU, Peng Q, Visessook N. *Foldable Intraocular Lenses: Evolution, Clinicopathologic Correlations, and Complications.* Thorofare, NJ: Slack; 2000.

Bahadur GG, Sinskey RM. *Manual of Cataract Surgery.* 2nd ed. Boston: Butterworth-Heinemann; 1999.

Buratto L, Werner L, Zanini M, Apple DJ. *Phacoemulsification: Principles and Techniques.* 2nd ed. Thorofare, NJ: Slack; 2003.

Chang D. *Phaco Chop: Mastering Techniques, Optimizing Technology, and Avoiding Complications.* Thorofare, NJ: Slack; 2004.

Fine IH. *Clear Corneal Lens Surgery.* Thorofare, NJ: Slack; 1999.

Gills JP, Fenzl R, Martin RG, eds. *Cataract Surgery: The State of the Art.* Thorofare, NJ: Slack; 1998.

Gills JP, Martin RG, Sanders DR, eds. *Sutureless Cataract Surgery: An Evolution Toward Minimally Invasive Technique.* Thorofare, NJ: Slack; 1992.

Harding J. *Cataract: Biochemistry, Epidemiology, and Pharmacology.* New York: Chapman & Hall; 2007.

Jaffe NS, Jaffe MS, Jaffe GF. *Cataract Surgery and Its Complications.* 6th ed. St Louis: Mosby; 1998.

Koch PS, Hoffman J. *Mastering Phacoemulsification: A Simplified Manual of Strategies for the Spring, Crack, and Stop and Chop Technique.* 4th ed. Thorofare, NJ: Slack; 1994.

Kohnen T, Koch DD, eds. *Essentials in Ophthalmology—Cataract and Refractive Surgery.* Germany: Springer-Verlag; 2006.

Pineda R, Espaillat A, Perez VL, Rowe S. *The Complicated Cataract: The Massachusetts Eye and Ear Infirmary Phacoemulsification Practice Handbook.* Thorofare, NJ: Slack; 2001.

Retzlaff JA, Sanders DR, Kraff M. *Lens Implant Power Calculation: A Manual for Ophthalmologists and Biometrists.* 3rd ed. Thorofare, NJ: Slack; 1990.

Seibel BS. *Phacodynamics: Mastering the Tools and Techniques of Phacoemulsification Surgery.* 4th ed. Thorofare, NJ: Slack; 2005.

Steinert RF, ed. *Cataract Surgery: Techniques, Complications, and Management.* 2nd ed. Philadelphia: Saunders; 2004.

Tasman W, Jaeger EA, eds. *Duane's Ophthalmology.* Philadelphia: Lippincott Williams & Wilkins; 2007.

Wilson ME Jr, Trivedi RH, Pandey SK. *Pediatric Cataract Surgery: Techniques, Complications, and Management.* Philadelphia: Lippincott Williams & Wilkins; 2005.

Related Academy Materials

Focal Points: Clinical Modules for Ophthalmologists

Individual modules are available in pdf format at aao.org/focalpointsarchive. Print modules are available only through an annual subscription.

Bohigian GM, Kamenetzky SA. Risk management in cataract surgery (Module 8, 2007).
Hill WE, Byrne SF. Complex axial length measurements and unusual IOL power calculations (Module 9, 2004).
Koch DD. Cataract surgery following refractive surgery (Module 5, 2001).
Maloney WF. Advances in small incision cataract surgery (Module 9, 2000).
Olson RJ. Strategies for complicated lens surgery, part 1: advanced cataract and pseudoexfoliation syndrome (Module 8, 2005).
Olson RJ. Strategies for complicated lens surgery, part 2: other conditions (Module 9, 2005).
Packer M, Fine IH, Hoffman RS. Refractive lens exchange (Module 6, 2007).
Rosenthal KJ. The capsular ring: indications and surgery (Module 7, 2002).
Rubenstein JB, Yeu E. Management of astigmatism in lens-based surgery (Module 3, 2008).
Stead SW, Bell SN. Ocular anesthesia (Module 3, 2001).
Wallace RB III. Multifocal and accommodating lens implementation (Module 11, 2004).

Print Publications

Arnold AC, ed. *Basic Principles of Ophthalmic Surgery* (2006).
Ford JG, Karp CL. *Cataract Surgery and Intraocular Lenses: A 21st-Century Perspective.* 2nd ed. (Ophthalmology Monograph 7, 2001).
Rockwood EJ, ed. *ProVision: Preferred Responses in Ophthalmology.* Series 4. Self-Assessment Program. 2-vol set (2007).
Wilson FM II, ed. *Practical Ophthalmology: A Manual for Beginning Residents.* 5th ed. (2005).

Online Materials

American Academy of Ophthalmology. Ophthalmic News and Education Network: Clinical Education Case Web site; http://www.aao.org/education/products/cases/index.cfm
American Academy of Ophthalmology. Ophthalmic News and Education Network: Clinical Education Course Web site; http://www.aao.org/education/products/courses/index.cfm

Basic and Clinical Science Course (Sections 1–13); http://www.aao.org/education/bcsc_online.cfm

Maintenance of Certification Exam Study Kit, Lens and Cataract, version 2.0 (2007); http://www.aao.org/moc

Rockwood EJ, ed. *ProVision: Preferred Responses in Ophthalmology.* Series 4. Self-Assessment Program. 2-vol set (2007); http://one.aao.org/CE/EducationalContent/Provision.aspx

Specialty Clinical Updates: Cataract/Anterior Segment, Cataract, Vol 1 (2003); http://www.aao.org/education/products/scu/index.cfm

CDs/DVDs

Basic and Clinical Science Course (Sections 1–13) (CD-ROM; 2008).

Front Row View: Video Collections of Eye Surgery. Series 1 (DVD; 2006).

Front Row View: Video Collections of Eye Surgery. Series 2 (DVD; 2007).

Lane SL, Fine IH, Masket S, Steinert RF. *LEO Clinical Update Course: Cataract* (CD-ROM; 2004).

Osher RH. *Challenging Cases in Cataract Surgery* (DVD, 2001; reviewed for currency 2007).

Osher RH. *Complications of Phacoemulsification* (DVD, 1999; reviewed for currency 2007).

Preferred Practice Patterns

Preferred Practice Patterns are available at http://one.aao.org/CE/PracticeGuidelines/PPP.aspx

Preferred Practice Patterns Committee, Cataract and Anterior Segment Panel. *Cataract in the Adult Eye* (2006).

Ophthalmic Technology Assessments

Ophthalmic Technology Assessments are available at http://one.aao.org/CE/PracticeGuidelines/Ophthalmic.aspx. Assessments are published in the Academy's journal, *Ophthalmology*. Individual reprints may be ordered at http://www.aao.org/store.

Ophthalmic Technology Assessment Committee. *Capsule Staining as an Adjunct to Cataract Surgery* (2006).

Ophthalmic Technology Assessment Committee. *Intracameral Anesthesia* (2001; reviewed for currency 2006).

Ophthalmic Technology Assessment Committee. *Intraocular Lens Implantation in the Absence of Ocular Support* (2003).

Complementary Therapy Assessments

Complementary Therapy Assessments are available at http://one.aao.org/CE/PracticeGuidelines/Therapy.aspx.

Complementary Therapy Task Force. *Antioxidant Vitamin and Mineral Supplements and Cataract Prevention and Progression* (2002).

To order any of these materials, please order online at www.aao.org/store, or call the Academy's Customer Service toll-free number 866-561-8558 in the U.S. If outside the U.S., call 415-561-8540 between 8:00 AM and 5:00 PM PST.

Credit Reporting Form

Basic and Clinical Science Course, 2009–2010
Section 11

The American Academy of Ophthalmology is accredited by the Accreditation Council for Continuing Medical Education to provide continuing medical education for physicians.

The American Academy of Ophthalmology designates this educational activity for a maximum of 30 *AMA PRA Category 1 Credits*™. Physicians should only claim credit commensurate with the extent of their participation in the activity.

If you wish to claim continuing medical education credit for your study of this Section, you may claim your credit online or fill in the required forms and mail or fax them to the Academy.

To use the forms:

1. Complete the study questions and mark your answers on the Section Completion Form.
2. Complete the Section Evaluation.
3. Fill in and sign the statement below.
4. Return this page and the required forms by mail or fax to the CME Registrar (see below).

To claim credit online:

1. Log on to the Academy website (www.aao.org/cme).
2. Select Review/Claim CME.
3. Follow the instructions.

Important: These completed forms or the online claim must be received at the Academy by June 2012.

I hereby certify that I have spent _____ (up to 30) hours of study on the curriculum of this Section and that I have completed the study questions.

Signature: ____
Date

Name: ____

Address: ____

City and State: ______________________ Zip: ______________________

Telephone: (_______) ______________________ Academy Member ID# ______________
area code

Please return completed forms to:
American Academy of Ophthalmology
P.O. Box 7424
San Francisco, CA 94120-7424
Attn: CME Registrar, Customer Service

Or you may fax them to: 415-561-8575

2009–2010
Section Completion Form

Basic and Clinical Science Course

Answer Sheet for Section 11

Question	Answer	Question	Answer	Question	Answer
1	a b c d e f	14	a b c d e	27	a b c d e
2	a b c d	15	a b c d e	28	a b c d e
3	a b c d	16	a b c d e	29	a b c d e
4	a b c d	17	a b c d e	30	a b c d e
5	a b c d e	18	a b c d	31	a b c d e
6	a b c d	19	a b c d	32	a b c d e
7	a b c d	20	a b c d	33	a b c d
8	a b c d	21	a b c d e	34	a b c d e
9	a b c d	22	a b c d	35	a b c d e
10	a b c d e	23	a b c d e	36	a b c d
11	a b c d	24	a b c d e	37	a b c d
12	a b c d	25	a b c d e	38	a b c d
13	a b c d e	26	a b c d e	39	a b c d

Section Evaluation

Please complete this CME questionnaire.

1. To what degree will you use knowledge from BCSC Section 11 in your practice?

   ☐ Regularly

   ☐ Sometimes

   ☐ Rarely

2. Please review the stated objectives for BCSC Section 11. How effective was the material at meeting those objectives?

   ☐ All objectives were met.

   ☐ Most objectives were met.

   ☐ Some objectives were met.

   ☐ Few or no objectives were met.

3. To what degree is BCSC Section 11 likely to have a positive impact on health outcomes of your patients?

   ☐ Extremely likely

   ☐ Highly likely

   ☐ Somewhat likely

   ☐ Not at all likely

4. After you review the stated objectives for BCSC Section 11, please let us know of any additional knowledge, skills, or information useful to your practice that were acquired but were not included in the objectives. [Optional]

5. Was BCSC Section 11 free of commercial bias?

   ☐ Yes

   ☐ No

6. If you selected "No" in the previous question, please comment. [Optional]

7. Please tell us what might improve the applicability of BCSC to your practice. [Optional]

Study Questions

Although a concerted effort has been made to avoid ambiguity and redundancy in these questions, the authors recognize that differences of opinion may occur regarding the "best" answer. The discussions are provided to demonstrate the rationale used to derive the answer. They may also be helpful in confirming that your approach to the problem was correct or, if necessary, in fixing the principle in your memory.

1. The normal, aging human crystalline lens
   a. develops an increasingly curved shape, resulting in more refractive power
   b. develops an increasingly flatter shape, resulting in less refractive power
   c. undergoes an increase in index of refraction as a result of decreasing presence of insoluble protein particles
   d. undergoes a decrease in index of refraction as a result of decreasing presence of insoluble protein particles
   e. a and c are correct
   f. a and d are correct

2. Terminal differentiation is the process whereby
   a. lens epithelial cells elongate into lens fibers
   b. the mass of cellular proteins is decreased
   c. glycolysis assumes a lesser role in metabolism
   d. cell organelles increase their metabolic activity

3. When the ciliary muscle contracts,
   a. the diameter of the muscle ring is reduced, thereby increasing tension on the zonular fibers, which allows the lens to become more spherical
   b. the diameter of the muscle ring is increased, thereby increasing tension on the zonular fibers, which allows the lens to become more spherical
   c. the diameter of the muscle ring is reduced, thereby relaxing tension on the zonular fibers, which allows the lens to become more spherical
   d. the diameter of the muscle ring is increased, thereby relaxing tension on the zonular fibers, which allows the lens to become more spherical

4. According to the pump-leak theory,
   a. sodium ions are actively pumped into the lens
   b. only active transport is involved in ion movement into the lens
   c. sodium flows in through the back of the lens with the concentration gradient
   d. ouabain can stimulate the pump cells

5. Which of the following systemic diseases is *not* associated with ectopia lentis?
   a. homocystinuria
   b. Ehlers-Danlos syndrome
   c. Marfan syndrome
   d. myotonic dystrophy
   e. sulfite oxidase deficiency

6. A lens coloboma
   a. is usually associated with previous lens trauma
   b. is typically located superiorly
   c. is typically associated with normal zonular attachments
   d. is often associated with cortical lens opacification

7. The epidemiology of cataracts suggests that
   a. they are more prevalent in those younger than 65 years
   b. they are more prevalent in men
   c. they occur only as a consequence of age
   d. they are the leading cause of reversible blindness

8. According to the results of epidemiologic studies, cataracts account for which of the following?
   a. the removal of 2 individuals from the workforce when 1 is blind, if the blind person requires the care of an able adult
   b. mobility problems, including falls
   c. the number of cataract surgeries performed worldwide will have to triple by the year 2020 in order to keep pace with the needs of the population
   d. all of the above

9. Which of the following statements about functional visual impairment caused by cataracts is *false*?
   a. "Second sight" is caused by lenticular myopia and improves near vision without correction.
   b. Monocular diplopia caused by cataract cannot be corrected by spectacles.
   c. Mild posterior subcapsular cataracts never cause visual symptoms.
   d. Cataract can cause greater impairment in contrast sensitivity than in Snellen acuity.

10. Which of the following statements about ectopia lentis in Marfan syndrome is *false*?
    a. The lens is usually subluxated in an inferior and nasal direction.
    b. Anterior dislocation is associated with pupillary block glaucoma.
    c. Posterior dislocation into the vitreous cavity can occur.
    d. It occurs in a majority of patients with Marfan syndrome.
    e. It can cause monocular diplopia.

11. Which agent is most appropriate for staining the anterior lens capsule in preparation for creating a capsulorrhexis in a patient with a poor red reflex?
    a. Fluorescein sodium
    b. Methylene blue
    c. Rose bengal
    d. Trypan blue

12. While cataract surgery by phacoemulsification is being performed on a patient with exfoliation syndrome, it is noted that the zonules are diffusely loose. If a small capsulorrhexis is performed, all of the following adverse situations may be accentuated *except*
    a. anterior capsular phimosis with further zonular loosening
    b. increased resistance to nuclear rotation
    c. increased difficulty with nuclear chopping
    d. more rapid opacification of posterior capsule

13. The surgeon may estimate the patient's postoperative visual acuity potential with all of the following methods *except*
    a. pinhole visual acuity
    b. potential acuity meter (PAM)
    c. laser interferometry
    d. contrast sensitivity testing
    e. blue-light entoptoscopy

14. If a patient has a dense white cataract and the posterior pole is not visible, which of the following would be *most* helpful for the clinician in deciding whether to perform surgery?
    a. specular microscopy
    b. B-scan ultrasonography
    c. laser interferometry
    d. Maddox rod test
    e. photostress recovery test

15. What consideration would be *least* important in the decision to perform cataract surgery?
    a. difficulties with activities of daily living
    b. dense nuclear sclerosis
    c. withdrawal from interactions with others
    d. recent fall after entering a darkened restaurant
    e. failure to pass a vision test at the driver's license bureau

16. Which of the following questions is (are) important to answer before a patient is scheduled for cataract surgery?
    a. Does the lens opacity correspond to the level of visual loss?
    b. Does the patient have a medical condition that would preclude surgery?
    c. Is the patient (or a person responsible for the patient) able to cooperate with the postoperative regimen and return for follow-up care?
    d. Will the patient's activities of daily living improve after successful surgery?
    e. All of the above.

17. A 56-year-old woman complains of increasing difficulty reading the newspaper in the morning, especially in bright sunlight. If her only ocular abnormality is cataract, which type of lens opacity is she most likely to have?
    a. posterior subcapsular
    b. nuclear
    c. cortical
    d. oil droplet
    e. anterior polar

18. Clear corneal incisions are associated with all of the following *except*
    a. more susceptible to wound burn
    b. more difficult to construct
    c. less likely to be watertight
    d. lower incidence of endophthalmitis

19. In cataract surgery in which the posterior lens capsule ruptures and vitreous presents in the anterior chamber, anterior vitrectomy is complete when
    a. vitreous is removed from the wound
    b. a posterior chamber IOL can be placed
    c. the surgeon can see the retina
    d. vitreous is removed anterior to the posterior lens capsule

20. The most common complication of retrobulbar anesthesia is
    a. perforation of the globe
    b. retrobulbar hemorrhage
    c. anesthesia of the opposite eye
    d. perforation of the optic nerve

21. Which of the following preoperative measures has proven most effective in reducing the risk of endophthalmitis?
    a. administering oral amoxicillin beginning 3 days before surgery
    b. prescribing topical antibiotics for 2 weeks following surgery
    c. decreasing the duration of surgery
    d. administering topical 5% povidone-iodine solution at the time of surgery
    e. injecting vancomycin into the infusion/irrigating solution

22. During phacoemulsification, when the surgeon notes a tear in the posterior capsule, the first priority is to
    a. finish phacoemulsification of the nucleus
    b. convert to extracapsular extraction
    c. stabilize the anterior chamber with OVD
    d. perform a vitrectomy

23. Appropriate management of severe retrobulbar hemorrhage includes all of the following *except*
    a. proceeding with surgery if the red reflex is maintained
    b. promptly applying firm direct pressure on the globe
    c. observing the optic nerve and fundus with an indirect ophthalmoscope
    d. administering carbonic anhydrase inhibitors or mannitol intravenously to reduce intraocular pressure (IOP)
    e. performing a lateral canthotomy if proptosis, increased IOP, and tight eyelids persist after other measures have been undertaken to relieve orbital swelling

24. If the posterior capsule ruptures and nuclear material falls back into the vitreous during phacoemulsification, the surgeon should
    a. immediately terminate the case
    b. send immediately for a vitreoretinal surgeon
    c. make every possible attempt to retrieve the lost piece of nucleus
    d. remove any remaining nuclear and cortical material from the posterior chamber and perform a vitrectomy
    e. never consider placement of an IOL in that case

25. All of the following reduce the risk of incision burns during phacoemulsification *except*
    a. higher aspiration flow rates and vacuum levels
    b. ophthalmic viscosurgical device (OVD) aspiration prior to applying ultrasound and use of lower power
    c. occlusion of the phaco tip
    d. loose fit between the phaco handpiece and the cataract incision
    e. use of cohesive OVDs

26. All of the following may result in a shallow or flat anterior chamber in the postoperative period after cataract surgery *except*
    a. wound leak
    b. pupillary block
    c. suprachoroidal effusion or hemorrhage
    d. posterior infusion syndrome
    e. ciliary block with aqueous misdirection

27. All of the following are risk factors for cystoid macular edema after cataract surgery *except*
    a. flexible open-loop anterior chamber IOL implantation
    b. ruptured posterior capsule
    c. marked postoperative inflammation
    d. vitreous loss
    e. diabetes mellitus

28. If ciliary block glaucoma is suspected as the source of a shallow anterior chamber after cataract surgery, all of the following maneuvers may be useful *except*
    a. miotic drops such as pilocarpine to constrict the pupil, deepen the anterior chamber, and open up the trabecular meshwork
    b. aqueous suppressants such as beta-blockers and carbonic anhydrase inhibitors to lower the IOP
    c. Nd:YAG laser disruption of the anterior vitreous face
    d. mechanical vitrectomy to decompress the vitreous and disrupt the anterior vitreous face
    e. laser iridotomy to eliminate the possibility of pupillary block

29. If the capsulorrhexis tear starts to extend too far peripherally, the following maneuver(s) may be used:
    a. Check for positive vitreous pressure and try to relieve any external pressure on the globe.
    b. Refill the anterior chamber with OVD.
    c. Insert a second instrument through the paracentesis site to press posteriorly on the lens.
    d. Use the bent cystitome to try to redirect the tear centrally.
    e. All of the above.

30. Evaluation of the cornea is important prior to cataract surgery. Which of the following statements is *true*?
    a. In order to speed visual rehabilitation, corneal transplant surgery should be combined with cataract extraction when guttae are present.
    b. Specular microscopy is the best means of determining how well the cornea will fare following cataract surgery.
    c. Normal corneal pachymetry measurements obtained in the early morning suggest that the cornea will probably remain clear following cataract surgery.
    d. Corneal pachymetry should be performed late in the day, after the cornea has had longer exposure to the environment.
    e. Other than determining lens implant power, keratometry does not have a role in the preoperative evaluation for cataract surgery.

31. Which of the following statements is *true* about the management of cataract associated with ocular trauma?
    a. After blunt or penetrating trauma in children, fibrin can be deposited on the anterior lens capsule that mimics the appearance of cataract.
    b. Cataracts associated with large corneal lacerations should be removed through the laceration to avoid making an additional corneoscleral wound.
    c. If a cataract does not develop in the injured eye within 10 days of the trauma, the patient is unlikely to develop a cataract later.
    d. Phacoemulsification through a small limbal incision is the best approach to the removal of any cataract associated with acute trauma.
    e. When a cataract is removed during the repair of a paracentral corneal laceration, the benefits of inserting an IOL at the time of surgery outweigh the risks.

32. A 3-year-old with a dense developmental cataract in the left eye demonstrates poor fixation OS and a left esotropia. The right eye appears normal. Which of the following statements is *true*?
    a. IOL implantation surgery should not be performed in children.
    b. The left esotropia should be repaired surgically prior to cataract surgery.
    c. Amblyopia therapy should begin prior to cataract surgery.
    d. Posterior capsulotomy should not be performed at the time of surgery because of the risk of retinal detachment.
    e. Cataract surgery with IOL implantation is a reasonable approach toward visual rehabilitation in this case.

33. A 50-year-old woman with myopia presents with complaints of monocular diplopia and difficulty driving at night. Her best-corrected visual acuity with a 2 D myopic shift is 20/30. On slit-lamp examination, she has minimal nuclear sclerosis. Which of the following would be most helpful to evaluate her symptoms?
    a. retinoscopy
    b. corneal topography
    c. fluorescein angiography
    d. MRI scan

34. A 76-year-old man complains of difficulty driving because of reduced vision. His best-corrected visual acuity is 20/70 OD and 20/40 OS. Goldmann visual fields are constricted, more in the OD than in the OS. A moderate nuclear cataract is present OD, and a mild one is seen OS. His IOP is 23 mm Hg OD and 18 mm Hg OS. He uses timolol 0.5% bid OD and dorzolamide tid OD. His cup–disc ratio is 0.8 OD and 0.6 OS. The fundus is otherwise normal. Which of the following statements is *true*?
    a. Cataract surgery in this patient carries a high risk of loss of fixation postoperatively.
    b. Cataract surgery combined with glaucoma filtering surgery is the only approach that should be considered for this patient.
    c. Medical glaucoma treatment should be maximized before cataract surgery is considered.
    d. The visual field constriction in this case is probably caused by glaucoma.
    e. Cataract surgery should be considered in order to improve his vision, and care should be taken to control IOP postoperatively.

35. Systemic use of α_{1A}-antagonists for the treatment of benign prostatic hypertrophy may cause intraoperative floppy iris syndrome (IFIS) by which of the following mechanisms?
    a. atrophy of the iris sphincter muscle
    b. competitive binding to the postsynaptic nerve endings of the iris dilator
    c. loss of iris stroma
    d. atrophy of the posterior pigment epithelium
    e. metabolic alkalosis of the aqueous humor

36. Epidemiologic studies have identified risk factors for nuclear opacification, which include
    a. current or past smoking
    b. non-Hispanic white race
    c. diabetes mellitus
    d. all of the above

37. Which manifestation of pseudoexfoliation syndrome is most related to cataract surgery complications?
    a. endothelial deposits on the iris and the lens capsule
    b. Sampaolesi line
    c. phacodonesis
    d. nuclear sclerosis

38. Which of the following statements is *true* regarding lens implant power calculations?
    a. Shorter axial length is obtained with immersion biometry as compared with contact biometry.
    b. Corneal thickness measurement is needed for regression formulas used to predict the appropriate IOL power.
    c. The calculated lens implant power for a sulcus-supported IOL is less than that for a lens positioned in the capsular bag.
    d. The calculations for IOL power will differ depending on the IOL material (eg, silicone, acrylic, or polymethylmethacrylate [PMMA]).

39. Which of the following statements about temporal clear corneal phacoemulsification is *false*?
    a. It is useful in a patient with a deep orbit.
    b. It cannot be used in combination with trabeculectomy.
    c. It is useful in a patient with a preexisting, functioning superior trabeculectomy.
    d. It can be performed with the patient under topical anesthesia.

Answers

1. **a.** With aging, the human lens develops an increasingly curved shape, which results in more refractive power. This change may be accompanied by—and sometimes offset by—a decrease in the index of refraction of the lens resulting from an increase in water-insoluble proteins.
2. **a.** Terminal differentiation involves elongation of the lens epithelial cells into lens fibers. This change is associated with a tremendous increase in the mass of cellular proteins in each cell. The cells lose organelles, including nuclei, mitochondria, and ribosomes. The loss of cell organelles is optically advantageous, and the cells now become more dependent on glycolysis for energy production.
3. **c.** The ciliary muscle is a ring, but upon contraction it does not have the effect that one would intuitively expect of a sphincter. When this muscle contracts, the diameter of the muscle ring is reduced, thereby relaxing tension on the zonular fibers, which allows the lens to become more spherical.
4. **c.** The combination of active transport and membrane permeability is referred to as the "pump-leak theory" of the lens. Potassium is actively transported into the anterior lens via the epithelium. It then diffuses out with the concentration gradient through the back of the lens, where there are no active transport mechanisms. Conversely, sodium flows in through the back of the lens with the concentration gradient and then is actively exchanged for potassium by the epithelium. Experimentally, ouabain can inhibit the sodium-potassium pumps.
5. **d.** Myotonic dystrophy is not associated with ectopia lentis.
6. **d.** A lens coloboma is a wedge-shaped defect or indentation of the lens periphery that occurs as an isolated anomaly or is secondary to the lack of ciliary body or zonular development. Lens colobomas are typically located inferiorly and may be associated with colobomas of the uvea. Cortical lens opacification or thickening of the lens capsule may appear adjacent to the defect.
7. **d.** Cataracts increase in prevalence with increasing age and are the leading cause of blindness worldwide. They can occur as a congenital condition or as a result of trauma, metabolic diseases, or medications. Major epidemiologic studies confirm an increased prevalence in women.
8. **d.** When an individual is incapacitated by blindness and requires the care of an able adult, the caregiver may be removed from the workforce as well. Reduced acuity is a primary factor in the decrease of mobility, and it contributes to falls. With the aging of the population in both the developed and the developing world, the number of individuals needing cataract surgery will increase from 40 million to 120 million in the next 2 decades.
9. **c.** Posterior subcapsular cataracts (even mild ones) can lead to severe visual impairment, especially when there is bright illumination and while the patient is reading.
10. **a.** In Marfan syndrome the lens is usually subluxated in a superior and temporal location.
11. **d.** Trypan blue is nontoxic and commercially available as a ready-made solution. Fluorescein is a very weak stain for all intraocular surfaces. Methylene blue is toxic to the corneal endothelium. Rose bengal is not approved for intraocular use and has been shown to be toxic to the corneal endothelial cells in animal studies.

12. **d.** Opacification of the posterior lens capsule is not dependent on CCC size. A small capsulorrhexis leaves more anterior capsule, which leads to greater resistance in nuclear rotation for quadrant removal techniques, as well as increased difficulty in chopping techniques. The zonular laxity allows the larger anterior capsule remaining to contract to a much smaller opening. YAG anterior capsular relaxing incisions can be made in the early postoperative period to reduce the anterior capsular phimosis, which can further reduce the zonular integrity.
13. **d.** Patients with cataracts may experience diminished contrast sensitivity, even when Snellen acuity is preserved. Thus, contrast sensitivity may be a very unreliable method for measuring visual potential. Although many patients find the blue-light entoptoscopy test difficult to comprehend, if they can see the shadows of white blood cells coursing through the perifoveal capillaries, macular function is probably intact.
14. **b.** B-scan ultrasonography is indicated to evaluate for occult tumors, retinal detachment, or posterior staphyloma or other posterior pathology that could affect visual outcome. Laser interferometry, Maddox rod testing, and photostress recovery are not reliable with such a dense cataract. Specular microscopy would be indicated if signs of corneal endothelial dysfunction were present.
15. **b.** The presence of dense nuclear sclerosis alone may not prevent the ophthalmologist, by means of a careful refraction, from improving acuity so that activities of daily living, interactions with others, stability in walking, and vision sufficient to drive (although perhaps in more limited circumstances) may be possible.
16. **e.** Each of these questions must bear on the decision to operate and be answered for each specific patient.
17. **a.** Posterior subcapsular cataracts create more difficulty with glare and near vision. Nuclear and cortical cataracts affect distance vision more than near vision. Progressive loss of vision from oil droplet or anterior polar cataracts is not often seen in this age group.
18. **d.** Studies have shown a higher incidence of endophthalmitis with clear corneal incisions although the mechanism has not been demonstrated. (McDonnell PJ, Taban M, Sarayba M, et al. Dynamic morphology of clear corneal cataract incisions. *Ophthalmology*. 2003;110:2342–2348.) Both poorly constructed incisions and wound burns can lead to a leaking wound, which many suspect may be the cause of increased infection rates. Experimental studies have demonstrated that transient reduction in postoperative IOP may also result in poor wound apposition in clear corneal incisions, with potential for fluid flow across the cornea and into the anterior chamber, with the attendant risk of endophthalmitis.
19. **d.** Loss of vitreous is not a problem for the eye; vitreous traction is. The goal of vitreous removal is to reduce the possibility of traction. The clinician may prevent traction by removing enough vitreous to keep it away from other intraocular structures, such as the lens implant, or away from the incision. Therefore, a vitrectomy is not complete until all vitreous is removed anterior to the posterior capsule. This ensures a lower risk of traction and is also the best way to decrease the risk of postoperative cystoid macular edema (CME).
20. **b.** The increasing preference for topical or sub-Tenon anesthesia for cataract surgery has been driven by the potential complications of anesthesia in which a needle is placed near the eye without visual confirmation of the needle's position. All of the answers are potential complications, but the most common complication is a retrobulbar hemorrhage. When this occurs, cataract surgery usually needs to be stopped and rescheduled, and other forms of anesthesia need to be considered.

21. **d.** Answers c and e are intraoperative measures, and controversy surrounds admixing antibiotics into the infusion solution. Oral antibiotics have poor ocular penetration and are not recommended.

22. **c.** Early detection of capsular rupture is critical to the satisfactory resolution of this unexpected occurrence. As soon as the surgeon notes a rupture or suspects one, he or she should freeze the action by instilling an OVD to keep the anterior chamber formed. This maneuver allows removal of the phaco handpiece, prevents further trauma to the capsule, and enables the surgeon to calmly assess the situation before proceeding any further. The next step is determined by the extent of the rupture, the amount of nucleus left to be removed, and the presence or absence of vitreous.

23. **a.** If a severe retrobulbar hemorrhage occurs, surgery should be canceled, despite an adequate red reflex. All of the other measures are appropriate in the presence of severe retrobulbar hemorrhage compromising optic nerve and retinal blood supply.

24. **d.** Capsular rupture during phacoemulsification presents a risk of nuclear material falling posteriorly into the vitreous cavity. The case does not need to be immediately terminated. Attempts to retrieve the nuclear remnant from deep in the vitreous are not recommended, as those maneuvers can result in more serious retinal complications. Nuclear and cortical material remaining in the posterior chamber should be removed and a vitrectomy performed via an anterior incision or the pars plana. Conversion of a small rent into a posterior continuous curvilinear capsulorrhexis may stabilize the posterior capsular opening. Surgeons familiar with pars plana techniques may attempt a posterior levitation maneuver for larger nuclear fragments present in the anterior or midvitreous. An IOL of choice may be implanted with due consideration to the integrity of the remaining capsule. The patient may be referred to a vitreoretinal surgeon, who can wait up to 7–14 days to remove retained lenticular material without jeopardizing the outcome.

25. **c.** Occlusion of the phaco tip reduces or interrupts fluid evacuation through the phaco handpiece. This results in an increased buildup of heat within the handpiece and a transfer of thermal energy to the incision. Use of lower ultrasound power reduces heat buildup. Aspiration of OVD, use of more easily aspirated cohesive OVDs, higher aspiration flow rates and vacuum levels, and a loose fit between the phaco handpiece and the incision all contribute to a more efficient fluid flow through the handpiece and/or the incision, reducing the transfer of thermal energy.

26. **d.** Posterior infusion syndrome causes shallowing of the anterior chamber during cataract surgery, not in the postoperative period. This rare complication typically occurs during hydrodissection, when fluid may be misdirected into the vitreous cavity, resulting in forward displacement of the lens. Wound leakage and suprachoroidal hemorrhage may result in a flat chamber during or following surgery. Suprachoroidal effusion, pupillary block, and ciliary block with aqueous misdirection occur in the postoperative period. Suprachoroidal effusion is often associated with hypotony and may be associated with a wound leak. Pupillary block and ciliary block, as well as suprachoroidal hemorrhage, are often associated with normal or elevated IOP.

27. **a.** Flexible open-loop anterior chamber IOL implantation is not associated with an increased risk of CME in the absence of other risk factors. CME is almost always the result of increased permeability of perifoveal capillaries, typically induced by release of inflammatory mediators. Diabetes mellitus, rupture of the posterior capsule, postoperative inflammation, and vitreous loss during surgery are each associated with an increased risk of CME.

28. **a.** Management of ciliary block glaucoma is directed at controlling the IOP, shrinking the expanded vitreous volume, and ultimately reestablishing the normal balance of aqueous circulation. Medical management consists of cycloplegia and mydriasis with atropine 1% and phenylephrine 10% to create a larger anterior hyaloid surface area for perfusion of posteriorly sequestered aqueous. IOP control with aqueous suppressants like beta-blockers, carbonic anhydrase inhibitors, and alpha agonists is very helpful. Miotics are expressly avoided, as they exacerbate the anterior displacement of the middle segment structures and may contribute to the initiating mechanism of the disease. If patients fail to respond to medical therapy, surgery is undertaken to reduce the expanded vitreous volume and disrupt the anterior vitreous face with either the Nd:YAG laser or mechanical vitrectomy.

29. **e.** All of these maneuvers may be helpful in redirecting a capsulorrhexis tear that is extending too far peripherally. Preserving an intact continuous-tear capsulorrhexis is very important to the ultimate success of phacoemulsification surgery.

30. **c.** Corneal thickness as measured by ultrasonic pachymetry is an important indicator of corneal endothelial function. Because the endothelium is under greatest stress after the eyelids have been closed during sleep, pachymetry should be performed in the early morning. Early-morning pachymetry is a better predictor of postoperative endothelial function than is specular microscopy. Keratometry can be helpful in determining the quality of the anterior refractive surface—that is, the tear layer. If epithelial irregularity within the visual axis is detected preoperatively, potential visual acuity after cataract surgery may be reduced.

31. **a.** The surgeon must distinguish carefully between an actual cataract and an apparent lens opacity due to fibrin coating on the anterior lens capsule of an otherwise clear lens. Cataracts should never be extracted through a corneal laceration; this procedure would cause additional injury to an already traumatized corneal endothelium. Traumatic cataracts can develop long after the actual ocular injury. The use of phacoemulsification through a limbal incision would not be preferred when the view through the cornea is inadequate. In this situation, cataract surgery should either be postponed or, if necessary, combined with penetrating keratoplasty. When the lens is subluxated as a result of zonular dehiscence, a pars plana approach is preferred. Insertion of an IOL as part of a combined cataract extraction and corneal laceration repair procedure is controversial. Preoperative biometry is usually impossible, or the measurements may be inaccurate, which can lead to significant anisometropia. Zonular status, as well as capsular integrity, may not be certain.

32. **e.** Lens implant surgery in a 3-year-old child with a monocular cataract is no longer considered controversial, assuming that the surgeon is familiar with the special techniques involved in performing such surgery in this age group. Strabismus surgery and amblyopia therapy should both be postponed until cataract surgery has cleared the visual axis. Posterior capsulotomy and anterior vitrectomy are usually performed at the time of surgery in a child this age. The posterior capsule usually opacifies in children and can become quite thick and fibrotic. Nd:YAG laser posterior capsulotomy is difficult to perform in this age group even if the capsule has not become fibrotic.

33. **a.** Patients with lens-induced myopia, symptoms of nighttime glare, and monocular diplopia often have a central nuclear sclerosis that, on slit-lamp examination, appears insignificant. Although the red reflex can be evaluated with the slit lamp, it is visualized more prominently with the retinoscope or the direct ophthalmoscope. When this finding is missed on initial evaluation, patients may unnecessarily undergo more expensive testing such as fluorescein angiography or magnetic resonance imaging.

34. **e.** Cataract surgery alone will address the patient's current visual needs. In this case, the visual field constriction is more likely to be the result of the cataract than of glaucoma. There is no mention of field loss approaching fixation, and with a cup–disc ratio of 0.8, fixation is not likely to be threatened by cataract surgery. Although combined glaucoma filtering and cataract surgery is a valid approach, it is not the *only* surgical approach in this case. Glaucoma filtering surgery could be performed as a subsequent procedure if needed. If combined surgery is performed, no additional glaucoma medications are needed preoperatively. With an IOP of 23 mm Hg, cataract surgery alone can probably be performed without additional medication. The surgeon must be prepared to treat a postoperative pressure spike if it occurs after surgery.

35. **b.** Systemic α_{1A}-antagonists competitively bind to the postsynaptic nerve endings of the iris dilator muscle for long periods. Atrophy of the iris dilator muscle results in intraoperative billowing of the iris and progressive miosis.

36. **d.** Current smoking, white race, and diabetes mellitus are all risk factors for nuclear opacification.

37. **c.** Phacodonesis is an ominous sign of zonular incompetence associated with pseudoexfoliation syndrome and requires special strategies to avoid dehiscence of the zonule or dislocation of the lens during surgery. Although the other choices are manifestations of pseudoexfoliation, they do not complicate cataract surgery.

38. **c.** The more anterior the position of the lens implant within the eye, the lower the dioptric power required. Measurements by the contact applanation method may result in falsely shorter axial length. Corneal thickness measurements are not part of the data needed for regression formulas. The material of the IOL does not affect the IOL power calculations. The *A* constant compensates for the lens location and light transmission.

39. **b.** A temporal incision for phacoemulsification can be coupled with a superior trabeculectomy in a 2-site procedure. A deep orbit may present challenges for the superior approach; the temporal approach obviates the need to work over a prominent brow. Keeping the incision away from a functioning filtering bleb reduces the risk of bleb failure. Topical anesthesia may be used with either a superior or a temporal approach.

Index

(*f* = figure; *t* = table)

A constant, in IOL power determination, 149
A-scan ultrasonography
  before cataract surgery, 88
  in IOL power determination, 149–150, 149*f*, 150
Abrasions, corneal, cataract surgery in diabetic patients and, 209
Accommodation, 22–23, 22*t*
  aging affecting, 22, 23, 29
  amplitude of, 23
  changes with, 22, 22*t*
Acid, cataract caused by, 57
ACIOL. *See* Intraocular lenses (IOLs), anterior chamber
Acne rosacea. *See* Rosacea
Acrylic, for foldable intraocular lenses, 146. *See also* Foldable intraocular lens
  for children, 204
  instrumentation for handling, 154
  posterior capsule opacification and, 183
AcrySof IQ intraocular lens, 148
AcrySof ReSTOR intraocular lens, 147, 148*f*
Active transport, in lens
  epithelium as site of, 19–20
  pump-leak theory and, 20–21, 20*f*
Activities of Daily Vision Scale (ADVS), 78, 157
ADVS. *See* Activities of Daily Vision Scale
Affinity constant (K_m), "sugar" cataract development and, 15
Age/aging
  accommodative response/presbyopia and, 22, 23, 29
  cataracts related to, 43–51. *See also* Age-related cataracts
  lens changes associated with, 7, 28–29, 43–51, 44*f*
  lens proteins affected by, 13, 43
Age-related cataracts, 43–51. *See also specific type*
  cortical, 45–46, 46*f*, 47*f*, 48*f*, 49*f*, 50*f*
  in diabetes, 59–60
  epidemiology of, 71–74
  genetic contributions to, 50–51
  nuclear, 43–44, 45*f*
  nutritional deficiency and, 62
  posterior subcapsular, 46–49, 51*f*
Age-Related Eye Disease Study (AREDS), 72
AK. *See* Astigmatic keratotomy
AL. *See* Axial length
Alcon Infiniti phacoemulsification system, 130
Aldose reductase
  in cataract formation, 15–16, 59
  in lens glucose/carbohydrate metabolism, 14*f*, 15
Aldose reductase inhibitors, cataract prevention/management and, 77
Alkalis (alkaline solutions), cataract caused by, 57
Alpha-antagonists, intraoperative floppy iris syndrome and, 79–80, 137, 173
Alpha-chymotrypsin, for ICCE, 95, 158
Alpha crystallins, 11–12, 11*f*
Alport disease/syndrome, lenticonus in, 30
Amblyopia
  aphakia correction in prevention of, 203–204
  in bilateral congenital cataracts, 199
  cataract surgery planning and, 199
Aminoglycosides, macular infarction and, 195
Amiodarone, lens changes caused by, 53
Amniotic membrane transplantation, for corneal edema after cataract surgery, 165
AMO Sovereign phacoemulsification system with WhiteStar, 130–131
Amplitude, of accommodation, 23
Anaerobic glycolysis, in lens glucose/carbohydrate metabolism, 13–14, 14*f*
Anesthesia (anesthetics), for cataract surgery, 100–104, 101*f*, 102*f*, 103*f*
  general, 103–104
    in arthritis patients, 207
  local (topical/regional), 102–103, 103*f*
  minimizing bleeding risk and, 205, 206
Angiographic cystoid macular edema, after cataract surgery, 193, 193*f*
Angle-closure glaucoma
  ciliary block (malignant/aqueous misdirection), cataract surgery and, 172, 174–175
  microspherophakia and, 33
  secondary, with pupillary block
    microspherophakia and, 33
    phacomorphic glaucoma and, 67
Aniridia, 33–34, 33*f*
Anisometropia
  asymmetric lens-induced myopia causing, 77
  second-eye cataract surgery for, 78
Ankylosing spondylitis, cataract surgery in patients with, 207, 207*f*
Anomalies, congenital. *See specific type and* Congenital anomalies
Anterior capsular fibrosis and phimosis, 184
  Nd:YAG laser capsulotomy for, 184. *See also* Nd:YAG laser therapy, capsulotomy
Anterior capsule opacity, 183
Anterior capsulotomy. *See* Capsulotomy, anterior
Anterior chamber
  evaluation of, before cataract surgery, 84
  flat or shallow
    cataract surgery and, 138, 170–172
      capsulorrhexis issues and, 138
      intraoperative complications, 170–171
      postoperative complications, 171–172
      preoperative considerations, 84
    posterior infusion syndrome and, 170–171
  phacoemulsification in, 124
  vitreous in, after cataract surgery, 178
Anterior chamber angle, developmental abnormalities of, cataract surgery and, 216
Anterior chamber intraocular lenses. *See* Intraocular lenses
Anterior lenticonus, 30
Anterior lentiglobus, 30

Anterior polar cataract (APC), 35, 36*f*
Anterior pole, 5, 6*f*, 7*f*, 8*f*
Anterior pupillary membrane, 29, 29*f*
Anterior segment dysgenesis syndrome, Peters anomaly and, 32
Anterior sutures, 9
Antibiotics, prophylactic, cataract surgery and, 132–134, 133*f*, 190–191
  macular infarction and, 195
Anticholinesterase agents. *See* Cholinesterase/acetylcholinesterase inhibitors
Anticoagulant therapy, cataract surgery and, 136, 187, 205–206
Antimetabolites, for combined glaucoma filtering and cataract surgery, 224
Antimicrobial prophylaxis, cataract surgery and, 132–134, 133*f*, 190–191
  macular infarction and, 195
Antiplatelet therapy, cataract surgery and, 136, 187
Aphakia
  congenital, 30
  contact lenses for correction of
    in children, 203–204
    as IOL alternative, 219
  intraocular lenses for correction of, 142–156. *See also* Intraocular lenses
    in children, 201, 204
  spectacle lenses for correction of, in children, 203
Aphakic spectacles
  for children, 203
  as IOL alternative, 219
Aquaporin 0 (major intrinsic protein/MIP), 12, 19
Aquaporins (water channels), 12, 19
Aqueous misdirection (malignant/ciliary block glaucoma; posterior aqueous diversion syndrome), cataract surgery and, 172, 174–175
Arachnodactyly, in Marfan syndrome, 40, 40*f*
AREDS (Age-Related Eye Disease Study), 72
Arthritis
  cataract surgery in patients with, 206–207, 207*f*
  rheumatoid, cataract surgery in patients with, corneal melting/keratolysis and, 210–211
Aspiration, in phacoemulsification, 106, 110–111, 110*f*, 111*f*, 112*f*
  strategies for, 122–123
Aspiration flow rate, in phacoemulsification, 106
  vacuum rise time and, 111, 112*f*
Aspirin, cataract surgery in patient taking, 206
Astigmatic keratotomy, cataract surgery and, 135
Astigmatism
  in cataract patient
    modification during surgery and, 134–136
    toric intraocular lenses for, 136
  after cataract surgery, 167
  surgical correction of, cataract surgery and, 134–136
  suture-induced, cataract surgery and, 167
Atopic dermatitis, cataracts associated with, 66
Atropine, accommodation affected by, 22
Axes, optic, 5, 6*f*
Axial length, in IOL power determination, 149–150

B-scan ultrasonography, before cataract surgery, 86, 216
Balanced salt solution (BSS)
  in ECCE, 97
  in phacoemulsification, 110
Baltimore Eye Survey, 73
Barbados Eye Study, 73
Barraquer erysiphake, 94, 95*f*
Basement membrane dystrophies, corneal epithelial, cataract surgery in patients with, 212, 212*f*
Bausch & Lomb Millennium phacoemulsification system, 131
Beaded filaments, 12
Beaver Dam Eye Study, 72, 72*t*
Behavioral/psychiatric disorders, cataract surgery in patients with, 81, 204–205
Benign prostatic hypertrophy, alpha-blockers/tamsulosin for, intraoperative floppy iris syndrome and, 79–80, 137, 173
Beta crystallins, 12
Betagamma crystallins, 11*f*, 12
Bimanual microphacoemulsification, 130–131
Biometry/biometrics
  before cataract surgery, 88
  in IOL power determination, 150
Biomicroscopy, slit-lamp, before cataract surgery, 83–85
  limitations of, 85
Birth defects. *See specific type and* Congenital anomalies
Bladder (Wedl) cells, 49, 182
Bleeding diathesis, cataract surgery in patients with, 205–206
Blepharitis, cataract surgery in patients with, 82, 210
Blindness, cataract causing, 71
Blue-dot (cerulean) cataract, 37, 38*f*
Blue-light entoptoscopy, before cataract surgery, 87
Blunt injury, lens injury/cataract caused by, 53–55, 54*f*
BMI. *See* Body mass index
BMP. *See* Bone morphogenetic protein
Body mass index (BMI), cataract risk and, 73
Bone morphogenetic protein, lens placode formation and, 25
Brightness acuity, evaluation of before cataract surgery, 81
Brown-McLean syndrome, 165
Brunescent cataracts, 44
  lens proteins in, 13
BSS. *See* Balanced salt solution
Bullous keratopathy, after cataract surgery, 163, 164*t*, 165, 165*f*
  IOL design and, 181
Burst mode phacoemulsification, 109

Ca^{2+}-ATPase (calcium pump), in calcium homeostasis in lens, 20*f*, 21
Calcium homeostasis, in lens, 20*f*, 21
Can-opener capsulotomy, 119, 120
  for ECCE, 160
Cannulas, for ECCE, 97–98
Cantholysis, lateral, bulbar hemorrhage release and, 100
Capsular block syndrome, 180–181
Capsular cataracts, 38
Capsular fibrosis, 184
  IOL decentration and, 179–180
  Nd:YAG laser capsulotomy for, 184. *See also* Nd:YAG laser therapy, capsulotomy

Capsular opacification, 182–183
in children, 202
IOL design considerations and, 182
Nd:YAG laser capsulotomy for, 182, 183. *See also* Nd:YAG laser therapy, capsulotomy
Capsular phimosis, 184
Nd:YAG laser capsulotomy for, 184. *See also* Nd:YAG laser therapy, capsulotomy
Capsular rupture, cataract surgery and, 140–141, 164*t*, 176–178
Capsular tension rings, for zonular incompetence, 138–139, 139*f*, 230, 231*f*
Capsule, lens. *See* Lens capsule
Capsule staining, for cataract surgery, 137
mature cataract/poor red reflex and, 215
Capsulectomy/vitrectomy, for pediatric cataract, 201
Capsulorrhexis
in children, 200
continuous-tear curvilinear, 119–120, 119*f*
capsule staining for, 137
mature cataract/poor red reflex and, 215
for ECCE, 160
issues associated with, 138
loose zonules and, 138, 230
mature cataract/poor red reflex and, 140, 214–215
Capsulotomy
anterior
can-opener, 119, 120
for ECCE, 160
in children, 200
for ECCE, 160
for phacoemulsification, 119, 120
Nd:YAG laser, 184–187, 185*f*, 186*f*
for capsular block syndrome, 181
in children, 201
complications of, 187
contraindications to, 184–185
indications for, 184
lens particle glaucoma and, 67
procedure for, 185–186, 185*f*, 186*f*
retinal detachment and, 187, 196–197
Carbohydrate metabolism, in lens, 13–16, 14*f*
Carotenoids (xanthophylls), cataract risk affected by, 62
Catalase, in lens, 16
Cataract
age-related, 43–51. *See also* Age-related cataracts
epidemiology of, 71–74
atopic dermatitis and, 66
brunescent, 44
lens proteins in, 13
capsular, 38
cerulean, 37, 38*f*
chemical injuries causing, 57
in children, 35*t*, 199–204. *See also* Cataract, congenital and infantile
clinical studies of impact of, 71–74
complete (total), 38
congenital and infantile, 34–39, 35*t*, 199–204
aniridia and, 33*f*, 34
bilateral, 199–200
surgical management of, 199–204. *See also* Cataract surgery, in children
unilateral, 200
contrast sensitivity affected by, 76, 82
contusion, 54, 54*f*
coronary, 37
cortical, 45–46, 46*f*, 47*f*, 48*f*, 49*f*, 50*f*
uveitis and, 64, 64*f*
visual acuity and, 76*t*
degenerative ocular disorders and, 68
diabetic, 59–60, 60*f*
"sugar," aldose reductase in development of, 15–16, 59
surgery for, 208–209
preoperative evaluation and, 85, 209
drug-induced, 52, 53
electrical injury causing, 58, 59*f*
epidemiology of, 71–74
evaluation of, 75–77, 76*t*
in galactosemia, 60–61, 61*f*
glassblowers', 56
glaucoma and, 67
in children, 202
management of, 221–224, 222*f*
history in, 75–77, 76*t*
surgery evaluation and, 79–80
hypermature, 46, 49*f*
phacolytic glaucoma and, 67
hypocalcemia and, 61
intralenticular foreign-body causing, 57
intumescent, 46
phacomorphic glaucoma and, 67, 68*f*
ischemia causing, 68
lamellar (zonular), 34, 36*f*
lens proteins and, 13
management of, 77–89. *See also* Cataract surgery
in children, 199–204
in glaucoma patient, 221–224, 222*f*
low vision aids in, 78
medical, 77
mature, 46, 48*f*
phacolytic glaucoma and, 67
surgery and, 139–140, 214–215
membranous, 39, 39*f*
metabolic, 59–61
morgagnian, 46, 50*f*
in myotonic dystrophy, 61
nuclear, 43–44, 45*f*
congenital, 37–38, 38*f*
postvitrectomy, 64
visual acuity and, 76*t*
nutritional disease and, 62
pediatric, 35*t*, 199–204. *See also* Cataract, congenital and infantile
perforating/penetrating injuries causing, 55, 55*f*, 56*f*
persistent fetal vasculature (persistent hyperplastic primary vitreous) and, 42, 201
polar, 35–37, 36*f*
surgery for removal of, 216–217
posterior lenticonus/lentiglobus and, 30
postvitrectomy, 64, 227
radiation-induced, 55–57
after refractive surgery, 215
rosette, 54, 54*f*
rubella, 39
in siderosis bulbi, 57

skin diseases and, 66
smoking/tobacco use and, 63
snowflake, 59–60, 60*f*
socioeconomic impact of, 71
steroid-induced, 52
subcapsular, posterior, 46–49, 51*f*
corticosteroids causing, 52
ischemia causing, 68
in myotonic dystrophy, 61
uveitis and, 63
visual acuity and, 75–76, 76*t*
"sugar," aldose reductase in development of, 15–16, 59
sunflower
in chalcosis, 58
in Wilson disease, 61
sutural (stellate), 37, 37*f*
tetanic, 61
total (complete), 38
traumatic, 40, 53–58, 54*f*, 228
surgery for, 228–231, 229*f*, 231*f*
treatment-induced, 64–65. *See also* Cataract, drug-induced
uveitis and, 63–64, 64*f*, 226–227
in Wilson disease, 61
zonular (lamellar), 34, 36*f*
Cataract surgery, 91–161. *See also specific procedure and* Phacoemulsification
in alpha-blocker patients, 79–80, 137, 173
ancient/medieval techniques for, 91–92, 91*f*, 92*f*
anesthesia for, 100–104, 101*f*, 102*f*, 103*f*
anterior capsule fibrosis and phimosis and, 184
in anticoagulated patient, 136, 187, 205–206
antimicrobial prophylaxis for, 132–134, 133*f*, 190–191
in arthritis patients, 206–207, 207*f*
astigmatism and
modification of preexisting, 134–136
suture-induced, 167
toric IOL for, 136
biometry before, 88
in bleeding diathesis, 205–206
Brown-McLean syndrome after, 165
bullous keratopathy after, 163, 164*t*, 165, 165*f*
IOL design and, 181
capsular block syndrome and, 180–181
capsular opacification and contraction and, 164*t*, 182–184
Nd:YAG laser capsulotomy for, 182, 183, 186. *See also* Nd:YAG laser therapy, capsulotomy
capsular rupture and, 140–141, 164*t*, 176–178
capsule staining and, 137
mature cataract/poor red reflex and, 215
capsulorrhexis in, 119–120, 119*f*, 160
capsule staining for, 137
mature cataract/poor red reflex and, 215
in children, 200
issues associated with, 138
loose zonules and, 138
in children, 199–204
aphakia correction and, 203–204
complications of, 202
planning, 199–200
postoperative care and, 202
prognosis for, 202–203
techniques for, 200–202
choroidal hemorrhage and. *See* Cataract surgery, suprachoroidal hemorrhage/effusion and
in chronic obstructive pulmonary disease, 207–208
chronic uveitis after, 164*t*, 175, 226
ciliary block (malignant) glaucoma and, 172, 174–175
in claustrophobic patient, 204
clear corneal incision for, 116–118, 116*f*, 117*f*
minimizing bleeding risk and, 206
communication with patient and, 205
complications of, 163–197, 164*t*. *See also specific type*
antimicrobial prophylaxis in prevention of, 132–134, 133*f*, 190–191
in children, 202
in glaucoma patient, 221–223
conjunctiva examination before, 83
corneal complications of ultrasound and, 166
corneal conditions and, 211–214
developmental abnormalities, 218–219, 220*f*
corneal edema and, 163–166
corneal melting/keratolysis after, 167–168
in patients with dry eye, 167, 210–211
corneal pachymetry before, 88
corneal topography before, 83, 88
cyclodialysis and, 174
cystoid macular edema and, 164*t*, 193–195, 193*f*
in glaucoma patient, 222
after Nd:YAG capsulotomy, 187
in dementia/mentally disabled patient, 205
Descemet's membrane detachment and, 166–167
developmentally abnormal eye and, 216–219, 217*f*, 218*f*, 219*f*
in diabetic patients, 208–209
preoperative evaluation and, 85, 209
economics of, 71
elevated intraocular pressure after, 164*t*, 172–173. *See also* Elevated intraocular pressure
abnormal angle structures/preexisting disease and, 216
in glaucoma patient, 222
endophthalmitis after, 164*t*, 190–192, 191*f*
prevention of, 132–134, 133*f*, 190–191
epithelial downgrowth and, 168–169
external eye disease and, 210–211
external eye examination before, 82–83
extracapsular cataract extraction (ECCE), 160–161. *See also* Extracapsular cataract extraction
early techniques for, 92–94, 93*f*
modern procedure for, 97–98, 98*f*
renaissance/rediscovery of, 97–98
transition to phacoemulsification from, 111–113
filtering bleb (inadvertent) after, 168
filtering surgery and
cataract surgery combined with, 223–224
cataract surgery following, 223
flat or shallow anterior chamber and, 138, 170–172
capsulorrhexis issues and, 138
intraoperative complications, 170–171
postoperative complications, 171–172
preoperative considerations, 84

fundus evaluation before, 85–86
in glaucoma patient, 221–224, 222*f*
complications of, 221–223
filtering surgery before, 223
filtering surgery combined with, 223–224
preoperative evaluation and, 80
globe exposure for, 113
hemorrhage and, 164*t*, 187–190
at-risk patients and, 219–221
high refractive error and, 224–226
clear lens extraction for, 225–226
history of use of
in recent past, 94–98, 95*f*, 98*f*
in remote past, 91–94, 91*f*, 92*f*, 93*f*, 94*f*
hyphema after, 190
hypotony as complication of, flat anterior chamber and, 171–172
in hypotony patients, 226
incision leak and, 168
flat anterior chamber and, 170, 171–172
incisions for. *See also* Incisions, for cataract surgery
for ECCE, 160
for ICCE, 158
modification of preexisting astigmatism and, 135
for phacoemulsification
clear corneal, 116–118, 116*f*, 117*f*
scleral tunnel, 113–115, 114*f*, 115*f*
indications for, 78–79
informed consent for, 88–89
intracapsular cataract extraction (ICCE), 157–159. *See also* Intracapsular cataract extraction
early techniques for, 94, 94*f*
modern advances in, 94–96, 95*f*
intraocular lens implantation and, 142–156. *See also* Intraocular lenses
in children, 201, 204
complications of, 164*t*, 178–182, 179*f*, 180*f*
iridodialysis and, 174
after keratoplasty, 213, 214
lens instability and, 138–139
loose zonules and, 138–139, 139*f*, 230, 231*f*
in glaucoma patient, 222–223
iris coloboma and, 216
macular function evaluation before, 87
macular infarction after, 195–196
mature cataract and, 139–140, 214–215
measurements taken before, 88
nucleus removal in
laser photolysis for, 132
phacoemulsification for, 104–131. *See also* Phacoemulsification
sutureless nonphaco surgery for, 131–132
water jet phacolysis for, 132
in obese patients, 209–210
ocular conditions and, 210–228
ocular hypotension after, 171–172
ophthalmic viscosurgical devices (viscoelastics) in, 98–100
outcomes of, 156–157
improving, 151–152
paracentesis for, 113
pars plana lensectomy, 142
patient preparation for, 88–89
in patient unable to communicate, 205
with penetrating keratoplasty and intraocular lens insertion (triple procedure), 156, 213–214
phacoemulsification, 104–131. *See also* Phacoemulsification
posterior capsule opacification and, 164*t*, 182–183
in children, 202
Nd:YAG laser capsulotomy for, 182, 183. *See also* Nd:YAG laser therapy, capsulotomy
posterior capsule rupture and, 140–141, 164*t*, 176–178
posterior misdirection of irrigation fluid (posterior infusion syndrome) and, 170–171
postoperative care and
in children, 202
after ECCE, 161
after ICCE, 159
potential acuity estimation before, 86
preoperative evaluation/preparation for, 79–81
in children, 199–200
psychosocial considerations in, 81, 204–205
pupillary capture and, 180, 180*f*
pupillary expansion and, 137–138
refraction before, 81
after refractive surgery, 215–216
intraocular lens power calculation and, 152–153
with refractive surgery, 134–136. *See also* Cataract surgery, astigmatism and
retained lens material and, 175–176
retinal detachment after, 164*t*, 196–197, 196*f*
in children, 202
in retinal disease, 227–228
retinal light toxicity and, 195
retrobulbar hemorrhage and, 188
scleral tunnel incisions for, 113–115, 114*f*, 115*f*
in children, 200
slit-lamp examination before, 83–85
specular microscopy before, 88
stromal/epithelial edema after, 163–166
suprachoroidal hemorrhage/effusion and, 164*t*, 188–189
delayed, 190
expulsive, 189
patients at risk for, 219–221
flat anterior chamber and, 170
sutureless nonphaco, 131–132
systemic conditions and, 205–210
in tamsulosin patient, 79–80, 137, 173
after trauma, 228–231, 229*f*, 231*f*
in triple procedure, 156, 213–214
ultrasound complications and, 166
uveitis and, 164*t*, 175, 226
in uveitis patient, 80, 226–227
visual function evaluation before, 81–82
visual function evaluation after, 156–157
vitreal complications of, 164*t*, 178
in glaucoma patient, 222–223
with ICCE, 158
prolapse, 178
vitreocorneal adherence, 165–166

vitreocorneal adherence after, 165–166
wound closure for
after ECCE, 161
for scleral tunnel incisions, 115, 115*f*, 200
zonular dehiscence/lens subluxation or dislocation and, 138–139, 139*f*, 230, 231*f*
Cation balance, in lens, maintenance of, 19–21, 20*f*
Cavitation, 104–105, 107, 107*f*
CCC. *See* Continuous-tear curvilinear capsulorrhexis
Cerulean cataract, 37, 38*f*
Chalcosis, 58
Chatter, 105, 108–109, 121
Chemical injury (burns), cataracts caused by, 57
Children
cataract surgery in, 199–204. *See also* Cataract surgery, in children
intraocular lens implantation in, 201, 204
Chlorpromazine, lens changes caused by, 52
Cholinesterase/acetylcholinesterase inhibitors, cataracts caused by, 53
Chondroitin sulfate, as viscoelastic, 98
Chopping techniques, in phacoemulsification, 127–129, 129*f*
instrument settings for, 122
Choroidal/suprachoroidal hemorrhage, 164*t*, 188–189
delayed, 190
expulsive, 189
patients at risk for, 219–221
flat or shallow anterior chamber and, 170
Chromophores, ultraviolet, intraocular lenses with, 148
Chronic obstructive pulmonary disease, cataract surgery in patients with, 207–208
Chymotrypsin (alpha-chymotrypsin), for ICCE, 95, 158
Cicatricial pemphigoid, cataract surgery in patients with, 211
Cigarette smoking, cataract development and, 63, 74
Ciliary block, after cataract surgery, flat anterior chamber and, 172
Ciliary block glaucoma (malignant glaucoma/aqueous misdirection), cataract surgery and, 172, 174–175
Ciliary muscle, in accommodation, 22, 22*t*
Claustrophobia, cataract surgery in patients with, 204
Clear corneal incision, 116–118, 116*f*, 117*f*
minimizing bleeding risk and, 206
Clear lens extraction, 225–226
Clopidogrel, cataract surgery in patient taking, 206
Closed-loop intraocular lenses, pseudophakic bullous keratopathy and, 181
CME. *See* Cystoid macular edema
Coagulation
disorders of, cataract surgery in patient with, 205–206
laboratory evaluation of, before cataract surgery, 206
Cohesive ophthalmic viscosurgical devices, 99
Colobomas
iris, cataract surgery in patients with, 216, 217*f*
lens, 31, 31*f*
Color vision, nuclear cataract affecting, 44
Communication, between clinician and patient, cataract surgery and, 205
Complete cataract, 38
Confrontation testing, before cataract surgery, 82
Congenital anomalies. *See also specific type*
cataract surgery in patients with, 216–219, 217*f*, 218*f*, 219*f*
of lens, 30–39
Congenital aphakia, 30. *See also* Aphakia
Congenital cataract, 34. *See also specific type and* Cataract, congenital and infantile
Congenital rubella syndrome, cataracts and, 39
Conjunctiva, examination of, before cataract surgery, 83
Conjunctival ballooning, cataract surgery and, 170
Conjunctival flaps
for corneal edema after cataract surgery, 165
for ICCE, 158
in scleral-tunnel incision for cataract surgery, 114
Consent, informed, for cataract surgery, 88–89
Contact lens method, for IOL power calculation after refractive surgery, 152
Contact lenses, for aphakia
in children, 203–204
as IOL alternative, 219
Continuous phacoemulsification, 108
Continuous-tear curvilinear capsulorrhexis, 119–120, 119*f*. *See also* Capsulorrhexis
capsule staining for, 137
mature cataract/poor red reflex and, 215
for ECCE, 160
loose zonules and, 138
Contrast sensitivity, testing, in cataract patient, 76, 82
Contusion cataract, 54, 54*f*
Contusion injury, lens damage caused by, 53–55, 54*f*
Copper
foreign body of, 58
sunflower cataract in Wilson disease and, 61
Cornea
abrasions of, cataract surgery in diabetic patients and, 209
congenital/developmental anomalies of, cataract surgery and, 218–219, 220*f*
disorders of
cataract surgery in patients with, 211–214, 218–219, 220*f*
intraocular lenses and, 218–219, 220*f*
edema of
after cataract surgery, 163–166
persistent, with vitreocorneal adherence, 165–166
intraocular lenses and, 181
epithelium of
defects of, after cataract surgery, 167, 211
protection of during cataract surgery in diabetic patients, 209
examination of, before cataract surgery, 83
flat (cornea plana), sclerocornea and, intraocular lens power and, 218, 220*f*
guttata/guttae
Brown-McLean syndrome and, 165
cataract surgery and, 83
melting of (keratolysis), cataract surgery and, 167–168
in patients with dry eye, 167, 210–211
opacification of, in Peters anomaly, 32

phacoemulsification/ultrasound complications affecting, 166
plana, sclerocornea and, intraocular lens power and, 218, 220*f*
thickness of, measurement of, before cataract surgery, 83, 88, 212–213
topography of, cataract surgery and, 83, 88
transplantation of
cataract surgery following, 213, 214
in triple procedure, 156, 213–214
Corneal dystrophies, cataract surgery in patients with, 212–214, 212*f*
Corneal incision, clear, 116–118, 116*f*, 117*f*
minimizing bleeding risk and, 206
Corneal melting (keratolysis), cataract surgery and, 167–168
in patients with dry eye, 167, 210–211
Coronary cataract, 37
Cortex, lens, 6*f*
Cortical cataracts, 45–46, 46*f*, 47*f*, 48*f*, 49*f*, 50*f*
uveitis and, 64, 64*f*
visual acuity and, 76*t*
Cortical spokes, 46, 47*f*
Corticosteroids (steroids)
cataracts caused by, 52
for postoperative cystoid macular edema, 194
Couching, 91–92, 91*f*, 92*f*
Cough, in COPD, cataract surgery and, 208
Coumadin. *See* Warfarin
Cranial nerve III (oculomotor nerve), in accommodation, 22
Cryoprobe, for lens extraction, 95, 95*f*, 158, 159*f*
Crystalens, 147, 148*f*
Crystallins, 11–12, 11*f*
alpha, 11–12, 11*f*
beta, 12
betagamma, 11*f*, 12
gamma, 12
CTRs. *See* Capsular tension rings
Cyclodialysis, after cataract surgery, 174
Cycloplegia/cycloplegics, 22
Cystitome, for ECCE, 97
Cystoid macular edema, postoperative, 164*t*, 193–195, 193*f*
in glaucoma patient, 222
after Nd:YAG capsulotomy, 187
Cytoskeletal (urea-soluble) lens proteins, 11*f*, 12

Deafness, cataract surgery in patients with, 205
Decentration, of intraocular lenses, 164*t*, 178–180, 179*f*
Degenerations, cataracts associated with, 68
Delayed suprachoroidal hemorrhage, after cataract surgery, 190
Dementia, cataract surgery in patients with, 205
Dermatitis, atopic, cataracts associated with, 66
Descemet's membrane/layer, detachment of, after cataract surgery, 166–167
Developmental defects. *See also specific type and* Congenital anomalies
of lens, 39–42
Diabetes mellitus, cataracts associated with, 59–60, 60*f*
"sugar," aldose reductase in development of, 15–16, 59
surgery for, 208–209
preoperative evaluation and, 85, 209
Diabetic retinopathy, proliferative, cataract surgery and, 208–209
Diaphragm pump, for phacoemulsification aspiration, 110, 111*f*
vacuum rise time for, 110, 112*f*
Diclofenac, corneal melting after cataract surgery and, 167
Diffusion, glucose transport into lens and, 13
Diplopia, monocular, in cataracts, 44, 45, 47, 77
Dipyridamole, cataract surgery in patient taking, 206
Dislocated lens, 40. *See also* Ectopia lentis
cataract surgery and, 230
traumatic, 54, 54–55, 54*f*
cataract surgery and, 230
Dispersive ophthalmic viscosurgical devices, 99
Doxazosin, cataract surgery complications and, 79–80
Drugs, lens changes caused by, 52–53, 52*f*
Dry eye syndrome, cataract surgery in patients with, 210–211
corneal melting/keratolysis and, 167, 210–211
Dulcitol (galactitol)
in cataract formation, 15, 61
in lens glucose/carbohydrate metabolism, 15
Duty cycle, in phacoemulsification, 105
Dysphotopsias, temporal, intraocular lens design and, 182
Dystrophies, corneal, cataract surgery in patients with, 212–214, 212*f*

ECCE. *See* Extracapsular cataract extraction
Echothiophate
cataract and, 53
inflammation after cataract surgery and, 222
Ectoderm, in lens development, 25, 26*f*
Ectopia lentis, 39–40
et pupillae, 42
in homocystinuria, 41
in hyperlysinemia, 41
in Marfan syndrome, 40, 40*f*
simple, 40
in sulfite oxidase deficiency, 41
traumatic, 40, 54–55, 54*f*
cataract surgery in patients with, 230
Edema, corneal. *See* Cornea, edema of
Effusion, suprachoroidal, 188–189
flat or shallow anterior chamber and, 170
Electrical injury, lens damage/cataracts caused by, 58, 59*f*
Electrolytes, in lens, maintenance of balance of, 19–21, 20*f*
Electroretinogram, before cataract surgery, 87
Elevated intraocular pressure
cataract surgery and, 164*t*, 172–173
abnormal angle structures and, 216
epithelial downgrowth and, 168–169
flat anterior chamber and, 172
in glaucoma patient, 222
patient with preexisting disease and, 216
retrobulbar hemorrhage and, 189
stromal/epithelial corneal edema and, 163
in glaucoma, phacolytic glaucoma and, 67
Nd:YAG laser capsulotomy and, 187
Elschnig pearls, 182–183

Embryonic nucleus, 9, 25–27, 27*f*
opacification of (congenital nuclear cataract), 37–38, 38*f*
Emulsification, locations of, 123–125, 124*f*, 125*f*
Endolenticular phacoemulsification, 129–130
Endophthalmitis, postoperative, 164*t*, 190–192, 191*f*
prevention of, 132–134, 133*f*, 190–191
sterile, 191
toxic anterior segment syndrome and, 169
Endophthalmitis Vitrectomy Study (EVS), 191–192
Endothelial dystrophies, cataract surgery in patients with, 212–213, 212*f*
Endothelial keratoplasty, cataract surgery following, 213
Energy delivery, for phacoemulsification, 108–109
advances in, 130–131
Enophthalmos, cataract surgery in patient with, 82
Entoptic images/phenomena, Purkinje's, evaluation of before cataract surgery, 87
Entoptoscopy, blue-light, before cataract surgery, 87
Epicapsular star, 31, 32*f*
Epimerase deficiency, galactosemia caused by, 60
cataract associated with, 61
Epithelial defects, corneal, after cataract surgery, 167, 211
Epithelial downgrowth (ingrowth), cataract surgery and, 168–169
Epithelial dystrophies, basement membrane, cataract surgery in patients with, 212, 212*f*
Epithelium
corneal, protection of during cataract surgery in diabetic patients, 209
lens, 6*f*, 8–9
active transport and, 19–20
development of, 26, 27*f*
opacification of (capsular cataract), 38
Equator, 5, 6*f*, 8, 8*f*
ERG. *See* Electroretinogram
Erysiphakes, 94, 95*f*
EVS (Endophthalmitis Vitrectomy Study), 191–192
Exfoliation. *See also* Pseudoexfoliation syndrome
infrared radiation/heat causing, 56
Expulsive choroidal/suprachoroidal hemorrhage, 164*t*, 189
patients at risk for, 219–221
External (outer) eye
cataract surgery in patients with disease of, 210–211
examination of, before cataract surgery, 82–83
Extracapsular cataract extraction (ECCE), 160–161. *See also* Cataract surgery
advantages of, 97
anterior capsulotomy in, 160
capsular opacification and, 182–183
Nd:YAG laser capsulotomy for, 182, 183. *See also* Nd:YAG laser therapy, capsulotomy
cystoid macular edema and, 193
early techniques for, 160–161
equipment for, 97–98, 98*f*
flat or shallow anterior chamber and, 170–172
intraoperative complications, 170–171
postoperative complications, 171–172
in glaucoma patient, vitreous loss/loose zonular fibers and, 222–223
incisions for, 160
intraocular lenses for, 143–144, 144, 161
lens particle glaucoma and, 67
nucleus removal in, 160–161
patient preparation for, 160
after posterior capsular rupture during phacoemulsification, 140, 141
postoperative course and, 161
procedure for, 97–98, 98*f*, 160–161
renaissance/rediscovery of, 97–98
retained lens fragments after, 175–176
retinal detachment and, 196
surgeon's transition to phacoemulsification and, 111–112
in triple procedure, 213
after vitrectomy, 228
vitreocorneal adherence/persistent corneal edema and, 165–166
wound closure and, 161
Eye
cataract surgery in patients with disorders of, 210–228
developmental abnormalities of, cataract surgery in patients with, 216–219, 217*f*, 218*f*, 219*f*
Eyedrops (topical medications), after cataract surgery, 134
corneal melting and, 167, 211
Eyelids, retraction of
after ECCE, 161
after ICCE, 159

Facial nerve block, for cataract surgery, 103, 103*f*
Facilitated diffusion, glucose transport into lens and, 13
Feiz and Mannis formula, for IOL power determination, 153
Fetal nucleus, 9, 27*f*, 28, 28*f*
opacification of (congenital nuclear cataract), 37–38, 38*f*
Fetal vasculature, persistent. *See* Persistent fetal vasculature
Fibrillin, defects in, in Marfan syndrome, 40
Filensin, 12
Filtering bleb, inadvertent, after cataract surgery, 168
Filtering procedures
cataract surgery after, 223
cataract surgery combined with, 223–224
Flaps, conjunctival
for corneal edema after cataract surgery, 165
for ICCE, 158
in scleral-tunnel incision for cataract surgery, 114
Flat anterior chamber. *See* Anterior chamber, flat or shallow
Flexible-loop anterior chamber intraocular lenses, 143, 145*f*
Flomax. *See* Tamsulosin
Floppy iris syndrome, intraoperative, alpha-blockers/tamsulosin and, 79–80, 137, 173
Foldable intraocular lenses, 145–146, 146*f*
implantation procedure for, 154
instrumentation for, 154
Followability, in phacoemulsification, 106
Foreign bodies
intralenticular, 57

intraocular, retained
cataract surgery and, 229
siderosis and, 57, 58*f*
Fornices, sterilization of during cataract surgery, 133
FOXC1 (FKHL7) gene, in Peters anomaly, 32
Free radicals (oxygen radicals), in lens, 16
Frequency, in phacoemulsification, 105
Fuchs heterochromic iridocyclitis/uveitis, cataracts in, 64, 64*f*
surgery and, 80
Fundus, evaluation of, before cataract surgery, 85–86

G6P. *See* Glucose-6-phosphate
Galactitol (dulcitol)
in cataract formation, 15, 61
in lens glucose/carbohydrate metabolism, 15
Galactokinase deficiency
cataract associated with, 61
galactosemia caused by, 60
Galactose
in cataract formation, 15, 60–61, 61*f*
in lens glucose/carbohydrate metabolism, 15
Galactose 1-phosphate uridyltransferase (Gal-1-PUT), galactosemia caused by defects in, 60
Galactosemia, 60–61, 61*f*
Gamma crystallins, 12
Gap junctions, in lens, 19
General anesthesia. *See also* Anesthesia
for cataract surgery, 103–104
in arthritis patients, 207
Genetic/hereditary factors, in age-related cataracts, 50–51
Geometrical optics, intraocular lenses and, 145
Germinative zone, 8, 8*f*
Glare
cataracts and, 45, 47, 76
intraocular lens design and, 182
Glare testing, in cataract evaluation, 76
Glassblowers' cataract, 56
Glaucoma
cataracts and, 67
in children, 202
management of, 221–224, 222*f*. *See also* Cataract surgery, in glaucoma patient
cataract surgery and, 223–224
ciliary block. *See* Aqueous misdirection
lens-induced, 67–68, 68*f*
lens particle, 67
microspherophakia and, 33
phacolytic, 67
phacomorphic, 67, 68*f*
Glaukomflecken, 68
Globe
exposure of for phacoemulsification, 113
stabilization of, for clear corneal incision, 116
Glucose
in cataract formation, 15, 59–60. *See also* Diabetes mellitus
metabolism of in lens, 13–16, 14*f*
Glucose-6-phosphate, in lens glucose/carbohydrate metabolism, 13, 14*f*, 15
Glutathione, oxidative changes in lens and, 13, 16
Glutathione peroxidase, in lens, 16
Glycolysis, in lens glucose/carbohydrate metabolism, 13–14, 14*f*
"Golden ring" sign, 121
Gonioscopy, before cataract surgery, 84
Gundersen flap, 165

Haigis formula, for IOL power determination, 151
Handpiece, phaco, 107, 108*f*
Healon 5, 99, 137
Hearing loss (deafness), cataract surgery in patients with, 205
Hemorrhages, cataract surgery and, 164*t*, 187–190
at-risk patients and, 219–221
flat anterior chamber and, 170
patient receiving anticoagulation therapy and, 136, 187, 205–206
retrobulbar, 188
suprachoroidal, 164*t*, 188–189
delayed, 190
expulsive, 189
patients at risk for, 219–221
flat anterior chamber and, 170
Hemostasis, disorders of, cataract surgery in patients with, 205–206
Heparin therapy, cataract surgery and, 206
Hepatolenticular degeneration (Wilson disease), 61
Heterochromia, in siderosis bulbi, 58*f*
Hexokinase, in lens glucose/carbohydrate metabolism, 13, 14*f*, 15
Hexose monophosphate shunt, in lens glucose/carbohydrate metabolism, 14*f*, 15
High hyperopia, cataract surgery in patients with, 225
clear lens extraction and, 225–226
High myopia, cataract surgery in patients with, 225
clear lens extraction and, 225–226
Historical methods, for IOL power calculation after refractive surgery, 152–153
History, in cataract, 75–77, 76*t*
evaluation for surgery and, 79–81
HMG-CoA (3-hydroxy-3-methylglutaryl coenzyme-A) reductase inhibitors, cataracts and, 53
HMP shunt. *See* Hexose monophosphate shunt
Hoffer Q formula, for IOL power determination, 151, 152–153
Holladay 2 formula, for IOL power determination, 151
Homocystinuria, 41
Honan balloon, 221
Horizontal phaco chop technique, in phacoemulsification, 127, 128
HPMC. *See* Hydroxypropyl methylcellulose
Hyaloid artery, tunica vasculosa lentis development and, 29, 29*f*
Hyaluronate/sodium hyaluronate, as viscoelastic, 98, 144
Hydrodelineation, in phacoemulsification, 121
Hydrodissection, in phacoemulsification, 120–121
3-Hydroxy-3-methylglutaryl coenzyme-A (HMG-CoA) reductase inhibitors, cataracts and, 53
Hydroxypropyl methylcellulose (HPMC), as viscoelastic, 98–99
Hyperbaric oxygen therapy, oxidative lens damage and, 16, 64–65
Hyperlysinemia, 41

Hypermature cataract, 46, 49*f*
phacolytic glaucoma and, 67
Hyperopia, high, cataract surgery in patients with, 225
clear lens extraction and, 225–226
Hyphema, after cataract surgery, 190
Hypocalcemia, cataracts associated with, 61
Hypopyon, after cataract surgery, 164*t*
Hypotony
cataract surgery in patients with, 226
during/after surgery, flat anterior chamber and, 171–172

ICCE. *See* Intracapsular cataract extraction
IFIS. *See* Intraoperative floppy iris syndrome
Immersion technique, in IOL power determination, 149–150, 149*f*
Incision leaks, after cataract surgery, 168
flat anterior chamber and, 170, 171–172
Incisions, for cataract surgery
clear corneal, 116–118, 116*f*, 117*f*
for ECCE, 160
wound closure and, 161
for ICCE, 158
minimizing bleeding and, 206
modification of preexisting astigmatism and, 135
for phacoemulsification
clear corneal, 116–118, 116*f*, 117*f*
scleral tunnel, 113–115, 114*f*, 115*f*
postoperative leaking and, 168
flat anterior chamber and, 170, 171–172
scleral tunnel, 113–115, 114*f*, 115*f*
in children, 200
wound closure and, 115, 115*f*, 200
self-sealing
beveled/biplanar, clear corneal incisions and, 116–117, 117*f*
scleral tunnel incisions and, 115
Infantile cataract, 34. *See also specific type and* Cataract, congenital and infantile
Inflammation (ocular), cataract surgery and, 164*t*, 175, 181, 226–227
in glaucoma patient, 221–222
trauma and, 228–229
Inflow, in phacoemulsification, 105
Informed consent, for cataract surgery, 88–89
Infrared radiation, lens affected by, 56
Instrumentation. *See* Ophthalmic instrumentation; Surgical instruments
Interferometry, laser, for potential acuity estimation before cataract surgery, 86
Intracameral lidocaine injections, for cataract surgery, 102
Intracapsular cataract extraction (ICCE), 157–159. *See also* Cataract surgery
advantages of, 96
contraindications to, 96
cystoid macular edema and, 193
disadvantages of, 96
early techniques for, 94, 94*f*
intraocular lenses for, 143, 144*f*
modern advances in, 94–96, 95*f*, 157–159
patient preparation for, 157–158
postoperative course for, 159
postoperative flat or shallow anterior chamber and, 171–172
procedure for, 158–159, 159*f*
retinal detachment and, 196
vitreocorneal adherence/persistent corneal edema and, 165–166
Intralenticular foreign bodies, 57
Intraocular lenses (IOLs). *See also* Cataract surgery
anterior chamber
after capsular rupture, 141, 177
closed-loop, pseudophakic bullous keratopathy and, 181
complications associated with, 143
contraindications to, 156
flexible-loop, 143, 145*f*
history of development of, 143, 145*f*
after ICCE, 159
implantation of, 155
secondary, 155–156
preoperative gonioscopy and, 84
capsular block syndrome and, 180–181
in children, 201, 204
closed loop, pseudophakic bullous keratopathy and, 181
complications of, 164*t*, 178–182, 179*f*, 180*f*
contraindications to, 156
corneal abnormalities and, 218–219, 220*f*
cystoid macular edema and, 194
decentration of, 164*t*, 178–180, 179*f*
developmentally abnormal eye and, 218–219, 219*f*, 220*f*
for diabetic patients, 209
dislocation of, 178–180, 179*f*
flexible-loop, 143, 145*f*
foldable, 145–146, 146*f*
implantation procedure for, 154
instrumentation for, 154
glare and, 182
history of, 142–144, 143*f*, 144*f*
implantation of, 142–156
anterior chamber, 155
after capsular rupture, 141, 177
complications of, 164*t*, 178–182, 179*f*, 180*f*
after ECCE, 161
after ICCE, 159
posterior chamber, 154–155
procedure for, 154–156
in children, 201, 204
secondary, 155–156
in children, 204
in keratoconus patient, 218–219
laser capsulotomy and, 185–186, 186*f*, 187
multifocal, 146–147, 148*f*
with penetrating keratoplasty and cataract surgery (triple procedure), 156, 213–214
piggyback, for keratoconus, 219
posterior chamber, 144–146, 146*f*
advantages of, 156
capsular block syndrome and, 180
after capsular rupture, 141
for cataract surgery after glaucoma filtering surgery, 223

for children, 204
for diabetic patients, 209
history of development of, 143–144
implantation procedure for, 154–155
after keratoplasty, 214
pupillary capture caused by anterior displacement of, 180, 180*f*
sutured, 155, 156
power determination for, 149–153, 149*f*
in children, 204
contact lens method for, 152
historical methods for, 152–153
improving outcomes of, 151–152
incorrect, 181–182
preventing errors in, 150–151
refraction and, 81
refractive surgery and, 152–153
regression formulas for, 151, 152–153
topographical method for, 152
triple procedure and, 214
pseudophakic bullous keratopathy and, 181
pupil evaluation and, 83
pupillary capture of, 180, 180*f*
for sclerocornea patient, 218, 220*f*
techniques of, 154
toric, 136
traumatic cataract and, 231
with UV chromophores, 148
in uveitis, 226
uveitis-glaucoma-hyphema (UGH) syndrome and, 181
Intraocular pressure
decreased, after cataract surgery, flat anterior chamber and, 171–172
elevated/increased. *See* Elevated intraocular pressure
Intraoperative floppy iris syndrome, alpha-blockers/tamsulosin and, 79–80, 137, 173
Intravitreal medications, corticosteroids, for cystoid macular edema, 194
Intumescent cortical cataract, 46
phacomorphic glaucoma and, 67, 68*f*
IOLMaster, 149, 150
Ionizing radiation, cataracts caused by, 55–56
Iridectomy
for ICCE, 158
peripheral, cataract surgery on inflamed eye and, 228
Iridocyclitis
Fuchs heterochromic, cataracts in, 64, 64*f*
intraocular lenses in patients with, 226
Iridodialysis, cataract surgery and, 174, 229, 229*f*
Iridodonesis, cataract surgery and, 84, 230
Iris
absence of (aniridia), 33–34, 33*f*
coloboma of, cataract surgery in patients with, 216, 217*f*
evaluation of, before cataract surgery, 84
prolapse of, cataract surgery and, 164*t*
traumatic damage to, cataract surgery and, 229–230, 229*f*
Iris clip intraocular lenses, pseudophakic bullous keratopathy and, 181
Iris hooks
for loose zonules, 138
for pupillary expansion, 137
Iris plane, phacoemulsification at, 124, 124*f*
Iris sphincter. *See* Sphincter muscle
Iron, foreign body of, siderosis caused by, 57, 58*f*
Irrigation, in phacoemulsification, 110, 122–123
posterior misdirection (posterior infusion syndrome) and, 170–171
with toxic solutions, corneal edema caused by, 163, 169
Irvine-Gass syndrome, 193. *See also* Cystoid macular edema
Ischemia, cataracts caused by, 68

Kalt forceps, 94, 94*f*
Kayser-Fleischer ring, 61
Kelman phaco tip, 107, 107*f*
Keratectomy, photorefractive (PRK). *See* Photorefractive keratectomy
Keratoconjunctivitis sicca, cataract surgery in patients with, 210–211
corneal melting/keratolysis and, 167, 210–211
Keratoconus, intraocular lens implantation and, 218–219
Keratolysis (corneal melting), cataract surgery and, 167–168
in patients with dry eye, 167, 210–211
Keratometry, before cataract surgery, 83, 211
IOL power determination and, 149
refractive surgery and, 152
Keratopathy, bullous, after cataract surgery, 163, 164*t*, 165, 165*f*
IOL design and, 181
Keratoplasty
for corneal edema after cataract surgery, 164–165, 166
endothelial, cataract surgery following, 213
penetrating
cataract surgery following, 214
cataract surgery and IOL implantation combined with (triple procedure), 156, 213–214
for corneal edema after cataract surgery, 164–165, 166
Keratorefractive surgery (KRS), cataract/cataract surgery and, 215–216
intraocular lens power calculation and, 152–153
Keratotomy
astigmatic, cataract surgery and, 135
radial, cataract surgery after, 215–216
intraocular lens power calculation and, 152–153
Ketorolac, for cystoid macular edema, after cataract surgery, 194
K_m (Michaelis/affinity constant), "sugar" cataract development and, 15
Kyphosis, cataract surgery in patients with, 207

Lamellae, zonular, 7
Lamellar (zonular) cataracts, 34, 36*f*
Laser capsulotomy (Nd:YAG), 184–187, 185*f*, 186*f*
for capsular block syndrome, 181
in children, 201
complications of, 187
contraindications to, 184–185
indications for, 184
lens particle glaucoma and, 67
procedure for, 185–186, 185*f*, 186*f*
retinal detachment and, 187, 196–197

Laser in situ keratomileusis (LASIK), cataract surgery after, 215–216
intraocular lens power calculation and, 152–153
Laser interferometry, for potential acuity estimation before cataract surgery, 86
Laser photolysis, 132
Laser pupilloplasty, for cataracts, 77
LASIK. *See* Laser in situ keratomileusis
Latanoprost, inflammation after cataract surgery and, 222
Lateral cantholysis, bulbar hemorrhage release and, 100
Lens (crystalline)
absence of, 30. *See also* Aphakia
aging changes in, 7, 13, 28–29, 43–51, 44*f*. *See also* Age-related cataracts
anatomy of, 5–9, 5*f*, 6*f*, 7*f*, 8*f*
biochemistry and metabolism of, 11–17
capsule of. *See* Lens capsule
carbohydrate metabolism in, 13–16, 14*f*
changing shape of. *See* Accommodation
chemical injuries affecting, 57
colobomas of, 31, 31*f*
coloration change in, 43, 44*f*
congenital anomalies and abnormalities of, 30–39
cortex of, 6*f*, 9
degenerative ocular disorders and, 68
development/embryology of, 25–42
congenital anomalies and abnormalities and, 30–39
developmental defects and, 39–42
normal, 25–30, 26–27*f*
diabetes mellitus affecting, 59–60, 60*f*
dislocated, 40. *See also* Ectopia lentis
traumatic, 54, 54–55, 54*f*
cataract surgery and, 230
disorders of, 43–69. *See also specific disorder and* Cataract
drug-induced changes in, 52–53, 52*f*
electrical injury of, 58, 59*f*
epithelium of, 6*f*, 8–9
active transport and, 19–20
development of, 26, 27*f*
opacification of (capsular cataract), 38
evaluation of, before cataract surgery, 84–85
foreign body in, 57
free radicals affecting, 16
glaucoma and, 67–68, 68*f*
in homocystinuria, 41
in hyperlysinemia, 41
ischemic damage to, 68
luxed/luxated, 40. *See also* Ectopia lentis
cataract surgery and, 230
in Marfan syndrome, 40, 40*f*
metabolic diseases affecting, 59–61
molecular biology of, 11–13
nucleus of, 6*f*, 9
congenital cataract of, 37–38, 38*f*
embryonic, 9, 25–27, 27*f*
opacification of (congenital nuclear cataract), 37–38, 38*f*
fetal, 9, 27*f*, 28
opacification of (congenital nuclear cataract), 37–38, 38*f*
opacification of. *See* Nuclear cataract
removal/disassembly of
in ECCE, 160–161
laser photolysis for, 132
in phacoemulsification
one-handed, 125, 126–130, 126*f*, 127*f*, 128*f*, 129*f*
two-handed, 126–130, 127*f*, 128*f*, 129*f*
sutureless nonphaco techniques for, 131–132
water jet phacolysis for, 132
rotation of in phacoemulsification, 121
nutritional diseases affecting, 62
oxidative damage to, 13, 16
perforating and penetrating injury of, 55, 55*f*, 56*f*
glaucoma and, 67
physiology of, 19–23
pseudoexfoliation syndrome and, 65–66, 65*f*
radiation affecting, 55–57
removal of. *See also* Cataract surgery; Lensectomy; Phacoemulsification
in early cataract surgery, 93, 94
retained, cataract surgery and, 175–176
size of, 7
skin diseases and, 66
subluxed/subluxated, 39–40. *See also* Ectopia lentis
traumatic, 54–55
cataract surgery and, 230
in sulfite oxidase deficiency, 41
sutures of, 9
development of, 28–29, 28*f*
opacification of (sutural/stellate cataract), 37, 37*f*
transport functions in, 19–21, 20*f*
traumatic damage to, 40, 53–58, 54*f*, 228
glaucoma and, 67
phacoantigenic uveitis and, 66
surgery and, 228–231, 229*f*, 231*f*
uveitis and, 63–64, 64*f*. *See also* Phacoantigenic endophthalmitis/uveitis
water and cation balance in, maintenance of, 19–21, 20*f*
zonular fibers/zonules of, 5, 6*f*, 8
development of, 29
loose, cataract surgery and, 138–139, 139*f*, 230, 231*f*
in glaucoma patient, 222–223
iris coloboma and, 216
Lens capsule, 6*f*, 7, 7*f*
development of, 25, 27, 27*f*
exfoliation of, infrared radiation/heat causing, 56
rupture of, cataract surgery and, 140–141, 164*t*, 176–178
staining, in cataract surgery, 137
mature cataract/poor red reflex and, 215
Lens crystallins. *See* Crystallins
Lens fibers
accommodation and, 22
development of, 8–9, 8*f*
primary fibers, 25–27, 27*f*
secondary fibers, 27–28, 27*f*
microspherophakia and, 32
zonular (zonules of Zinn), 5, 6*f*, 8
development of, 29
loose, cataract surgery and, 138–139, 139*f*, 230, 231*f*
in glaucoma patient, 222–223
iris coloboma and, 216
Lens-induced glaucoma, 67–68, 68*f*
Lens Opacities Classification System III (LOCS III), 73

Lens particle glaucoma, 67
Lens pit, formation of, 25, 26*f*
Lens placode, 25, 26*f*
Lens proteins, 11, 11*f*
  aging affecting, 13, 43
  crystallins, 11–12, 11*f*. *See also* Crystallins
  cytoskeletal and membrane, 11*f*, 12
  in phacoantigenic endophthalmitis/uveitis, 66
  in phacolytic glaucoma, 67
  urea-insoluble (membrane structural), 11*f*, 12
  urea-soluble (cytoskeletal), 11*f*, 12
  water-insoluble, 11, 11*f*, 12
    age affecting, 13, 43
  water-soluble, 11, 11*f*. *See also* Crystallins
    conversion of to water-insoluble, 13
Lens vesicle, formation of, 25, 26*f*
Lensectomy
  in children, 201
  clear lens extraction, 225–226
  in Marfan syndrome, 41
  pars plana, 142
Lenticonus, 30–31
  posterior/lentiglobus, 30–31, 30*f*
Lenticular myopia (myopic shift), 43, 77
Lentiglobus, 30–31, 30*f*
Leukomas, in Peters anomaly, 32
Lidocaine, for cataract surgery, 102
Light, pupillary response to, evaluation of, before cataract surgery, 82–83
Light toxicity/photic damage/phototoxicity, cataract surgery and, 195
Limbal relaxing incisions, cataract surgery and, 135
Lipid peroxidation, in lens opacification, 16
Load, in phacoemulsification, 105
Local anesthesia. *See* Anesthesia (anesthetics), local
LOCS III (Lens Opacities Classification System III), 73
Longitudinal Study of Cataract, 73
Low vision aids, 78
LRI. *See* Limbal relaxing incisions
LSC (Longitudinal Study of Cataract), 73
Lutein, cataract risk affected by, 62
Luxed/luxated lens, 40. *See also* Ectopia lentis
  cataract surgery and, 230

Macula, evaluation of function of, before cataract surgery, 87
Macular degeneration, cataract surgery in patients with, 85, 227
Macular edema, cystoid, cataract surgery and, 164*t*, 193–195, 193*f*
  in glaucoma patient, 222
  Nd:YAG capsulotomy and, 187
Macular infarction, after cataract surgery, 195–196
Maddox rod testing, before cataract surgery, 87
Major intrinsic protein (MIP/aquaporin 0), 12, 19
Malignant glaucoma. *See* Aqueous misdirection
Malondialdehyde (MDA), oxidative lens damage and, 16
Marfan syndrome, 40–41, 40*f*
Mature cataract, 46, 48*f*
  phacolytic glaucoma and, 67
  surgery and, 139–140, 214–215
Mazzocco foldable intraocular lens, 145, 146*f*
McCannel sutures (transcorneal iris fixation sutures), for intraocular lens decentration, 179, 179*f*
Megalophthalmos, intraocular lens implantation and, 218, 219*f*
Meibomianitis, cataract surgery in patients with, 210
Membrane structural (urea-insoluble) lens proteins, 11*f*, 12
Membranous cataract, 39, 39*f*
Meridians, 5
Mesodermal dysgenesis, Peters anomaly and, 32
Metabolic disorders, cataracts and, 59–61
Metallosis, lens damage/cataracts caused by, 57–58, 58*f*
Methionine, in homocystinuria, 41
Methylcellulose, hydroxypropyl (HPMC), as viscoelastic, 98–99
Michaelis constant (K_m), "sugar" cataract development and, 15
Microphacoemulsification, bimanual, 130–131
Microphthalmia (microphthalmos), intraocular lens implantation and, 218
Microscope
  operating, phototoxicity and, 195
  specular, examination with before cataract surgery, 88
Microspherophakia, 32–33, 33*f*
Microwave radiation, cataract development and, 57
Millennium phacoemulsification system, 131
Miosis/miotic agents
  cataracts caused by, 53
  for glaucoma, cataract/cataract surgery and, 221, 222
MIP. *See* Major intrinsic protein
Mitomycin C, for combined glaucoma filtering and cataract surgery, 224
Mittendorf dot, 29, 31
Monocular diplopia, in cataracts, 44, 45, 47, 77
Morgagnian cataract, 46, 50*f*
Morgagnian globules, 46
Motility examination. *See* Ocular motility, assessment of
Multifocal lenses, intraocular, 146–147, 148*f*
Multiplanar incisions, for clear corneal incision, 116, 116*f*
Mydriasis/mydriatics, for pupillary capture, 180
Myopia
  cataract causing, 43, 77
  lenticular (myopic shift), 43, 77
Myopic shift, in cataracts (lenticular myopia), 43, 77
Myotonic dystrophy, lens disorders/cataracts in, 61, 62*f*

Na^+,K^+-ATPase (sodium-potassium pump), in lens active transport, 20
  pump-leak theory and, 20*f*, 21
NADP, in lens glucose/carbohydrate metabolism, 14*f*, 15
NADPH, in lens glucose/carbohydrate metabolism, 14*f*, 15
Nanophthalmos, cataract surgery in patients with, 217, 218*f*
Nd:YAG laser therapy
  capsulotomy, 184–187, 185*f*, 186*f*
    for capsular block syndrome, 181
    for capsule opacification, 182, 183
    in children, 201
    complications of, 187
    contraindications to, 184–185
    indications for, 184
    lens particle glaucoma and, 67

procedure for, 185–186, 185*f*, 186*f*
retinal detachment and, 187, 196–197
photolysis, 132
"Near clear" incision, 117–118
Nerve block, facial, 103, 103*f*
Neurocristopathy, Peters anomaly and, 32
Nicotinamide-adenine dinucleotide phosphate, in lens glucose/carbohydrate metabolism, 14*f*, 15
Noninfectious (sterile) endophthalmitis, postoperative, 191
toxic anterior segment syndrome and, 169
Nonsteroidal anti-inflammatory drugs (NSAIDs), corneal melting after cataract surgery associated with, 167, 211
Nuclear cataracts, 43–44, 45*f*
congenital, 37–38, 38*f*
postvitrectomy, 64, 227
visual acuity and, 76*t*
Nuclear disassembly techniques
one-handed, 125, 126*f*
two-handed, 126–130, 127*f*, 128*f*, 129*f*
Nuclear sclerosis, 43
Nucleus, lens. *See* Lens (crystalline), nucleus of
Nutritional deficiency, cataract formation and, 62

Obesity, cataract surgery and, 209–210
Obstructive pulmonary disease, cataract surgery in patients with, 207–208
Occlusion, in phacoemulsification, 106
Ocular history, cataract surgery evaluation and, 80
Ocular hypotension. *See* Hypotony
Ocular motility, assessment of, before cataract surgery, 82
Ocular trauma. *See* Trauma
Oculomotor nerve. *See* Cranial nerve III
Oil droplet appearance
in galactosemia, 60, 61*f*
in lenticonus and lentiglobus, 30–31
One-handed nucleus disassembly, 125, 126*f*
Opacities, fundus evaluation with, 86
Operating microscope, phototoxicity and, 195
Ophthalmic instrumentation, phototoxicity from, cataract surgery and, 195
Ophthalmic viscosurgical devices (viscoelastic agents), 98–100
for capsular rupture during surgery, 140, 177
characteristics of, 99–100
in children, 200
elevated intraocular pressure and, 172
for inflamed eye, 229
for intraoperative floppy iris syndrome, 173
IOL implantation and, 154, 155, 161
in phacoemulsification, 104, 123
physical properties of, 99
for pupil expansion, 137–138
for shallow anterior chamber, 138
Ophthalmoscopy, before cataract surgery, 85
Optic axis, 5, 6*f*
Optic cup, development of, 25
Optic nerve (cranial nerve II), evaluation of, before cataract surgery, 85–86
Optic vesicle, lens development and, 25, 26*f*
Optical clarity, of ophthalmic viscosurgical device, 100
Optical coherence biometry
before cataract surgery, 88
in IOL power determination, 150
OVDs. *See* Ophthalmic viscosurgical devices
Oxygen radicals. *See* Free radicals
Oxygen therapy, hyperbaric, oxidative lens damage and, 16, 64–65

Pachymetry (pachymeter), before cataract surgery, 88, 212–213
PAM. *See* Potential acuity meter
Panel control ultrasound, for phacoemulsification, 108
Paracentesis, in phacoemulsification, 113
Parasympatholytic agents, accommodation affected by, 22
Parasympathomimetic agents, accommodation affected by, 22
Pars plana lensectomy, 142
Pars plana vitrectomy
for capsular rupture during cataract surgery, 140, 177
cataract surgery after, 227–228
for postoperative endophthalmitis, 192
for retained lens fragments after phacoemulsification, 176
Pars planitis, intraocular lenses in patients with, 226
PAX6 gene mutation
in aniridia, 33–34
in Peters anomaly, 32
PCIOL. *See* Intraocular lenses (IOLs), posterior chamber
Pemphigoid, cataract surgery in patients with, 211
Penetrating injuries, lens damage caused by, 55
glaucoma and, 67
Penetrating keratoplasty. *See* Keratoplasty, penetrating
Pentose phosphate pathway (hexose monophosphate shunt), in lens glucose/carbohydrate metabolism, 14*f*, 15
Perforating injuries, lens damage caused by, 55, 55*f*, 56*f*
glaucoma and, 67
Peribulbar anesthesia, 100–102, 102*f*
anticoagulation therapy and, 205, 206
Peristaltic pump, for phacoemulsification aspiration, 110, 110*f*
vacuum rise time for, 110, 112*f*
Peroxidation, lipid, in lens opacification, 16
Persantine. *See* Dipyridamole
Persistent fetal vasculature (persistent hyperplastic primary vitreous), 42, 201
Peters anomaly, 32
PEX syndrome. *See* Pseudoexfoliation syndrome
PFV. *See* Persistent fetal vasculature
Phaco chop technique ("stop and chop" phaco), 127–129, 129*f*
Phaco fracture technique, 126–127, 127*f*, 128*f*
Phaco handpiece, 107, 108*f*
Phaco tip, 107, 107*f*, 108*f*, 109*f*
Phacoantigenic endophthalmitis/uveitis (lens-induced granulomatous/phacoanaphylactic endophthalmitis/phacoanaphylaxis), 66–67
Phacoemulsification, 104–131. *See also* Cataract surgery
anterior capsulotomy for, 119, 120
in anterior chamber, 124

aspiration system for, 110–111, 110*f*, 111*f*, 112*f*
strategies for use of, 122–123
burst mode, 109
capsular opacification and, 182–183
Nd:YAG laser capsulotomy for, 182, 183. *See also* Nd:YAG laser therapy, capsulotomy
capsular rupture during, 140–141, 176–178
capsulorrhexis in, 119–120, 119*f*
capsule staining for, 137
issues associated with, 138
loose zonules and, 138
clear corneal incision for, 116–118, 116*f*, 117*f*
continuous, 108
corneal complications of, 166
cystoid macular edema after, 193
endolenticular, 129–130
expulsive hemorrhage risk and, 220–221
flat or shallow anterior chamber and
intraoperative complications, 170–171
postoperative complications, 171–172
foldable intraocular lenses for, 145–146. *See also* Foldable intraocular lenses
in glaucoma patient
combined with filtering surgery, 224
after filtering surgery, 223
vitreous loss/loose zonular fibers and, 222–223
globe exposure for, 113
in high refractive error patient, 225
hydrodelineation in, 121
hydrodissection in, 120–121
instrumentation for, 106–107, 107*f*, 108*f*, 109*f*
settings for, 121–122
at iris plane, 124, 124*f*
irrigation in, 110
posterior misdirection (posterior infusion syndrome) and, 170–171
strategies for, 122–123
toxic solutions exposure and, corneal edema caused by, 163, 169
locations of, 123–125, 124*f*, 125*f*
mature cataract and, 139–140
nuclear rotation in, 121
nucleus disassembly/removal in
chopping techniques for, 127–129, 129*f*
endolenticular technique for, 129–130
one-handed, 125, 126*f*
phaco fracture technique for, 126–127, 127*f*, 128*f*
two-handed, 126–130, 127*f*, 128*f*, 129*f*
panel control ultrasound and, 108
paracentesis for, 113
after pars plana vitrectomy, 227–228
in posterior chamber, 124–125, 125*f*
for posterior polar cataract, 217
power delivery and, 108–109
advances in, 130–131
procedure for, 113–130
pulsed, 109
retained lens fragments after, 175–176
retinal detachment and, 196
scleral tunnel incisions for, 113–115, 114*f*, 115*f*
supracapsular, 125
surgeon-controlled ultrasound and, 108
surgeon's transition to, 111–113
in triple procedure, 213–214
ultrasonics terminology and, 104–105
ultrasound complications and, 166
vacuum terminology and, 106
after vitrectomy, 227–228
vitreocorneal adherence/persistent corneal edema and, 165–166
in zonular dehiscence/lens subluxation or dislocation, 230
Phacolysis, water jet, 132
Phacolytic glaucoma, 67
Phacomorphic glaucoma, 67, 68*f*
Phakinin, 12
Phenothiazines, lens changes caused by, 52, 52*f*
Phosphofructokinase, in lens glucose/carbohydrate metabolism, 13, 14*f*
Phospholine. *See* Echothiophate
Photic damage/phototoxicity/light toxicity, ophthalmic instrumentation causing, cataract surgery and, 195
Photolysis, laser, 132
Photorefractive keratectomy (PRK), cataract surgery after, 215–216
intraocular lens power calculation and, 152–153
Photostress recovery test, before cataract surgery, 87
PHPV (persistent hyperplastic primary vitreous). *See* Persistent fetal vasculature
Piezoelectric crystal, in phacoemulsification handpiece, 105
Piggybacking, with intraocular lenses, for keratoconus, 219
Pigmentations/pigment deposits, lens, drugs causing, 52, 52*f*
Pilocarpine
accommodation affected by, 22
cataracts caused by, 53
PITX2 gene, in Peters anomaly, 32
Placode, lens, 25, 26*f*
Plavix. *See* Clopidogrel
Pleomorphism, specular photomicroscopy in evaluation of, before cataract surgery, 88
PMMA. *See* Polymethylmethacrylate
Polar cataracts, 35–37, 36*f*
surgery for removal of, 216–217
Polymegethism, specular photomicroscopy in evaluation of, before cataract surgery, 88
Polymethylmethacrylate (PMMA), intraocular lenses made from, 142–143, 143*f*
implantation procedure for, 154
instrumentation for handling, 154
posterior capsule opacification and, 183
Polyol (sorbitol) pathway
in cataract formation, 15, 59–60
in lens glucose/carbohydrate metabolism, 14*f*, 15
Polyopia, in cataracts, 77
Posterior capsular opacification (PCO), 182–183
in children, 202
Nd:YAG laser capsulotomy for, 182, 183. *See also* Nd:YAG laser therapy, capsulotomy
Posterior capsular rupture, cataract surgery and, 140–141, 164*t*, 176–178
Posterior chamber, phacoemulsification in, 124–125, 125*f*

Posterior chamber intraocular lenses. *See* Intraocular lenses
Posterior corneal defects/depression. *See* Peters anomaly
Posterior infusion syndrome, 170–171
Posterior lenticonus/lentiglobus, 30–31, 30*f*
Posterior polar cataract, 35–37
  surgery for removal of, 216–217
Posterior pole, 5, 8*f*
Posterior subcapsular cataract, 46–49, 51*f*
  corticosteroids causing, 52
  ischemia causing, 68
  in myotonic dystrophy, 61
  uveitis and, 63
  visual acuity and, 75–76, 76*t*
Posterior sutures, 9
Posterior synechiae
  traumatic, cataract surgery and, 228
  in uveitis, lens changes/cataract and, 63–64
Postoperative care
  in children, 202
  after ECCE, 161
  after ICCE, 159
Postoperative endophthalmitis, 164*t*, 190–192, 191*f*
  prevention of, 132–134, 133*f*, 190–191
Postvitrectomy cataract, 64
Potassium balance, in lens, pump-leak theory of maintenance of, 20*f*, 21
Potential acuity meter (PAM), for patient evaluation before cataract surgery, 86, 216, 227
Power, in phacoemulsification, 105
  delivery of, 108–109
    advances in, 130–131
Power (optical), intraocular lens, determination of, 149–153, 149*f*
  in children, 204
  contact lens method for, 152
  developmentally abnormal eye and, 218–219, 220*f*
  historical methods for, 152–153
  improving outcomes of, 151–152
  incorrect, 181–182
  preventing errors in, 150–151
  refraction and, 81
  refractive surgery and, 152–153
  regression formulas for, 151, 152–153
  topographical method for, 152
  triple procedure and, 214
Power prediction formulas, for IOLs, 151, 152–153
Prazosin, cataract surgery complications and, 79–80
Prematurity, retinopathy of, cataract surgery in patients with, 217
Preoperative assessment/preparation, 79–81
  antimicrobial prophylaxis and, 132–133
  in children, 199–200
  in diabetic patient, 85, 209
  for ECCE, 160
  for ICCE, 157–158
Presbyopia, 23
Primary aphakia, 30. *See also* Aphakia
Primary coloboma, lens, 31. *See also* Coloboma
Primary lens fibers, development of, 25–27, 27*f*
Primary vitreous, persistent hyperplasia of. *See* Persistent fetal vasculature
PRK. *See* Photorefractive keratectomy
Propionibacterium acnes, chronic uveitis after cataract surgery caused by, 175
Prostaglandins, inflammation after cataract surgery and, 222
PSC. *See* Posterior subcapsular cataract
Pseudoexfoliation syndrome, 65–66, 65*f*
Pseudophakic bullous keratopathy, after cataract surgery, 163, 164*t*, 165, 165*f*
  IOL design and, 181
Pseudoplasticity, of ophthalmic viscosurgical device, 99
Pulmonary diseases, obstructive, cataract surgery in patients with, 207–208
Pulsed phacoemulsification, 109
Pump-leak theory, 20–21, 20*f*
Pupil size, cataract surgery and, 83, 223
Pupillary block
  after cataract surgery, flat anterior chamber and, 172
  intumescent cataract causing, phacomorphic glaucoma and, 67, 68*f*
  microspherophakia causing, 33
Pupillary capture, after cataract surgery, 180, 180*f*
Pupillary defects, relative afferent, cataract surgery on patient with, 83
Pupillary expansion, for cataract surgery, 137–138
Pupillary light reflex (pupillary response to light), evaluation of before cataract surgery, 82–83
Pupillary membrane, anterior, 29, 29*f*
Pupilloplasty, for cataracts, 77
  trauma and, 228
Pupils
  in ectopia lentis et pupillae, 42
  examination of, before cataract surgery, 82–83
  small, in glaucoma patient, cataract surgery and, 223
  trauma affecting, cataract surgery and, 228
Purkinje's entoptic phenomenon, evaluation of, before cataract surgery, 87
Pyridoxine (vitamin B_6), for homocystinuria, 41

Race, cataract development and, 74
Radial keratotomy (RK), cataract surgery after, 215–216
  intraocular lens power calculation and, 152–153
Radiation, cataracts caused by, 55–57
Red reflex
  in complete cataract, 38
  in lenticonus and lentiglobus, 30–31
  poor, cataract surgery and, 214–215
Refraction, before cataract surgery, 81
  IOL power determination and, 81
Refractive errors, high, cataract surgery in patient with, 224–226
Refractive index, of lens, 7
Refractive surgery, cataract/cataract surgery and, 215–216
  intraocular lens power calculation and, 152–153
  preoperative evaluation/planning and, 80
Regression formulas, for IOL power determination, 151, 152–153
Relative afferent pupillary defect, cataract surgery on patient with, 83
Relaxing incisions, limbal, 135
Retained lens material, cataract surgery and, 175–176

Retina
examination of, before cataract surgery, 85, 86, 87
oxidative lens damage during surgery on, 16
photic injury of, during cataract surgery, 195
Retinal detachment, after cataract surgery, 164*t*, 196–197, 196*f*
in children, 202
family history as risk factor and, 80
Nd:YAG laser capsulotomy and, 187, 196–197
Retinal disease, cataract surgery in patients with, 227–228
Retinitis pigmentosa, cataract surgery in patients with, 227
Retinopathy of prematurity, cataract surgery in patients with, 217
Retrobulbar anesthesia, 100, 101*f*
anticoagulation therapy and, 205, 206
hemorrhage and, 188
Retrobulbar hemorrhage, after cataract surgery, 188
ReZoom intraocular lens, 147, 148*f*
Rheumatoid arthritis, cataract surgery in patients with, corneal melting/keratolysis and, 167, 210–211
Riders, 34
Ridley intraocular lens, 142, 143*f*
Rise time, in phacoemulsification, 106, 111, 112*f*
RK. *See* Radial keratotomy
ROP. *See* Retinopathy of prematurity
Rosacea, cataract surgery in patients with, 82, 210, 210*f*
Rosette cataract, 54, 54*f*
RP. *See* Retinitis pigmentosa
Rubella, congenital, cataracts and, 39

Scleral support ring, for ICCE, 158
Scleral tunnel incisions, 113–115, 114*f*, 115*f*
in children, 200
closure of, 115, 115*f*, 200
Sclerocornea, intraocular lens implantation and, 218, 220*f*
Sclerosis, nuclear, 43
Sclerostomy, with cataract surgery, 224
Sculpting, instrument settings for, 122
Second sight, 43, 77
Secondary aphakia, 30. *See also* Aphakia
Secondary coloboma, lens, 31. *See also* Coloboma
Secondary lens fibers, development of, 27–28, 27*f*
microspherophakia and, 32
Seidel test, 171
Self-sealing incision
beveled/biplanar, clear corneal incision and, 116–117, 117*f*
scleral tunnel incisions and, 115
Shallow anterior chamber. *See* Anterior chamber, flat or shallow
Siderosis/siderosis bulbi, 57, 58*f*
Silicone foldable intraocular lenses, 146. *See also* Foldable intraocular lenses
instrumentation for handling, 154
posterior capsule opacification and, 183
Simple diffusion, glucose transport into lens and, 13
Simvastatin, cataract risk and, 53
Sjögren syndrome, cataract surgery in patients with, corneal melting/keratolysis and, 167, 210–211
Skin disorders, cataracts associated with, 66
Slit-lamp biomicroscopy/examination. *See* Biomicroscopy, slit-lamp
Smith-Indian operation, 94
Smoking, cataract development and, 63, 74
Snellen acuity. *See also* Visual acuity
Snowflake cataract, 59–60, 60*f*
Social history, cataract surgery evaluation and, 81
Sodium balance, in lens, pump-leak theory of maintenance of, 20*f*, 21
Sodium hyaluronate, as viscoelastic, 96, 144
Sodium-potassium pump (Na^+,K^+-ATPase), in lens active transport, 20
pump-leak theory and, 20*f*, 21
Soemmering ring, 182
SofPort Advanced Optics intraocular lens, 148
Sonic WAVE phacoemulsification system, 131
Sorbitol/sorbitol pathway
in cataract formation, 15, 59–60
in lens glucose/carbohydrate metabolism, 14*f*, 15
Sovereign phacoemulsification system with WhiteStar, 130–131
Space maintenance, by ophthalmic viscosurgical device, 99–100
Spectacle lenses (spectacles), aphakic. *See* Aphakic spectacles
Specular microscopy/photomicroscopy, before cataract surgery, 88
Sphincter muscle, damage to, cataract surgery and, 229
Spondylitis, ankylosing, cataract surgery in patients with, 207, 207*f*
SRK formulas, for IOL power selection, 151
STAAR Surgical Sonic WAVE phacoemulsification system, 131
Staphylococcus epidermidis
chronic uveitis after cataract surgery caused by, 175
postoperative endophthalmitis caused by, 192
Statins, cataracts and, 53
Stellate (sutural) cataracts, 37, 37*f*
Sterile (noninfectious) endophthalmitis, postoperative, 191
toxic anterior segment syndrome and, 169
Steroids. *See* Corticosteroids
"Stop and chop" phaco (phaco chop technique), 127–129, 129*f*
Stroke (phacoemulsification), 105
Stromal edema, after cataract surgery, 163–166
Subcapsular cataract, posterior, 46–49, 51*f*
corticosteroids causing, 52
ischemia causing, 68
in myotonic dystrophy, 61
uveitis and, 63
visual acuity and, 75–76, 76*t*
Subconjunctival lidocaine, for cataract surgery, 102
Subluxed/subluxated lens, 39–40. *See also* Ectopia lentis
traumatic, 54–55
cataract surgery and, 230
Sub-Tenon lidocaine, for cataract surgery, 102, 103*f*
Sub-Tenon's approach, for periocular corticosteroid injection, in cystoid macular edema, after cataract surgery, 194
"Sugar" cataracts, aldose reductase in development of, 15–16, 59
Sulfite oxidase deficiency, 41

Sulfur metabolism, in sulfite oxidase deficiency, 41
Sunflower cataract
in chalcosis, 58
in Wilson disease, 61
Sunglasses, ultraviolet-absorbing, cataract prevention and, 57
Sunlight. *See* Ultraviolet light
Superoxide dismutase, in lens, 16
Supracapsular phacoemulsification, 125
Suprachoroidal/choroidal hemorrhage, 164*t*, 188–189
delayed, 190
expulsive, 189
patients at risk for, 219–221
flat or shallow anterior chamber and, 170
Suprachoroidal effusion, 188–189
flat or shallow anterior chamber and, 170
Surface ectoderm, lens development and, 25, 26*f*
Surface tension, of ophthalmic viscosurgical device, 99
Surge, in phacoemulsification, 106
Surgeon-controlled ultrasound, for phacoemulsification, 108
Surgical instruments, for phacoemulsification, 106–107, 107*f*, 108*f*, 109*f*
settings for, 121–122
Sutural cataracts, 37, 37*f*
Sutureless nonphaco cataract surgery, 131–132
Sutures (lens), 9
development of, 28–29, 28*f*
opacification of (sutural/stellate cataract), 37, 37*f*
Sutures (surgical), for cataract surgery, astigmatism and, 167
Swinging flashlight test, before cataract surgery, 83
Synechiae, posterior
traumatic, cataract surgery and, 228
in uveitis, lens changes/cataract and, 63–64

Tamsulosin, intraoperative floppy iris syndrome and, 79–80, 137, 173
TAP. *See* Tap/biopsy of vitreous
Tap/biopsy of vitreous (TAP), for endophthalmitis after cataract surgery, 192
TASS. *See* Toxic Anterior Segment Syndrome
Tear film (tears), evaluation of, before cataract surgery, 82
TECNIS intraocular lens, 148
Temporal approach clear ("near clear") technique, for cataract surgery, 117–118
Temporal dysphotopsias, intraocular lens design and, 182
Tension rings, capsular, for zonular incompetence, 138–139, 139*f*, 230, 231*f*
Terazosin, cataract surgery complications and, 79–80
Tetanic cataract, 61
TGF-β. *See* Transforming growth factor-beta
Thioridazine, lens changes caused by, 52
Tobacco use, cataract development and, 63, 74
Topical anesthesia, for cataract surgery, 102–103, 103*f*
Topographical method, for IOL power calculation after refractive surgery, 152
Toric intraocular lenses, 136
Total cataract, 38
Toxic anterior segment syndrome (TASS), 169
Toxic solutions, exposure to during cataract surgery, corneal edema caused by, 163, 169
Trabeculectomy, with cataract surgery, 224
Transcorneal iris fixation sutures (McCannel sutures), for intraocular lens decentration, 179, 179*f*
Transforming growth factor-beta, in pseudoexfoliation syndrome, 66
Transport mechanisms, lens, 19–21, 20*f*
Trauma
cataract surgery after, 228–231, 229*f*, 231*f*
ectopia lentis caused by, 40
cataract surgery in patients with, 230
lens damage/cataracts caused by, 40, 53–58, 54*f*, 228
glaucoma and, 67
phacoantigenic uveitis and, 66
surgery for, 228–231, 229*f*, 231*f*
Triamcinolone, for cystoid macular edema, after cataract surgery, 194
Triple procedure, 156, 213–214
Tunica vasculosa lentis, 29, 29*f*
remnant of
epicapsular star, 31, 32*f*
Mittendorf dot, 29, 31
Tuning, in phacoemulsification, 105
Twin studies, in age-related cataract, 50
Two-handed nucleus disassembly, 126–130, 127*f*, 128*f*, 129*f*

UDP galactose 4-epimerase deficiency, galactosemia caused by, 60
cataract associated with, 61
UGH syndrome. *See* Uveitis-glaucoma-hyphema (UGH) syndrome
Ultrasonic, definition of, 105
Ultrasonography/ultrasound
before cataract surgery, 86, 88, 216
in IOL power determination, 149–150, 149*f*, 150
for phacoemulsification
corneal complications of, 166
panel control, 108
surgeon-controlled, 108
terminology related to, 104–105
Ultraviolet-absorbing lenses, cataract prevention and, 57
Ultraviolet chromophores, intraocular lenses with, 148
Ultraviolet light (ultraviolet radiation), cataracts associated with exposure to, 57
Urea-insoluble (membrane structural) lens proteins, 11*f*, 12
Urea-soluble (cytoskeletal) lens proteins, 11*f*, 12
Uveitis
cataracts and, 63–64, 64*f*, 226–227
after cataract surgery, 164*t*, 175, 181
surgery in patients with, 80, 226–227, 228–229
lens-induced/phacoantigenic/phacoanaphylactic, 66–67
Uveitis-glaucoma-hyphema (UGH) syndrome, intraocular lens implantation and, 181

Vacuum, phacoemulsification
definition of, 106
settings for, 121–122
terminology related to, 106

Vacuum rise time, in phacoemulsification, 106, 111, 112*f*
Venting, in phacoemulsification, 106
Venturi pump, for phacoemulsification aspiration, 110, 111*f*
  vacuum rise time for, 110, 112*f*
VER. *See* Visual evoked response
Vertical chopping techniques, in phacoemulsification, 128
VF-14. *See* Visual Function Index
Vimentin, 12
Viscoelasticity, definition of, 99
Viscoelastics, 98–100. *See also* Ophthalmic viscosurgical devices
Viscomydriasis, 100
  for pupil expansion, 137–138
Viscosity, of ophthalmic viscosurgical device, 99
Viscosurgical devices, ophthalmic (viscoelastic agents), 98–100. *See also* Ophthalmic viscosurgical devices
Vision rehabilitation, for cataract patient, 78
Visual acuity
  in cataract, 75–76, 76*t*
    bilateral congenital cataracts, 199
    preoperative evaluation and, 80, 81, 216
  after cataract surgery, 156
    in children, 203
    cystoid macular edema and, 193
    with ECCE, 161
    endophthalmitis and, 192
    with ICCE, 159
    incorrect lens power and, 181–182
  testing, before cataract surgery, 81, 216
Visual axis, Nd:YAG laser capsulotomy location and, 185
Visual evoked response, before cataract surgery, 87
Visual field defects, in glaucoma, cataract/media opacities and, 221, 222*f*
Visual field testing, before cataract surgery, 82
Visual function, measuring
  before cataract surgery, 81–82
  after cataract surgery, 156–157
Visual Function Index (VF-14), 78, 156–157
Visual loss/impairment. *See also* Visual acuity
  cataract and, 75–76, 76*t*
Vitamin B_6 (pyridoxine), for homocystinuria, 41
Vitamin E, cataract surgery in patient taking, 206
Vitamin deficiency, cataracts caused by, 62
Vitamin supplements, cataract prevention and, 62, 77
Vitrectomy
  anterior
    for capsular rupture during cataract surgery, 140, 141, 177
    for pediatric cataract, 201
  for capsular rupture during cataract surgery, 140, 177, 178
  cataract caused by, 64
  cataract surgery after, 80, 227–228
  for cystoid macular edema, postoperative, 194
  for endophthalmitis, postoperative, 192
  oxidative lens damage and, 16
  pars plana. *See* Pars plana vitrectomy
  for pediatric cataract, 201
  for retained lens fragments after phacoemulsification, 176
  for vitreocorneal adherence/persistent corneal edema, 165–166
  for vitreous prolapse, 178
Vitreocorneal adherence, after cataract surgery, 165–166
Vitreous
  cataract surgery complications and, 164*t*, 178
    in glaucoma patient, 222–223
    with ICCE, 158
    prolapse, 178
    vitreocorneal adherence, 165–166
  primary, persistent hyperplasia of. *See* Persistent fetal vasculature
  tap/biopsy of, for endophthalmitis after cataract surgery, 192
Vitreous biopsy, in infectious endophthalmitis, after cataract surgery, 192
Vitreous wick syndrome, 178
von Graefe knife, 94
Vossius ring, 53–54

WAGR syndrome, 34
Warfarin/warfarin derivatives, cataract surgery in patient taking, 206
Water and electrolyte balance, in lens, maintenance of, 19–21, 20*f*
Water-insoluble lens proteins, 11, 11*f*, 12
  aging affecting, 13, 43
Water jet phacolysis, 132
Water-soluble lens proteins, 11, 11*f*. *See also* Crystallins
  conversion of to water-insoluble, 13
Wedl (bladder) cells, 49, 182
Weill-Marchesani syndrome, microspherophakia in, 32
Wilms tumor, aniridia and, 34
Wilson disease (hepatolenticular degeneration), 61
Wound closure
  after ECCE, 161
  scleral tunnel incisions and, 115, 115*f*, 200

Xalatan. *See* Latanoprost
Xylocaine. *See* Lidocaine

Y-sutures, lens, 9
  development of, 28–29, 28*f*
  opacification of (sutural/stellate cataract), 37, 37*f*

Zeaxanthin, cataract risk affected by, 62
Zinn, zonules of. *See* Zonular fibers, lens
Zonular (lamellar) cataracts, 34, 36*f*
Zonular dehiscence, cataract surgery and, 138–139, 139*f*, 230, 231*f*
  in glaucoma patient, 222–223
  iris coloboma and, 216
  traumatic, 230, 231*f*
Zonular fibers, lens (zonules of Zinn), 5, 6*f*, 8
  development of, 29
  loose, cataract surgery and, 138–139, 139*f*, 230, 231*f*
    in glaucoma patient, 222–223
    iris coloboma and, 216
Zonular lamella, 7
Zonules of Zinn. *See* Zonular fibers, lens